The Occupational
Therapy Assistant

The Occupational Therapy Assistant

Resources for Practice & Education

Edited by

Teri L. Black, COTA, ROH, and

Kathryn Melin Eberhardt, MAEd, COTA/L, ROH

AOTA
PRESS

The American
Occupational Therapy
Association, Inc.

Vision Statement

AOTA advances occupational therapy as the pre-eminent profession in promoting the health, productivity, and quality of life of individuals and society through the therapeutic application of occupation.

Mission Statement

The American Occupational Therapy Association advances the quality, availability, use, and support of occupational therapy through standard-setting, advocacy, education, and research on behalf of its members and the public.

AOTA Staff

Frederick P. Somers, *Executive Director*

Christopher M. Bluhm, *Chief Operating Officer*

Audrey Rothstein, *Director, Marketing and Communications*

Chris Davis, *Managing Editor, AOTA Press*

Carrie Mercadante, *Production Editor*

Denise A. Rotert, MA, OTR/L, *Senior Associate, Academic Affairs,*
    Education and Professional Development

Robert A. Sacheli, *Manager, Creative Services*

Sarah E. Ely, *Book Production Coordinator*

Marge Wasson, *Marketing Manager*

Elizabeth Sarcia, *Marketing Specialist*

The American Occupational Therapy Association, Inc.

4720 Montgomery Lane

Bethesda, MD 20814

Phone: 301-652-AOTA (2682)

TDD: 800-377-8555

Fax: 301-652-7711

www.aota.org

To order: 1-877-404-AOTA (2682)

Disclaimers

This publication is designed to provide accurate and authoritative information in regard to the subject matter covered. It is sold or distributed with the understanding that the publisher is not engaged in rendering legal, accounting, or other professional service. If legal advice or other expert assistance is required, the services of a competent professional person should be sought.

—From the Declaration of Principles jointly adopted by the American Bar Association and a Committee of Publishers and Associations.

It is the objective of the American Occupational Therapy Association to be a forum for free expression and interchange of ideas. The opinions expressed by the contributors to this work are their own and not necessarily those of either the editors or the American Occupational Therapy Association.

ISBN: 1-56900-207-X

Library of Congress Control Number: 2005926580

Cover design by Sarah E. Ely

Text design and composition by Grammarians, Inc.

Printed by Victor Graphics

Contents

INTRODUCTION

Brief History of the Occupational Therapy Assistant

The year 2008 marks the 50th anniversary of the occupational therapy assistant (OTA) working in the occupational therapy profession. Since then, occupational therapy assistants have provided very valuable service and contributed to the expansion of occupational therapy.

Occupational therapists Ruth Brunyate Wiemer, Colonel Ruth Robinson, Marion Crampton, and Mildred Schwagmeyer are credited with creating the OTA's role, which was conceptualized and defined through official American Occupational Therapy Association (AOTA) structures of the Board of Management, the Delegate Assembly (now the Representative Assembly, or RA), and a Committee on the Recognition of Occupational Therapy Assistants, starting in 1956.

Robinson, AOTA president from 1955 to 1958, assisted in the development of the OTA's role, responsibilities, and job duties. Her passion was critical to the recognition of the assistant level in the profession: "Recognition of the certified occupational therapy assistant through certification made me the proudest" (Robinson & Wiemer, 1993). Her long-standing support was evident in her continued involvement as a member of the Committee on Occupational Therapy Assistants in 1964.

Wiemer anticipated career mobility and changes in the future of the occupational therapy profession and believed that the role of occupational therapy assistants would develop into a working relationship with occupational therapists, which would have positive outcomes for clients. In a training for occupational therapy assistants in Detroit, Michigan, in 1964, she said,

> Able seaman far outnumber captains and commodores, yet ships do not sink, and new ships, from sail to nuclear power, have evolved to meet

man's need. So, too, the varied level of our profession can be coordinated to achieve efficiency and growth. (Wiemer, 2001)

Her leadership and vision for occupational therapy assistants had great emotional influence, and her powerful message was the cornerstone of a lifelong professional relationship. She believed that, when assistants were created, there would be room for both levels, a belief that holds true today.

The assistant level in the occupational therapy profession was first considered after World War II, when there was a shortage of occupational therapists in psychiatric hospitals to provide direct occupational therapy intervention. Occupational therapy assistants were officially created in 1958 to alleviate occupational therapist shortages in psychiatric programs. "The standards for the training and recognition of occupational therapy assistants in psychiatry, which were adopted by [AOTA] in October 1958, were developed from guidelines which had a favorable vote of a majority of state associations in January 1956." There was consensus that assistants should be trained in one specialty area and that 3 months was adequate time to complete the training objectives.

Educational opportunities were implemented to train individuals with in-depth knowledge in providing direct occupational therapy services. The U.S. military provided the first in-service training. In 1960, the Westboro State Hospital in Massachusetts began one of the first formal educational training programs for occupational therapy assistants. The first program in the United States leading to an associate's degree was founded in 1965 at Mt. Aloysius College in Pennsylvania. OTA education evolved from these early programs of 3 months to 1-year programs and now are conducted in a 2-year associate-degree programs accredited by the Accreditation Council for Occupational Therapy Education (Mt. Aloysius College, n.d.). In general, the education of the occupational therapy assistant underwent the following changes:

Portions of this introduction are taken from Alterio, C., & Black, T., (2005, March 7). OT assistants: The foundation for the future. *OT Practice*, pp. 16–19.

- The assistant level was officially created in 1958 to alleviate the occupational therapy shortage in psychiatric programs (12-week training programs).
- In 1960, training in general practice was added.
- In 1961, 3-month programs for nursing home practice were added.
- By 1972, OTA programs ranged from 9 months to 2 years.
- AOTA adopted the "Essentials for an Approved Education Program" in 1975, and most programs then went to 2-year associate degrees.
- The certification exam was required after 1977.
- Today, 37 states have comprehensive practice and supervision requirements.

Indeed, occupational therapy assistants have had many advances and milestones since our creation.

We also have had some challenges along the way. Originally, occupational therapy assistants were not allowed to serve as AOTA representatives on committees or commissions, to vote in AOTA elections or on proposals, or to receive the *American Journal of Occupational Therapy.* Motions to allow us to participate more fully in the organization were defeated by the RA in the mid-1960s. It was not until 1975 that many of these rights were granted to occupational therapy assistants. In addition, awards were established that recognized the achievements of occupational therapy assistants. Today, we are involved in all aspects of AOTA membership, serving on commissions and committees, in the RA, and on the Board of Directors. Occupational therapy assistants also are eligible for the OTA Award of Excellence, the Roster of Honor, and the Terry Brittell OTA/OT Partnership Award.

As occupational therapy practice has grown, occupational therapy assistants have grown along with it, and now we are in almost every practice area. Our greatest value is that we extend occupational therapy services in all the places where we work. Individuals for whom we provide intervention receive more services because our role exists. Occupational therapy assistants are educators in OTA and occupational therapy programs and also are authors, presenters, and occupational therapy regulatory board members.

Practice settings have changed considerably over time as well. Occupational therapy assistants have roots in mental health and geriatric practice; now we are in a vast array of practice settings, with skilled-nursing facilities and schools the largest areas. We also are prepared to function in today's ever-changing health care marketplace and are poised to serve in many emerging practice areas. As our history shows, the assistant role was created to meet unserved needs, and we believe that will hold true well into the future.

How to Use This Book

This collection of regulatory and reimbursement information, standards, guidelines, and language is designed to be comprehensive resource manual for occupational therapy assistants and occupational therapists. Part I provides an overview of state and professional regulations, and Part II discusses supervision, roles, and responsibilities. Part III explains reimbursement, and Part IV details ethical jurisdiction. Part V is a collection of additional resources.

In today's fast-paced, complex practice environment when questions often arise about roles, responsibilities, and supervision of occupational therapy assistants, this guide can provide practitioners with the resources needed for quick, accurate answers. It is hoped that occupational therapy practitioners will use this guide often to help facilitate ethical, legal, best, and evidence-based practice.

The intent of this manual is to provide current (as of print time) practice resources. Readers are encouraged to stay informed by visiting the AOTA Web site at www.aota.org; the "Members-Only" section contains the most up-to-date information on occupational therapy assistant roles and responsibilities, supervision issues, and more.

—*Kathryn Melin Eberhardt, MAEd, COTA/L, ROH*
    Academic Fieldwork Coordinator, Occupational Therapy
        Assistant Program
    South Suburban College
    South Holland, Illinois

—*Teri L. Black, COTA, ROH*
    OT Assistant Program
    Madison Area Technical College
    Madison, Wisconsin

References

American Occupational Therapy Association. (1956). Board minutes, Report of Speaker of House of Delegates. *American Journal of Occupational Therapy, 10,* 163.

Mt. Aloysius College. (n.d.). Occupational therapy assistant. Retrieved June 1, 2004, from http://www.mtaloy.edu/occtal.html.

Robinson, R., & Wiemer, R.W. (1993). AOTA's role in the development of the COTA. In S. E. Ryan (Ed.), *The certified occupational therapy assistant* (2nd ed., pp. 22–23). Thorofare, NJ: Slack.

Wiemer R. W. (2001). AOTA's role in the development of the COTA. In S. E. Ryan (Ed.), *The certified occupational therapy assistant: Principles, concepts, and techniques* (3rd ed., p. 21). Thorofare, NJ: Slack

PART I

State and Professional Regulations

To practice in compliance with the law, occupational therapy practitioners must have a thorough understanding of all the applicable state laws and regulatory statutes, in addition to rules that implement the law and reimbursement requirements. Regulatory language that delineates supervision and practice parameters for occupational therapy assistants must be followed. Currently, not every state has specific language that guides occupational therapy assistant practice. Readers whose states do not have these regulations can use the appropriate reimbursement language. Also, the American Occupational Therapy Association (AOTA) offers requirements that practitioners are ethically bound to follow to maintain a professional standard of practice. However, these professional guidelines are not laws and rules that practitioners are legally required to follow.

When trying to decide which supervisory language to use, a good unwritten rule is to follow the more restrictive one. For example, a client is covered under Medicare Part A, and the state regulatory rules state only that the occupational therapy assistant must meet certain requirements but give no guidance as to how much supervision is required. In this case, the occupational therapy team should follow the Medicare requirement when the assistant is seeing that client, and the team can also follow the AOTA *Guidelines for Supervision, Roles, and Responsibilities During the Delivery of OT Services* (see Chapter 4). As always, when there is doubt, readers should contact their state's regulatory or licensing board or organization for specific interpretations of the rules.

Both occupational therapists and occupational therapy assistants share equal responsibility in knowing the laws and rules and how to follow them in all practice settings. This can be a complex process if a team is working in several practice areas at one time. Practicing ethically and within the laws and rules can be challenging, but a creative team committed to understanding the complexities and also to good communication can provide services optimally. To assist in this process, this section offers the following resources:

• Chapter 1. Definition of Occupational Therapy Practice for the AOTA Model Practice Act
• Chapter 2. Scope of Practice
• Chapter 3. State Regulation of Occupational Therapy Assistants.

Chapter 1

Definition of Occupational Therapy Practice for the AOTA Model Practice Act

The practice of occupational therapy means the therapeutic use of everyday life activities (occupations) with individuals or groups for the purpose of participation in roles and situations in home, school, workplace, community, and other settings. Occupational therapy services are provided for the purpose of promoting health and wellness and to those who have or are at risk for developing an illness, injury, disease, disorder, condition, impairment, disability, activity limitation, or participation restriction. Occupational therapy addresses the physical, cognitive, psychosocial, sensory, and other aspects of performance in a variety of contexts to support engagement in everyday life activities that affect health, well-being, and quality of life.

The practice of occupational therapy includes

A. Methods or strategies selected to direct the process of interventions, such as
   1. Establishment, remediation, or restoration of a skill or ability that has not yet developed or is impaired
   2. Compensation, modification, or adaptation of activity or environment to enhance performance
   3. Maintenance and enhancement of capabilities without which performance in everyday life activities would decline
   4. Health promotion and wellness to enable or enhance performance in everyday life activities
   5. Prevention of barriers to performance, including disability prevention.

B. Evaluation of factors affecting activities of daily living (ADL), instrumental activities of daily living (IADL), education, work, play, leisure, and social participation, including
   1. Client factors, including body functions (such as neuromuscular, sensory, visual, perceptual, cognitive) and body structures (such as cardiovascular, digestive, integumentary, genitourinary systems)
   2. Habits, routines, roles, and behavior patterns
   3. Cultural, physical, environmental, social, and spiritual contexts and activity demands that affect performance
   4. Performance skills, including motor, process, and communication/interaction skills.

C. Interventions and procedures to promote or enhance safety and performance in activities of daily living (ADL), instrumental activities of daily living (IADL), education, work, play, leisure, and social participation, including
   1. Therapeutic use of occupations, exercises, and activities
   2. Training in self-care, self-management, home management, and community/work reintegration
   3. Development, remediation, or compensation of physical, cognitive, neuromuscular, sensory functions and behavioral skills
   4. Therapeutic use of self, including one's personality, insights, perceptions, and judgments, as part of the therapeutic process
   5. Education and training of individuals, including family members, caregivers, and others
   6. Care coordination, case management, and transition services
   7. Consultative services to groups, programs, organizations, or communities
   8. Modification of environments (home, work, school, or community) and adaptation of processes, including the application of ergonomic principles
   9. Assessment, design, fabrication, application, fitting, and training in assistive technology, adaptive devices, and orthotic devices and training in the use of prosthetic devices
   10. Assessment, recommendation, and training in techniques to enhance functional mobility, including wheelchair management
   11. Driver rehabilitation and community mobility
   12. Management of feeding, eating, and swallowing to enable eating and feeding performance
   13. Application of physical agent modalities and use of a range of specific therapeutic procedures (such as wound care management; techniques to enhance sensory, perceptual, and cognitive processing; manual therapy techniques) to enhance performance skills.

Adopted by the Representative Assembly 5/21/04 (Agenda A11, Charge 60)

Chapter 2

Scope of Practice

Statement of Purpose

The purpose of this document is to define the scope of practice in occupational therapy in order to

1. Delineate the domain of occupational therapy practice that directs the focus and actions of services provided by occupational therapists and occupational therapy assistants.
2. Delineate the dynamic process of occupational therapy evaluation and intervention services to achieve outcomes that support the participation of clients in their everyday life activities (occupations).
3. Describe the education and certification requirements to practice as an occupational therapist and occupational therapy assistant.
4. Inform consumers, health care providers, educators, the community, funding agencies, payers, referral sources, and policymakers regarding the scope of occupational therapy.

Introduction

The occupational therapy scope of practice is based on the American Occupational Therapy Association (AOTA) document *Occupational Therapy Practice Framework: Domain and Process* (AOTA, 2002) and on the *Philosophical Base of Occupational Therapy*, which states that "the understanding and use of occupations shall be at the central core of occupational therapy practice, education, and research" (AOTA, 2003a, Policy 1.11). Occupational therapy is a dynamic and evolving profession that is responsive to consumer needs and to emerging knowledge and research.

This scope of practice document is designed to support and be used in conjunction with the *Definition of Occupational Therapy Practice for the Model Practice Act* (AOTA, 2004a). While this scope of practice document helps support state laws and regulations that govern the practice of occupational therapy, it does not supersede those existing laws and other regulatory requirements. Occupa-

tional therapists and occupational therapy assistants are required to abide by statutes and regulations when providing occupational therapy services. State laws and other regulatory requirements typically include statements about educational requirements to practice occupational therapy, procedures to practice occupational therapy legally within the defined area of jurisdiction, the definition and scope of occupational therapy practice, and supervision requirements.

AOTA (1994) states that a referral is not "required for the provision of occupational therapy services" (p. 1034); however, a referral may be indicated by some state laws and other regulatory requirements. The AOTA 1994 document *Statement of Occupational Therapy Referral* states that "occupational therapists respond to requests for services, whatever their sources. They may accept and enter cases at their own professional discretion and based on their own level of competency" (p. 1034). Occupational therapy assistants provide services under the supervision of an occupational therapist. State laws and other regulatory requirements should be viewed as minimum criteria to practice occupational therapy. Ethical guidelines that ensure safe and effective delivery of occupational therapy services to clients always influence occupational therapy practice (AOTA, 2000).

Definition of *Occupational Therapy*

AOTA's *Definition of Occupational Therapy for the Model Practice Act* defines *occupational therapy* as

> the therapeutic use of everyday life activities (occupations) with individuals or groups for the purpose of participation in roles and situations in home, school, workplace, community, and other settings. Occupational therapy services are provided for the purpose of promoting health and wellness and to those who have or are at risk for developing an illness, injury, disease, disorder, condition, impairment, disability, activity limitation, or participation restriction. Occupational therapy addresses the physical, cognitive,

psychosocial, sensory, and other aspects of performance in a variety of contexts to support engagement in everyday life activities that affect health, well-being, and quality of life." (AOTA, 2004a)

Scope of Practice—*Domain* and *Process*

The scope of practice includes the domain and process of occupational therapy services. These concepts are intertwined with the domain defining the focus of occupational therapy (see Figure 1) and the process defining the delivery of occupational therapy (see Figure 2). The domain of occupational therapy is the everyday life activities (occupations) that people find meaningful and purposeful. Within this domain, occupational therapy services enable clients to engage (participate) in their everyday life activities in their desired roles, context, and life situations. Clients may be individuals, groups, communities, or populations. The occupations in which clients engage occur throughout the life span and include

- Activities of daily living (self-care activities)
- Education (activities to participate as a learner in a learning environment)
- Instrumental activities of daily living (multistep activities to care for self and others, such as household management, financial management, and child care)
- Leisure (nonobligatory, discretionary, and intrinsically rewarding activities)
- Play (spontaneous and organized activities that promote pleasure, amusement, and diversion)
- Social participation (activities expected of individuals or individuals interacting with others)
- Work (employment-related and volunteer activities).

Within this domain of practice, occupational therapists and occupational therapy assistants consider the repertoire of occupations in which the client engages, the performance skills and patterns the client uses, the contexts influencing engagement, the features and demands of the activity, and the client's body functions and structures. Occupational therapists and occupational therapy assis-

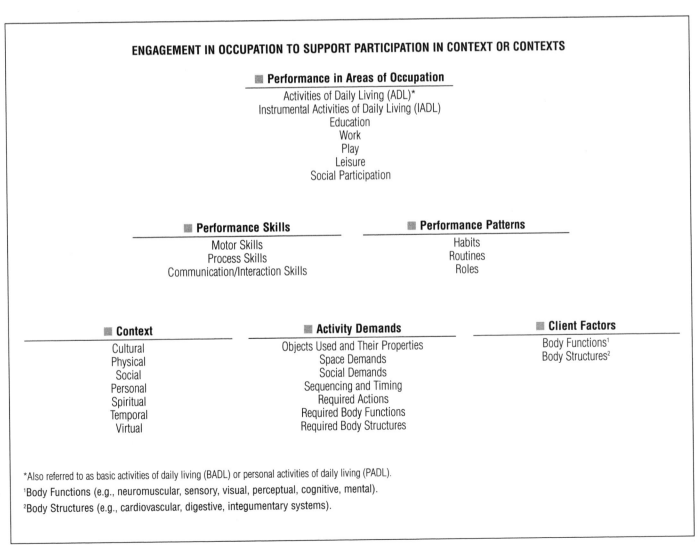

ENGAGEMENT IN OCCUPATION TO SUPPORT PARTICIPATION IN CONTEXT OR CONTEXTS

▨ **Performance in Areas of Occupation**
Activities of Daily Living (ADL)*
Instrumental Activities of Daily Living (IADL)
Education
Work
Play
Leisure
Social Participation

▨ **Performance Skills**
Motor Skills
Process Skills
Communication/Interaction Skills

▨ **Performance Patterns**
Habits
Routines
Roles

▨ **Context**
Cultural
Physical
Social
Personal
Spiritual
Temporal
Virtual

▨ **Activity Demands**
Objects Used and Their Properties
Space Demands
Social Demands
Sequencing and Timing
Required Actions
Required Body Functions
Required Body Structures

▨ **Client Factors**
Body Functions[1]
Body Structures[2]

*Also referred to as basic activities of daily living (BADL) or personal activities of daily living (PADL).
[1] Body Functions (e.g., neuromuscular, sensory, visual, perceptual, cognitive, mental).
[2] Body Structures (e.g., cardiovascular, digestive, integumentary systems).

Figure 1. Domain of Occupational Therapy. (AOTA, 2002, p. 611)

tants use their knowledge and skills to help clients "attain and resume daily life activities that support function and health" throughout the lifespan (AOTA, 2002, p. 610). Participation in activities and occupations that are meaningful to the client involves emotional, psychosocial, cognitive, and physical aspects of performance. This participation provides a means to enhance health, well-being, and life satisfaction.

The domain of occupational therapy practice complements the World Health Organization's (WHO) conceptualization of participation and health articulated in the *International Classification of Functioning, Disability, and Health (ICF)* (WHO, 2001). Occupational therapy incorporates the basic constructs of *ICF*, including environment, participation, activities, and body structures and functions, when addressing the complexity and richness of occupations and occupational engagement.

The process of occupational therapy relates to service delivery (see Figure 2) and includes evaluating, intervening, and targeting outcomes. Occupation remains central to the occupational therapy process. It is client-centered, involving collaboration with the client throughout each aspect of service delivery. During the evaluation, the therapist develops an occupational profile, analyzes the client's ability to carry out everyday life activities, and determines the client's occupational needs, problems, and priorities for intervention. Evaluation and intervention may address one or more of the domains (see Figure 1) that influence occupational performance. Intervention includes planning and imple-

menting occupational therapy services and involves therapeutic use of self, activities, and occupations, as well as consultation and education. The occupational therapist and occupational therapy assistant utilize occupation-based theories, frames of reference, evidence, and clinical reasoning to guide the intervention (AOTA, 2002).

The outcome of occupational therapy intervention is directed toward "engagement [of the client] in occupations that support participation in [daily life situations] (AOTA, 2002, p. 618). Outcomes of the intervention determine future actions with the client. Outcomes include the client's occupational performance, role competence and adaptation, health and wellness, quality of life and satisfaction, and prevention initiatives (AOTA, 2002, p. 619).

Occupational Therapy Practice

Occupational therapists and occupational therapy assistants are experts at analyzing the performance skills and patterns necessary for people to engage in their everyday activities in the context in which those activities and occupations occur. The occupational therapist assumes responsibility for the delivery of all occupational therapy services and for the safety and effectiveness of occupational therapy services provided. The occupational therapy assistant delivers occupational therapy services under the supervision of and in partnership with the occupational therapist (AOTA, 2004b).

The practice of occupational therapy includes
A. Strategies selected to direct the process of interventions, such as
  1. Establishment, remediation, or restoration of a skill or ability that has not yet developed or is impaired.
  2. Compensation, modification, or adaptation of activity or environment to enhance performance.
  3. Maintenance and enhancement of capabilities without which performance in everyday life activities would decline.
  4. Health promotion and wellness to enable or enhance performance in everyday life activities.
  5. Prevention of barriers to performance, including disability prevention.
B. Evaluation of factors affecting activities of daily living (ADL), instrumental activities of daily living (IADL), education, work, play, leisure, and social participation, including
  1. Client factors, including body functions (e.g., neuromuscular, sensory, visual, perceptual, cognitive) and body structures (e.g., cardiovascular, digestive, integumentary, genitourinary systems).

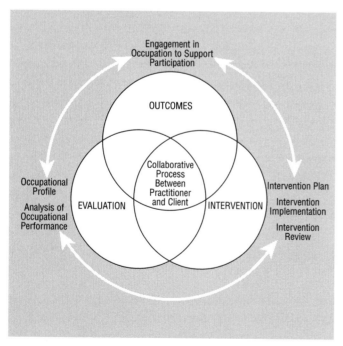

Figure 2. Collaborative Process Model. Illustration of the framework emphasizing client–practitioner interactive relationship and interactive nature of the service delivery process (AOTA, 2002, p. 614).

2. Habits, routines, roles, and behavior patterns.

3. Cultural, physical, environmental, social, and spiritual contexts and activity demands that affect performance.

4. Performance skills, including motor, process, and communication/interaction skills.

C. Interventions and procedures to promote or enhance safety and performance in activities of daily living (ADL), instrumental activities of daily living (IADL), education, work, play, leisure, and social participation, including

1. Therapeutic use of occupations, exercises, and activities.

2. Training in self-care, self-management, home management, and community/work reintegration.

3. Development, remediation, or compensation of physical, cognitive, neuromuscular, sensory functions, and behavioral skills.

4. Therapeutic use of self, including one's personality, insights, perceptions, and judgments, as part of the therapeutic process.

5. Education and training of individuals, including family members, caregivers, and others.

6. Care coordination, case management, and transition services.

7. Consultative services to groups, programs, organizations, or communities.

8. Modification of environments (home, work, school, or community) and adaptation of processes, including the application of ergonomic principles.

9. Assessment, design, fabrication, application, fitting, and training in assistive technology, adaptive devices, and orthotic devices, and training in the use of prosthetic devices.

10. Assessment, recommendation, and training in techniques to enhance functional mobility, including wheelchair management.

11. Driver rehabilitation and community mobility.

12. Management of feeding, eating, and swallowing to enable eating and feeding performance.

13. Application of physical agent modalities, and use of a range of specific therapeutic procedures (e.g., wound care management; techniques to enhance sensory, perceptual, and cognitive processing; manual therapy techniques) to enhance performance skills. (AOTA, 2004a)

Site of Intervention

Along the continuum of service, occupational therapy services may be provided to clients throughout the life span in a variety of settings. The settings may include, but are not limited to, the following:

- Institutional settings (inpatient) (e.g., acute rehabilitation, psychiatric hospital, community and specialty-focused hospitals, nursing facilities, prisons)
- Outpatient settings (e.g., hospitals, clinics, medical and therapy offices)
- Home and community settings (e.g., home care, group homes, assisted living, schools, early intervention centers, day care centers, industry and business, hospice, sheltered workshops, wellness and fitness centers, community mental health facilities)
- Research facilities.

Education and Certification Requirements

To practice as an occupational therapist, the individual

- Must have graduated from an occupational therapy program accredited by the Accreditation Council for Occupational Therapy Education (ACOTE®) or predecessor organizations, and
- Must have successfully completed a period of supervised fieldwork experience required by the recognized educational institution where the applicant met the academic requirements of an educational program for occupational therapists that is accredited by ACOTE® or predecessor organizations (AOTA, 2003b, Policy 5.3).

To practice as an occupational therapy assistant, the individual

- Must have graduated from an associate- or certificate-level occupational therapy assistant program accredited by ACOTE® or predecessor organizations, and
- Must have successfully completed a period of supervised fieldwork experience required by the recognized educational institution where the applicant met the academic requirements of an educational program for occupational therapy assistants that is accredited by ACOTE® or predecessor organizations (AOTA, 2003b, Policy 5.3).

AOTA supports licensure of qualified occupational therapists and occupational therapy assistants (AOTA, 2003b, Policy 5.3). State and other legislative or regulatory agencies may impose additional requirements to practice as an occupational therapist and occupational therapy assistants in their area of jurisdiction.

References

American Occupational Therapy Association. (1994). Statement of occupational therapy referral. *American Journal of Occupational Therapy, 48,* 1034.

American Occupational Therapy Association. (2000). Occupational therapy code of ethics. *American Journal of Occupational Therapy, 54,* 614–616.

American Occupational Therapy Association. (2002). Occupational therapy practice framework: Domain and process. *American Journal of Occupational Therapy, 56,* 609–639.

American Occupational Therapy Association. (2003a). Policy 1.11: The philosophical base of occupational therapy. *Policy Manual* (2003 ed.). Bethesda, MD: Author.

American Occupational Therapy Association. (2003b). Policy 5.3: Licensure. *Policy Manual* (2003 ed.). Bethesda, MD: Author.

American Occupational Therapy Association. (2004a). Definition of occupational therapy practice for the AOTA Model Practice Act. (Available from the State Affairs Group, American Occupational Therapy Association, 4720 Montgomery Lane, Bethesda, MD 20814)

American Occupational Therapy Association. (2004b). Guidelines for supervision, roles, and responsibilities during the delivery of occupational therapy services. *American Journal of Occupational Therapy, 58*(November/December).

World Health Organization. (2001). *International Classification of Functioning, Disability, and Health (ICF).* Geneva: Author.

Additional Reading

American Occupational Therapy Association. (1993). Occupational therapy roles. *American Journal of Occupational Therapy, 47,* 1087–1099.

American Occupational Therapy Association. (1994). Statement of occupational therapy referral. *American Journal of Occupational Therapy, 48,* 1034.

American Occupational Therapy Association. (1998). Guidelines to the occupational therapy code of ethics. *American Journal of Occupational Therapy, 2,* 881–884.

American Occupational Therapy Association. (1999). The guide to occupational therapy practice. *American Journal of Occupational Therapy, 53,* 247–322.

Moyers, P. (1999). The guide to occupational therapy practice. *American Journal of Occupational Therapy, 53,* 247–322.

Youngstrom, M. J. (2002). Introduction to the occupational therapy practice and framework: Domain and process. *OT Practice,* CE-1–CE-7.

Authors

THE COMMISSION ON PRACTICE

Sara Jane Brayman, PhD, OTR/L, FAOTA, *Chairperson*

Gloria Frolek Clark, MS, OTR/L, FAOTA

Janet V. DeLany, DEd, OTR/L

Eileen R. Garza, PhD, OTR, ATP

Mary V. Radomski, MA, OTR/L, FAOTA

Ruth Ramsey, MS, OTR/L

Carol Siebert, MS, OTR/L

Kristi Voelkerding, BS, COTA/L

Patricia D. LaVesser, PhD, OTR/L, *SIS Liaison*

Lenna King, *ASD Liaison*

Deborah Lieberman, MHSA, OTR/L, FAOTA, *AOTA Headquarters Liaison*

for

THE COMMISSION ON PRACTICE

Sara Jane Brayman, PhD, OTR/L FAOTA, *Chairperson*

Adopted by the Representative Assembly 2004C23

Originally published as American Occupational Therapy Association. (2004). Scope of practice. *American Journal of Occupational Therapy, 58,* 673–677.

State/Citation	Scope of Practice Language
Alabama Ala. Code, §34-39-3	*Occupational therapy.* The application of purposeful activity in which one engages for evaluation, treatment, and consultation related to problems interfering with functional performance in persons impaired or threatened by physical illness or injury; psychosocial dysfunction; congenital dysfunction; developmental and learning dysfunction; the aging process; environmental deprivation or anticipated dysfunction; in order to maximize independence, prevent disability, and maintain health. Specific occupational therapy services include, but are not limited to, evaluation techniques such as assessment of sensory motor abilities; assessment of the development of self-care activities and capacity for independence; assessment of the capacity for work readiness and work tasks; assessment of play and leisure performance; and assessment of environmental areas for the handicapped. Specific occupational therapy treatment techniques include activities of daily living (ADL); the design, fabrication, and application of selected splints or orthotics, or both; sensorimotor activities and exercise; the use of specifically designed goal oriented arts and crafts; design, fabrication, selection, and use of adaptive equipment; therapeutic activities, modalities, and exercises to enhance functional performance; work readiness evaluation and training. An occupational therapist or occupational therapy assistant is qualified to perform the above activities for which they have received training and any other activities for which appropriate training or education, or both, has been received. Notwithstanding any other provision of this chapter, no occupational therapy treatment programs to be rendered by an occupational therapist, occupational therapy assistant, or occupational therapy aide shall be initiated without the referral of a licensed physician or dentist who shall establish a medical diagnosis of the condition for which the individual will receive occupational therapy services. In cases of long-term or chronic disease, disability, or dysfunction, or any combination of the foregoing, requiring continued occupational therapy services, the person receiving occupational therapy services must be reevaluated by a licensed physician or dentist at least annually for confirmation or modification of the medical diagnosis. Occupational therapists employed by state agencies and those employed by the public schools and colleges of this state who provide screening and rehabilitation services for the educationally related needs of the students are exempt from this referral requirement.
Alaska Alaska Stat., §08.84	"Occupational therapy" means, for compensation, the use of purposeful activity, evaluation, treatment, and consultation with human beings whose ability to cope with the tasks of daily living are threatened with, or impaired by developmental deficits, learning disabilities, aging, poverty, cultural differences, physical injury or illness, or psychological and social disabilities to maximize independence, prevent disability, and maintain health; "occupational therapy" includes (A) developing daily living, play, leisure, social, and developmental skills; (B) facilitating perceptual-motor and sensory intergrative functioning; (C) enhancing functional performance, prevocational skills, and work capabilities using specifically designed exercises, therapeutic activities and measure, manual intervention, and appliances; (D) design, fabrication, and application of splints or selective adaptive equipment; (E) administering and interpreting standardized and nonstandardized assessments, including sensory, manual muscle, and range of motion assessments, necessary for planning effective treatment; and (F) adapting environments for the disabled.
Arizona Ariz. Rev. Stat., §32-3401	*Occupational therapy* means the use of occupational therapy services with individuals who are limited by physical injury or illness, psychosocial dysfunction, developmental or learning disabilities, socioeconomic and cultural differences or the aging process in order to achieve optimum functional performance, maximize independence, prevent disability and maintain health including evaluation, treatment and consultation.
Arkansas Ark. Code, §17-88-102	"Occupational therapy" means the evaluation and treatment of individuals whose ability to cope with the tasks of living is threatened or impaired by developmental deficits, the aging process, poverty or cultural differences, environmental or sensory deprivation, physical injury or illness, or psychological and social disability. (A) The treatment utilizes task-oriented activities to prevent or correct physical or emotional deficits or to minimize the disabling effect of these deficits in the life of the individual so that he might perform tasks normally performed at his stage of development. (B) Specific occupational therapy techniques include, but are not limited to: (i) Instruction in activities of daily living, design, fabrication, application, recommendation, and instruction in the use of selected orthotic or prosthetic devices and other adaptive equipment; (ii) Perceptual-motor and sensory integrative activities; (iii) The use of specifically designed crafts; (iv) Exercises to enhance functional performance; and (v) Prevocational evaluation and treatment. (C) The techniques are applied in the treatment of individual patients or clients, in groups, or through social systems.

(Continued)

State/Citation	Scope of Practice Language
California California Code, §2570.2	(i) "Occupational therapy services" means the services of an occupational therapist or the services of an occupational therapy assistant under the appropriate supervision of an occupational therapist. (k) "Practice of occupational therapy" means the therapeutic use of purposeful and meaningful goal-directed activities (occupations) which engage the individual's body and mind in meaningful, organized, and self-directed actions that maximize independence, prevent or minimize disability, and maintain health. Occupational therapy services encompass occupational therapy assessment, treatment, education of, and consultation with individuals who have been referred for occupational therapy services subsequent to diagnosis of disease or disorder (or who are receiving occupational therapy services as part of an Individualized Education Plan (IEP) pursuant to the federal Individuals with Disabilities Education Act (IDEA)). Occupational therapy assessment identifies performance abilities and limitations that are necessary for self-maintenance, learning, work, and other similar meaningful activities. Occupational therapy treatment is focused on developing, improving, or restoring functional daily living skills (excluding speech-language skills); designing or fabricating selective temporary orthotic devices, and applying or training in the use of assistive technology or orthotic and prosthetic devices (excluding gait training). Occupational therapy consultation provides expert advice to enhance function and quality of life. Consultation or treatment may involve modification of tasks or environments to allow an individual to achieve maximum independence. Services are provided individually, in groups, or through social groups.
Colorado N/A	Trademark law does not provide a definition of occupational therapy.
Connecticut Conn. Gen. Stat., §20-74a	"Occupational therapy" means the evaluation, planning and implementation of a program of purposeful activities to develop or maintain adaptive skills necessary to achieve the maximal physical and mental functioning of the individual in his daily pursuits. The practice of "occupational therapy" includes, but is not limited to, evaluation and treatment of individuals whose abilities to cope with the tasks of living are threatened or impaired by developmental deficits, the aging process, learning disabilities, poverty and cultural differences, physical injury or disease, psychological and social disabilities, or anticipated disfunction, using (A) such treatment techniques as task-oriented activities to prevent or correct physical or emotional deficits or to minimize the disabling effect of these deficits in the life of the individual, (B) such evaluation techniques as assessment of sensory motor abilities, assessment of the development of self-care activities and capacity for independence, assessment of the physical capacity for prevocational and work tasks, assessment of play and leisure performance, and appraisal of living areas for the handicapped, (C) specific occupational therapy techniques such as activities of daily living skills, the fabrication and application of splinting devices, sensory motor activities, the use of specifically designed manual and creative activities, guidance in the selection and use of adaptive equipment, specific exercises to enhance functional performance and treatment techniques for physical capabilities for work activities. Such techniques are applied in the treatment of individual patients or clients, in groups or through social systems. Occupational therapy also includes the establishment and modification of peer review.
Delaware Del. Code Ann. Title 24, 2002	"Occupational therapy services" shall mean, but are not limited to: a. The assessment, treatment and education of or consultation with the individual, family or other persons; or b. Interventions directed toward developing, improving or restoring daily living skills, work readiness or work performance, play skills or leisure capacities, or enhancing educational performance skills; or c. Providing for the development, improvement or restoration of sensorimotor, oral-motor, perceptual or neuromuscular functioning, or emotional, motivational, cognitive or psychosocial components of performance. These services may require assessment of the need for use of interventions such as the design, development, adaptation, application or training in the use of assistive technology devices; the design, fabrication or application of rehabilitative technology such as selected orthotic devices; training in the use of assistive technology, orthotic or prosthetic devices; the application of thermal agent modalities, including, but not limited to, paraffin, hot and cold packs and fluido therapy, as an adjunct to, or in preparation for, purposeful activity; the use of ergonomic principles; the adaptation of environments and processes to enhance functional performance; or the promotion of health and wellness. "Practice of occupational therapy" shall mean the use of goal-directed activities with individuals who are limited by physical limitations due to injury or illness, psychiatric and emotional disorders, developmental or learning disabilities, poverty and cultural differences or the aging process, in order to maximize independence, prevent disability and maintain health.
District of Columbia D.C. Code Ann. §2-1705.2	The term "occupational therapy" means the evaluation and treatment of individuals whose ability to cope with the tasks of living are threatened or impaired by developmental deficits, the aging process, poverty and cultural differences, physical injury or illness, or psychological and social disability. The treatment utilizes task oriented activities to prevent or correct physical or emotional deficits on the individual, with special emphasis on the developmental and functional skills needed throughout life. Specific therapeutic and diagnostic techniques used in occupational therapy include, but are not limited to, self-care and other activities of daily living, developmental oriented tasks, training in basic work habits, perceptual-motor and sensory motor activities, prevocational evaluation and treatment, fabrication and application of splints, selection and use of adaptive equipment, and exercises and exercises and other modalities to enhance functional performance. Such techniques are applied in the treatment of individual patients or clients, in groups, or through social systems.

State/Citation	Scope of Practice Language
Florida Fla. Stat. §468.203	"Occupational therapy" means the use of purposeful activity or interventions to achieve functional outcomes. (a) For the purposes of this subsection: 1. "Achieving functional outcomes" means to maximize the independence and the maintenance of health of any individual who is limited by a physical injury or illness, a cognitive impairment, a psychosocial dysfunction, a mental illness, a developmental or a learning disability, or an adverse environmental condition. 2. "Assessment" means the use of skilled observation or the administration and interpretation of standardized or nonstandardized tests and measurements to identify areas for occupational therapy services. (b) Occupational therapy services include, but are not limited to: 1. The assessment, treatment, and education of or consultation with the individual, family, or other persons. 2. Interventions directed toward developing daily living skills, work readiness or work performance, play skills or leisure capacities, or enhancing educational performance skills. 3. Providing for the development of: sensory-motor, perceptual, or neuromuscular functioning; range of motion; or emotional, motivational, cognitive, or psychosocial components of performance. These services may require assessment of the need for use of interventions such as the design, development, adaptation, application, or training in the use of assistive technology devices; the design, fabrication, or application of rehabilitative technology such as selected orthotic devices; training in the use of assistive technology; orthotic or prosthetic devices; the application of physical agent modalities as an adjunct to or in preparation for purposeful activity; the use of ergonomic principles; the adaptation of environments and processes to enhance functional performance; or the promotion of health and wellness. (c) The use of devices subject to 21 C.F.R. s. 801.109 and identified by the board is expressly prohibited except by an occupational therapist or occupational therapy assistant who has received training as specified by the board. The board shall adopt rules to carry out the purpose of this provision.
Georgia Ga. Code §43-28-3	"Occupational therapy" includes but is not limited to the following: (A) Evaluation and treatment of individuals whose abilities to cope with the tasks of living are threatened or impaired by developmental deficiencies, the aging process, learning disabilities, poverty and cultural differences, physical injury or disease, psychological and social disabilities, or anticipated dysfunction. The treatment utilizes task oriented activities to prevent or correct physical, cognitive, or emotional deficiencies or to minimize the disabling effect of these deficiencies in the life of the individual; (B) Such evaluation techniques as assessment of sensory motor abilities, assessment of the development of self-care activities and capacity for independence, assessment of the physical capacity for prevocational and work tasks, assessment of play and leisure performance, and appraisal of living areas for persons with disabilities; and (C) Specific occupational therapy techniques, such as activity analysis, activities of daily living skills, the fabrication and application of splints and adaptive devices, sensory motor activities, the use of specifically designed manual and creative activities, guidance in the selection and use of adaptive equipment, specific exercises and physical agent modalities to enhance physical functional performance, work capacities, and treatment techniques for physical capabilities and cognitive retraining. Such techniques are applied in the treatment of individual patients or clients, in groups, or through social systems.
Hawaii N/A	Registration law does not provide a definition of occupational therapy.
Idaho Idaho Code §54-3702	"Occupational therapy" is the use of purposeful, goal-oriented activity with individuals who are limited by physical injury or illness, psychosocial dysfunction, developmental or learning disabilities/deficits, poverty or cultural difficulties or the aging process in order to achieve optimum functional performance, independence, prevent further disability and maintain health. The practice of occupational therapy encompasses the evaluation, consultation and treatment of individuals whose abilities to cope with the tasks of daily living are threatened or impaired by physical injury or illness, psychosocial dysfunction, developmental or learning disabilities/deficits, poverty or cultural difficulties or the aging process and includes a treatment program through the use of specific techniques which enhance functional performance and includes the evaluation/assessment of the patient/clients self-care, work and leisure skills, cognition, perception; sensory and motor performance; play skills; vocational and prevocational capacities; need for adaptive equipment; application of selected prosthetic or orthotic devices; and the administration of standardized and nonstandardized assessments.
Illinois 225 Illinois Compiled Statutes 75/2.2	"Occupational Therapy" means the evaluation of functional performance ability of persons impaired by physical illness or injury, emotional disorder, congenital or developmental disability, or the aging process, and the analysis, selection and application of occupations or goal directed activities, for the treatment or prevention of these disabilities to achieve optimum functioning. Occupational therapy services include, but are not limited to activities of daily living (ADL); the design fabrication and application of splints, administration and interpretation of standardized tests to identify dysfunctions, sensory-integrative and perceptual motor activities, the use of task oriented activities, guidance in the selection and use of assistive devices, goal oriented activities directed toward enhancing functional performance, prevocational evaluation and vocational training, and consultation in the adaptation of physical environments for the handicapped. These services are provided to individuals or groups through medical, health, educational, and social systems. An occupational therapist may evaluate a person but shall obtain a referral by a physician before treatment is administered by the occupational therapist. An occupational therapist shall refer to a licensed physician, dentist, or podiatrist any patient whose medical condition should, at the time of evaluation or treatment, be determined to be beyond the scope of practice of the occupational therapist.

(Continued)

State/Citation	Scope of Practice Language
Indiana Ind. Code §25-23.5-1-5	"Occupational therapy" means the functional assessment of learning and performance skills and the analysis, selection, and adaptation of exercises or equipment for a person whose abilities to perform the requirements of daily living are threatened or impaired by physical injury or disease, mental illness, a developmental deficit, the aging process, or a learning disability. The term consists primarily of the following functions: (1) Planning and directing exercises and programs to improve sensory-integration and motor functioning at a level of performance neurologically appropriate for a person's stage of development. (2) Analyzing, selecting, and adapting functional exercises to achieve and maintain a person's optimal functioning in daily living tasks and to prevent further disability.
Iowa Iowa Code §148B.2	"Occupational therapy" means the therapeutic application of specific tasks used for the purpose of evaluation and treatment of problems interfering with functional performance in persons impaired by physical illness or injury, emotional disorder, congenital or developmental disability, or the aging process in order to achieve optimum function, for maintenance of health and prevention of disability.
Kansas Kan. Stat. Ann. §65-5402	"Occupational therapy" is a health care profession whose practitioners, other than occupational therapy practitioners working with the educationally handicapped in a school system, are employed under the supervision of a physician and whose practitioners provide therapy, rehabilitation, diagnostic evaluation, care and education of individuals who are limited by physical injury or illness, psychosocial dysfunction, developmental or learning disabilities or the aging process in order to maximize independence, prevent disability and maintain health. Specific occupational therapy services include: (1) Administering and interpreting tests necessary for effective treatment planning; (2) Developing self-care and daily living skills such as feeding, dressing, hygiene and homemaking; (3) Designing, fabricating, applying or training, or any combination thereof, in the use of selected orthotics, upper extremity prosthetics or adaptive equipment; (4) Developing sensory integrative skills and functioning; (5) Using therapeutic activity and exercise to enhance functional or motor performance, or both; (6) Developing prevocational/vocational work capacities and play/leisure skills; and (7) Adapting environment for the disabled.
Kentucky Ky. Rev. Stat. Ann. §319A.010	"Occupational therapy" means the use of goal directed activities with individuals who are limited by physical limitations due to injury or illness, psychiatric and emotional disorders, developmental or learning disabilities, poverty and cultural differences or the aging process, in order to maximize independence, prevent disability and maintain health. The practice encompasses evaluation, treatment and consultation. Occupational therapy services include: teaching daily living skills; developing perceptual-motor skills and sensory integrative functioning; developing play skills and prevocational and leisure capacities; designing, fabricating, or applying selective orthotic and prosthetic devices or selective adaptive equipment; using specifically designed crafts and therapeutic activities to enhance functional performance; administering and interpreting tests such as manual muscle and range of motion; using and administering certain modalities, specifically hot and cold water, hot packs and cold packs, neutral warmth, quick icing, and paraffin to the hand; and consulting in the adaptation of the environment for individuals with disabilities. These services shall be provided individually, in groups, or through medical, health, educational and social systems. The practice of occupational therapy shall not include gait training; the use or application of electromodalities; accessory joint mobilizations; assessment of integrity and pathology of muscle, soft tissue and joint capsule; and postural or biomechanical analysis; fluidotherapy, diathermy (shortwave, microwave or infrared), ultrasound or whirlpools.
Louisiana La. Rev. Stat. Ann §37:3001	"Occupational therapy" means the application of any activity in which one engages for the purposes of evaluation, interpretation, treatment planning, and treatment of problems interfering with functional performance in persons impaired by physical illness or injury, emotional disorders, congenital or developmental disabilities or the aging process, in order to achieve optimum functioning and prevention and health maintenance. The occupational therapist may enter a case for the purposes of providing consultation and indirect services and evaluating an individual for the need of services. Implementation of direct occupational therapy to individuals for their specific medical condition or conditions shall be based on a referral or order from a physician licensed to practice in the state of Louisiana. Practice shall be in accordance with published standards of practice established by the AOTA, and the essentials of accreditation established by the agencies recognized to accredit specific facilities and programs. Specific occupational therapy services include, but are not limited to, activities of daily living; the design, fabrication and application of prescribed temporary splints, sensorimotor activities; the use of specifically designed crafts; guidance in the selection and use of adaptive equipment; therapeutic activities to enhance functional performance; pre-vocational evaluation and training and consultation concerning the adaption of physical environments for the handicapped. These services are provided to individuals or groups through medical, health, educational and social systems.

State/Citation	Scope of Practice Language
Maine Me. Rev. Stat. Ann. §2272	*Occupational therapy.* "Occupational therapy" means the assessment, planning and implementation of a program of purposeful activities to develop or maintain adaptive skills necessary to achieve the maximal physical and mental functioning of the individual in the individual's daily pursuits. The practice of "occupational therapy" includes, but is not limited to, assessment and treatment of individuals whose abilities to cope with the tasks of living are threatened or impaired by developmental deficits, the aging process, learning disabilities, poverty and cultural differences, physical injury or disease, psychological and social disabilities or anticipated dysfunction, using: A. Treatment techniques such as task-oriented activities to prevent or correct physical or emotional deficits or to minimize the disabling effect of these deficits in the life of the individual. B. Assessment techniques such as assessment of cognitive and sensory motor abilities, assessment of the development of self-care activities and capacity for independence, assessment of the physical capacity for prevocational and work tasks, assessment of play and leisure performance and appraisal of living areas for the disabled; and C. Specific occupational therapy techniques such as daily living skill activities, the fabrication and application of splinting devices, sensory motor activities, the use of specifically designed manual and creative activities, guidance in the selection and use of adaptive equipment, specific exercises to enhance functional performance and treatment techniques for physical capabilities for work activities. The techniques may be applied in the treatment of individuals or groups.
Maryland Md. Ann. Code Art. Health Occ., §10-101	"Practice occupational therapy" means to evaluate, treat, and consult regarding problems that interfere with the functional and occupational performance of an individual who is impaired by physical, emotional, or developmental disability. "Practice occupational therapy" includes: (i) selecting, designing, making, and using splints and adaptive equipment; (ii) using therapeutic activities; (iii) using developmental, perceptual-motor, and sensory integrative activities; (iv) using activities of daily living; (v) prevocational evaluating and training; (vi) consulting about the adaption of environments for the handicapped; and (vii) performing and interpreting manual muscle and range of motion tests.
Massachusetts Mass. Gen. L. Ch. 112 , §23A	"Occupational therapy," the application of principles, methods and procedures of evaluation, problem identification, treatment, education, and consultation which utilizes purposeful activity in order to maximize independence, prevent or correct disability, and maintain health. These services are used with individuals, throughout the life span, whose abilities to interact with their environment are limited by physical injury or illness, disabilities, poverty and cultural differences or the aging process. Occupational therapy includes but is not limited to: (1) administering and interpreting tests necessary for effective treatment planning; (2) developing daily living skills, perceptual motor skills, sensory integrative functioning, play skills and prevocational and vocational work capacities; (3) designing, fabricating or applying selected orthotic and prosthetic devices or selected adaptive equipment; (4) utilizing designated modalities, superficial heat and cold, and neuromuscular facilitation techniques to improve or enhance joint motion muscle function; (5) designing and applying specific therapeutic activities and exercises to enhance or monitor functional or motor performance and to reduce stress; and (6) adapting environments for the handicapped. These services are provided to individuals or groups through medical, health, educational, industrial or social systems. Occupational therapy shall also include delegating of selective forms of treatment to occupational therapy assistants and occupational therapy aides; provided, however, that the occupational therapist so delegating shall assume the responsibility for the care of the patient and the supervision of the occupational therapy assistant or the occupational therapy aide.
Michigan Mich. Stat. Ann. §14.15(18301)	"Certified occupational therapist" means an individual who diminishes or corrects pathology in order to promote and maintain health through application of the art and science of directing purposeful activity designed to restore, reinforce, and enhance the performance of individuals and who is registered in accordance with this article.

(Continued)

State/Citation	Scope of Practice Language
Minnesota Authorizing Statute Minn. Stat. §214.13	214.13 *Human services occupations.* Subdivision 1. Application for credential. The commissioner of health shall promote the recognition of human services occupations useful in the effective delivery of human services. The commissioner shall coordinate the development of a credentials policy among the health-related licensing boards consistent with Section 214.001.
Regulation Minn. R. 4666	*Occupational therapy.* "Occupational therapy" means the use of purposeful activity to maximize the independence and the maintenance of health of an individual who is limited by a physical injury or illness, a cognitive impairment, a psychosocial dysfunction, a mental illness, a developmental or learning disability, or an adverse environmental condition. The practice encompasses evaluation, assessment, treatment, and consultation. Occupational therapy services may be provided individually, in groups, or through social systems. Occupational therapy includes those services described in Part 4666.0040. 4666.0040 SCOPE OF PRACTICE. The practice of occupational therapy by an occupational therapist or occupational therapy assistant includes, but is not limited to, intervention directed toward: A. assessment and evaluation, including the use of skilled observation or the administration and interpretation of standardized or nonstandardized tests and measurements, to identify areas for occupational therapy services; B. providing for the development of sensory integrative, neuromuscular, or motor components of performance; C. providing for the development of emotional, motivational, cognitive, or psychosocial components of performance; D. developing daily living skills; E. developing feeding and swallowing skills; F. developing play skills and leisure capacities; G. enhancing educational performance skills; H. enhancing functional performance and work readiness through exercise, range of motion, and use of ergonomic principles; I. designing, fabricating, or applying rehabilitative technology, such as selected orthotic and prosthetic devices, and providing training in the functional use of these devices; J. designing, fabricating, or adapting assistive technology and providing training in the functional use of assistive devices; K. adapting environments using assistive technology such as environmental controls, wheelchair modifications, and positioning; L. employing physical agent modalities, in preparation for or as an adjunct to purposeful activity, within the same treatment session or to meet established functional occupational therapy goals, consistent with the requirements of part 4666.1000; and M. promoting health and wellness.
Mississippi Miss. Code of 1972 §73-24-3	"Occupational therapy" is the use of purposeful activity with individuals who are limited by physical injury or illness, psychosocial dysfunction, developmental or learning disabilities, or the aging process in order to maximize independence, prevent disability and maintain health. The practice encompasses evaluation, treatment and consultation. Specific occupational therapy services include: teaching daily living skills; developing perceptual-motor skills and sensory integrative functioning; developing play skills and prevocational and leisure capacities; designing, fabricating or applying selected splints or selective adaptive equipment; using specifically designed activities and exercises to enhance functional performance; administering and interpreting tests such as manual muscle and range of motion; and adapting environments for the handicapped. These services are provided individually, in groups, or through social systems, i.e., schools, nursing homes, etc.
Missouri Mo. Rev. Stat. §324.050	"Occupational therapy," the use of purposeful activity or interventions designed to achieve functional outcomes which promote health, prevent injury or disability and which develop, improve, sustain or restore the highest possible level of independence of any individual who has an injury, illness, cognitive impairment, psychosocial dysfunction, mental illness, developmental or learning disability, physical disability or other disorder or condition. It shall include assessment by means of skill observation or evaluation through the administration and interpretation of standardized or nonstandardized tests and measurements. Occupational therapy services include, but are not limited to: (a) The assessment and provision of treatment in consultation with the individual, family or other appropriate persons; (b) Interventions directed toward developing, improving, sustaining or restoring daily living skills, including self-care skills and activities that involve interactions with others and the environment, work readiness or work performance, play skills or leisure capacities or enhancing educational performances skills; (c) Developing, improving, sustaining or restoring sensorimotor, oral-motor, perceptual or neuromuscular functioning; or emotional, motivational, cognitive or psychosocial components of performance; and (d) Education of the individual, family or other appropriate persons in carrying out appropriate interventions. Such services may encompass assessment of need and the design, development, adaptation, application or training in the use of assistive technology devices; the design, fabrication or application of rehabilitative technology such as selected orthotic devices; training in the use of orthotic or prosthetic devices; the application of ergonomic principles; the adaptation of environments and processes to enhance functional performance; or the promotion of health and wellness.

State/Citation	Scope of Practice Language
Montana Mont. Code Ann. §37-24-103	"Occupational therapy" means the use of purposeful activity and interventions to achieve functional outcomes to maximize the independence and the maintenance of health of an individual who is limited by physical injury or illness, psychosocial dysfunction, mental illness, developmental or learning disability, the aging process, cognitive impairment, or an adverse environmental condition. The practice encompasses assessment, treatment, and consultation. Occupational therapy services may be provided individually, in groups, or through social systems. Occupational therapy interventions include but are not limited to: (a) teaching daily living skills; (b) developing perceptual-motor skills and sensory integrative functioning; (c) developing play skills and leisure capacities and enhancing educational performance skills; (d) designing, fabricating, or applying splints or selective adaptive equipment and training in the use of upper extremity prosthetics or upper extremity orthotic devices; (e) providing for the development of emotional, motivational, cognitive, psychosocial, or physical components of performance; (f) providing assessment and evaluation, including the use of skilled observation or the administration and interpretation of standardized or nonstandardized tests and measurements to identify areas for occupational therapy services; (g) adapting environments for the disabled, including assistive technology, such as environmental controls, wheelchair modifications, and positioning; (h) developing feeding and swallowing skills; (i) enhancing and assessing work performance and work readiness through occupational therapy intervention, including education and instruction, activities to increase and improve general work behavior and skill, job site evaluation, on-the-job training and evaluation, development of work-related activities, and supported employment placement; (j) providing neuromuscular facilitation and inhibition, including the activation, facilitation, and inhibition of muscle action, both voluntary and involuntary, through the use of appropriate sensory stimulation, including vibration or brushing, to evoke a desired muscular response; (k) employing physical agent modalities as defined in this section; and (l) promoting health and wellness.
Nebraska Neb. Rev. Stat. §71-6103	"Occupational therapy" shall mean the use of purposeful activity with individuals who are limited by physical injury or illness, psychosocial dysfunction, developmental or learning disabilities, or the aging process in order to maximize independence, prevent disability, and maintain health. Occupational therapy shall encompass evaluation, treatment, and consultation. Occupational therapy may include teaching daily living skills, developing perceptual-motor skills and sensory integrative functioning, developing prevocational capacities, designing, fabricating, or applying selected orthotic and prosthetic devices or selective adaptive equipment, using specifically designed therapeutic media and exercises to enhance functional performance, administering and interpreting tests such as manual muscle and range of motion, and adapting environments for the handicapped.
Nevada Nev. Rev. Stat. §640A.050	"Occupational therapy" means the application of purposeful activity in the evaluation, teaching and treatment, in groups or on an individual basis, of patients who are handicapped by age, physical injury or illness, psychosocial dysfunction, developmental or learning disability, poverty or aspects of culture, to increase their independence, alleviate their disability and maintain their health. The term includes: 1. Teaching patients skills for daily living; 2. Assisting patients in the development of cognitive and perceptual motor skills, and in the integration of sensory functions; 3. Assisting patients in learning to play and to use their leisure time constructively; 4. Assisting patients in developing functional skills necessary to be considered for employment; 5. Assessing the need for, designing, constructing and training patients in the use and application of selected orthotic devices and adaptive equipment; 6. Assessing the need for prosthetic devices for the upper body and training patients in the functional use of prosthetic devices; 7. Teaching patients crafts and exercises designed to enhance their ability to function normally; 8. Administering to patients manual tests of their muscles and range of motion, and interpreting the results of those tests; 9. Incorporating into the treatment of patients the safe and appropriate use of physical therapeutic modalities and techniques which have been acquired through an appropriate program of education approved by the board pursuant to subsection 2 of NRS 640A.120, or through a program of continuing education or higher education; and 10. Adapting the environment of patients to reduce the effects of handicaps.
New Hampshire N.H. Rev. Stat. Ann. §326-C:1	"Occupational therapy" means the therapeutic use of self-care, work and play activities to increase independent function in activities of daily living, to enhance development, and to prevent disability. The term may include the adaptation of task or environment to achieve maximum independence and to enhance the quality of life. Specific occupational therapy techniques include, but are not limited to, the fabrication and application of splints, perceptual-motor and sensory integrative activities, the use of specifically designed crafts, guidance in the selection and use of adaptive equipment, exercises to increase functional performance, and prevocational evaluation and treatment.

(Continued)

State/Citation	Scope of Practice Language
New Jersey N.J. Rev. Stat. §45:9-37.53	"Occupational therapy" means the evaluation, planning and implementation of a program of purposeful activities to develop or maintain functional skills necessary to achieve the maximal physical or mental functioning, or both, of the individual in his daily occupational performance. The tasks of daily living may be threatened or impaired by physical injury or illness, developmental deficits, sensorimotor dysfunction, psychological and social dysfunction, the aging process, poverty, or cultural deprivation. Occupational therapy utilizes task oriented activities adapted to prevent or correct physical or emotional deficits as well as to minimize the disabling effects of those deficits on the life of the individual. Occupational therapy services include the use of specific techniques which enhance functional performance and include, but are not limited to, the evaluation and assessment of an individual's self care, lifestyle performance patterns, work skills, performance related cognitive, sensory, motor, perceptual, affective, interpersonal and social functioning, vocational and prevocational capacities, the design, fabrication and application of adaptive equipment or prosthetic or orthotic devices, excluding dental devices, the administration of standardized and nonstandardized assessments, and consultation concerning the adaptation of physical environments for the handicapped. These services are provided to individuals or groups through medical, health, educational and social systems.
New Mexico N.M. Stat. Ann. §61-12A-3	"Occupational therapy" means the use of purposeful activity or intervention designed to achieve functional outcomes that promote health, prevent injury or disability and develop, improve, sustain or restore to the highest possible level of independence a person who has an injury, illness, psychosocial dysfunction, mental illness, developmental or learning disability, physical disability or other disorder or condition;
N.M. Stat. Ann. §61-12A-3	A. Occupational therapy services include the assessment, reassessment, planning and discontinuation of: (1) the provision of treatment in consultation with the individual, family or other appropriate persons; (2) treatment directed toward developing, improving or restoring daily living skills, including self-care skills and activities that involve interactions with others and the environment, work readiness or work performance, play skills or leisure capacities or enhancing educational performance skills; (3) the development, improvement or restoration of sensorimotor, perceptual or neuromuscular functioning; or emotional, motivational, cognitive or psychosocial components of performance; and (4) education of individuals, families or the appropriate persons in carrying out appropriate treatment objectives. B. The services provided for in Subsection A of this section shall encompass the assessment of needs and the design, development, adaptation, application or training in the use of assistive technology devices; the design, fabrication or application of rehabilitative technology such as selected orthotic devices; training in the use of orthotic devices; the application and training in the use of physical agent modalities as an adjunct to or in preparation for purposeful activity; the application of ergonomic principles; the adaptation of environments and processes to enhance functional performance; and the promotion of health and wellness
New York Statute N.Y. Education Law §7901	The practice of the profession of occupational therapy is defined as the functional evaluation of the client and the planning and utilization of a program of purposeful activities to develop or maintain adaptive skills, designed to achieve maximal physical and mental functioning of the patient in his or her daily life tasks. Such treatment program shall be rendered on the prescription or referral of a physician or nurse practitioner.
Regulation N.Y. Comp. Codes R. & Regs. Tit. 8, §76.7	*Definition of occupation therapy practice.* (a) A functional evaluation within the meaning within the meaning of Education Law, Section 7901 may include screening, observing, consulting, administering and/or interpreting standardized and nonstandardized assessment tools, and simulating and analyzing activities or environments for the purpose of: (1) assessing levels of functional abilities and deficits resulting from developmental deficits, injury, disease, or any limiting condition; and/or (2) identifying areas of functional abilities and deficits resulting from developmental deficit, injury, disease or any limiting condition; and/or (3) determining the need for the types of initial and/or subsequent occupational therapy. (b) Purposeful activity is defined as goal-directed behavior aimed at the development of functional daily living skills in the categories of self-care, work, homemaking or play/leisure. (c) A treatment program within the meaning of Education Law, section 7901 shall be consistent with the statutory scope of practice and may: (1) Include the therapeutic use of goal-directed activities, exercises, or techniques to maximize the client's physical and/or mental functioning in life tasks. Treatment is directed toward maximizing functional skill and task-related performance for the development of a client's vocational, avocational, daily living or relating capacities. (2) Relate to physical, perceptual, sensory, neuromuscular, sensory-integrative, cognitive or psychosocial skills. (3) Include, where appropriate for such purposes, and under appropriate conditions, modalities and techniques based on approaches taught in an occupational therapy curriculum and included in a program of professional education in occupational therapy registered by the department, and consistent with areas of individual competence. These approaches are based on:

State/Citation	Scope of Practice Language

New York (Continued)

(i) The neurological and physiological sciences as taught in a registered occupational therapy professional education program. Modalities and techniques may be based on, but not limited to, any one or more of the following:

    (a) sensory integrative approaches;

    (b) developmental approaches;

    (c) sensorimotor approaches;

    (d) neurophysiological treatment approaches;

    (e) muscle reeducation;

    (f) superficial heat and cold; or

    (g) cognitive and perceptual remediation.

(ii) The behavioral and social sciences as taught in a registered occupational therapy professional education program. Modalities and techniques may be based on, but not limited to, any one or more of the following:

    (a) behavioral principles;

    (b) work-related programs and simulation;

    (c) group dynamics and process; or

    (d) leisure/avocational activities.

(iii) The biomechanical sciences as taught in a registered occupational therapy professional education program. Modalities and techniques may be based on, but not limited to, any one or more of the following:

    (a) passive, active assistive, and active range of motion;

    (b) muscle strengthening and conditioning;

    (c) positioning;

    (d) participation in design, fabrication, and/or application, and patient education related to orthotics and adaptive equipment;

    (e) evaluation of appropriateness, participation in design concept, application and patient education related to prosthetics;

    (f) daily life tasks;

    (g) adapting the client's environment; or

    (h) work-related programs.

North Carolina
N.C. Gen. Stat. §90-270.67

"Occupational therapy" means a health care profession providing evaluation, treatment and consultation to help individuals achieve a maximum level of independence by developing skills and abilities interfered with by disease, emotional disorder, physical injury, the aging process, or impaired development. Occupational therapists use purposeful activities and specially designed orthotic and prosthetic devices to reduce specific impairments and to help individuals achieve independence at home and in the work place.

North Dakota
Enacted 1999 H.B. 1467,
Chapter 394

"Occupational therapy practice" means the use of occupation and purposeful activity or intervention designed to achieve functional outcomes that promote health, prevent injury or disability and which develop, improve, sustain, or restore the highest possible level of independence of any individual who has an injury, illness, cognitive impairment, psychosocial dysfunction, mental illness, developmental or learning disability, physical disability or other disorder or condition, and occupational therapy education. Occupational therapy encompasses evaluation, treatment, consultation, research, and education. Occupational therapy practice includes evaluation by skilled observation, administration, and interpretation of standardized and nonstandardized tests and measurements. The occupational therapy practitioner designs and implements interventions directed toward developing, improving, sustaining, and restoring sensorimotor, neuromuscular, emotional, cognitive, or psychosocial performance components. Interventions include activities that contribute to optimal occupational performance including self-care; daily living skills; skills essential for productivity, functional communication and mobility; positioning; social integration; cognitive mechanisms; enhancing play and leisure skills; and the design, provision, and training in the use of assistive technology, devices, orthotics, or prosthetics or environmental adaptations to accommodate for loss of occupational performance. Therapy may be provided individually, or in groups, to prevent secondary conditions, promote community integration, and support the individual's health and well-being within the social and cultural contexts of the individual's natural environment.

Ohio
OH Rev. Code §4755.01

"Occupational therapy" means the evaluation of learning and performance skills and the analysis, selection, and adaptation of activities for an individual whose abilities to cope with daily living, perform tasks normally performed at his stage of development, and perform vocational tasks are threatened or impaired by developmental deficiencies, the aging process, environmental deprivation, or physical, psychological, or social injury or illness, through specific techniques which include:

(1) Planning and implementing activities and programs to improve sensory and motor functioning at the level of performance normal for the individual's stage of development;

(2) Teaching skills, behaviors, and attitudes crucial to the individual's independent, productive, and satisfying social functioning;

(3) Designing, fabricating, applying, recommending, and instructing in the use of selected orthotic or prosthetic devices and other equipment which assists the individual to adapt to his potential or actual impairment;

(4) Analyzing, selecting, and adapting activities to maintain the individual's optimal performance of tasks and to prevent further disability.

(Continued)

State/Citation	Scope of Practice Language
Oklahoma Okla. Stat. Tit. 59, §59-888.3	"Occupational therapy" is a health profession for which practitioners provide assessment, treatment, and consultation through the use of purposeful activity with individuals who are limited by or at risk of physical illness or injury, psycho-social dysfunction, developmental or learning disabilities, poverty and cultural differences or the aging process, in order to maximize independence, prevent disability, and maintain health. Specific occupational therapy services include but are not limited to the use of media and methods such as instruction in daily living skills and cognitive retraining, facilitating self-maintenance, work and leisure skills, using standardized or adapted techniques, designing, fabricating, and applying selected orthotic equipment or selective adaptive equipment with instructions, using therapeutically applied creative activities, exercise, and other media to enhance and restore functional performance, to administer and interpret tests which may include sensorimotor evaluation, psycho-social assessments, standardized or nonstandardized tests, to improve developmental skills, perceptual motor skills, and sensory integrative function, and to adapt the environment for the handicapped. These services are provided individually, in groups, or through social systems.
Oregon Or. Rev. Stat. §675.210	"Occupational therapy" means the analysis and use of purposeful activity with individuals who are limited by physical injury or illness, developmental or learning disabilities, psycho-social dysfunctions or the aging process in order to maximize independence, prevent disability and maintain health. The practice of occupational therapy encompasses evaluation, treatment and consultation. Specific occupational therapy services includes but is not limited to: Activities of daily living (ADL); perceptual motor and sensory integrated activity; development of work and leisure skills; the design, fabrication or application of selected orthotics or prosthetic devices; the use of specifically designed crafts; guidance in the selection and use of adaptive equipment; exercises to enhance functional performance; prevocational evaluation and training; performing and interpreting manual muscle and range of motion test; and appraisal and adaptation of environments for people with mental and physical disabilities. The services are provided individually, in groups, or through social systems.
Pennsylvania Pa. Act 140 of 1982 Occupational Therapy Practice Act	*Occupational therapy.* The evaluation of learning and performance skills and the analysis, selection and adaptation of activities for an individual whose abilities to cope with the activities of daily living, to perform tasks normally performed at a given stage of development and to perform essential vocational tasks which are threatened or impaired by that person's developmental deficiencies, aging process, environmental deprivation or physical, psychological, injury or illness, through specific techniques which include: (1) Planning and implementing activity programs to improve sensory and motor functioning at the level of performance normal for the individual's stage of development. (2) Teaching skills, behaviors and attitudes crucial to the individual's independent, productive and satisfying social functioning. (3) The design, fabrication and application of splints, not to include prosthetic or orthotic devices, and the adaptation of equipment necessary to assist patients in adjusting to a potential or actual impairment and instructing in the use of such devices and equipment. (4) Analyzing, selecting and adapting activities to maintain the individual's optimal performance of tasks to prevent disability. "Occupational therapy" is the field of study which makes use of evaluative methods and of functional, motor and sensorial selected activities specifically for the purpose of promoting and conserving the health, to avoid disabilities, evaluate the conduct and to treat or train patients with physical or psychosocial disabilities.
Puerto Rico P.R. Laws Ann. Tit. 20, §1031	"Occupational therapy" (OT) is the use of purposeful activity or interventions designed to achieve functional outcomes which promote health, prevent injury or disability, and develop, improve, sustain, or restore the highest possible level of independence of any individual who has an injury, illness, cognitive impairment, sensory impairment, psychosocial dysfunction, mental illness, developmental or learning disability, physical disability, or other disorder or condition.
Rhode Island R.I. Gen. Laws §5-40.1-3	Occupational therapy includes evaluation by means of skilled observation of functional performance and/or assessment through the administration and interpretation of standardized or nonstandardized tests and measurements. Occupational therapy services includes, but are not limited to: (a) The evaluation and provision of treatment in consultation with the individual, family or other appropriate persons; (b) Interventions directed toward developing, improving, sustaining or restoring daily living skills, including self-care skills and activities that involve interactions with others and the environment, work readiness or work performance, play skills or leisure capacities or educational performance skills; (c) Developing, improving, sustaining or restoring sensorimotor, oral-motor, perceptual or neuromuscular functioning; or emotional, motivational, cognitive or psychosocial components of performance; and (d) Education of the individual, family or other appropriate persons in carrying out appropriate interventions. These services may encompass evaluation of need and the design, development, adaptation, application or training in the use of assistive technology devices; the design, fabrication or application of rehabilitative technology, such as selected orthotic devices; training in the functional use of orthotic or prosthetic devices; the application of therapeutic activities, modalities, or exercise as an adjunct to or in preparation for functional performance; the application of ergonomic principles; the adaptation of environments and processes to enhance daily living skills; or the promotion of health and wellness.

State/Citation	Scope of Practice Language
South Carolina S.C. Code Ann. §40-36-20	"Occupational therapy" means the functional evaluation and treatment of individuals whose ability to cope with the tasks of living are threatened or impaired by developmental deficits, the aging process, poverty and cultural differences, physical injury or illness, or psychological or social disability. The treatment utilizes occupational, namely goal-oriented activities, to prevent or correct physical or emotional deficits or to minimize the disabling effect of these deficits in the life of the individual. Specific occupational therapy techniques include, but are not limited to, activities of daily living (ADL), the fabrication and application of splints, sensory-motor activities, the use of specifically designed crafts, guidance in the selection and use of adaptive equipment, exercises to enhance functional performance, prevocational evaluation and treatment and consultation concerning adaption of physical environments for the handicapped. These techniques are applied in the treatment of individual patients or clients, in groups, or through social systems.
South Dakota S.D. Codified Laws §36-31-1	"Occupational therapy," the evaluation, planning and implementation of a program of purposeful activities to develop or maintain adaptive skills necessary to achieve the maximal physical and mental functioning of the individual in his daily pursuits. The practice of "occupational therapy" includes, but is not limited to, consultation, evaluation and treatment individuals whose abilities to cope with the tasks of living are threatened or impaired by developmental deficits, the aging process, learning disabilities, poverty and cultural differences, physical injury or disease, psychological and social disabilities or anticipated dysfunction. Occupational therapy services include such treatment techniques as task-oriented activities to prevent or correct physical or emotional deficits or to minimize the disabling effect of these deficits in the life of the individual; such evaluation techniques as assessment of sensory integration and motor abilities, assessment of development of self-care and feeding, activities and capacity for independence, assessment of the physical capacity for prevocational and work tasks, assessment of play and leisure performance, and appraisal of living areas for the handicapped; and specific occupational therapy techniques such as activities of daily living skills, designing, fabricating or applying selected orthotic devices or selecting adaptive equipment, sensory integration and motor activities, the use of specifically designed manual and creative activities, specific exercises to enhance functional performance and treatment techniques for physical capabilities for work activities. Such techniques are applied in the treatment of individual patients or clients, in groups, or through social systems.
Tennessee Enacted 1999 H.B. 1245, Chapter 415	"Occupational therapy" means the screening, evaluation, assessment, planning, implementation and discharge planning of a program of purposeful, meaningful and functional activities with individuals who are limited by physical injury or illness, psychosocial dysfunction, developmental or learning disabilities, environmental deprivation, poverty or cultural difficulties, or the aging process, in order to improve, sustain, or restore the highest level of independence possible for the individual. The practice of occupational therapy includes, but is not limited to: (A) The evaluation and provision of treatment in consultation with the individual, family and other appropriate persons; (B) Selection and administration of standardized and nonstandardized tests and measurements; (C) The interpretation of assessments in relation to performance areas and performance components; (D) Selection and teaching of selected life tasks and activities in the performance areas of: activities of daily living, work and productive activities, and play or leisure; (E) The grading and adapting of purposeful activity for therapeutic intervention; (F) Development, improvement, retention, and restoration of sensorimotor, cognitive, and psychosocial performance components; (G) Consideration of the performance contexts in which the individual must perform, including the temporal and environmental aspects; (H) Fostering of prevention, health maintenance, and safety programs, including family or caretaker training; (I) Reevaluation for effect of occupational therapy intervention and need for continued or changed treatment; (J) Termination of occupational therapy services including determination of discharge, summary of occupational therapy outcome, and appropriate recommendations and referrals to maximize treatment gains; (K) Management of occupational therapy services including the planning, organizing, staffing, coordinating, directing, or controlling of individuals and organizations; and (L) Administration, interpretation and application of research to occupational services. Occupational therapy services may encompass evaluation of need and the design, development, adaptation, application and training in the use of assistive technology devices; the design, fabrication, or application of rehabilitative technology such as selective orthotic devices; training in the use of orthotic or prosthetic devices; the application of physical agent modalities as an adjunct to or in preparation for purposeful activity with proper training; the application of ergonomic principles; the adaptation of environments and processes to enhance functional performance; or the promotion of health and wellness. Occupational therapy services may be provided in many settings including, but not limited to, hospitals, nursing homes, mental health facilities, industrial settings, community programs, community services, home health, outpatient rehabilitation facilities, and schools. Additionally, occupational therapists may be certified in areas of specialization such as, but not limited to, hand therapy, neurodevelopmental treatment, sensory integration, pediatrics, and neurorehabilitation through programs approved by the AOTA or other nationally recognized organizations.

(Continued)

State/Citation	Scope of Practice Language
Texas Tex. Occ. Code Ann. §8851	"Occupational therapy" means the evaluation and treatment of individuals whose ability to perform the tasks of living is threatened or impaired by developmental deficits, the aging process, environmental deprivation, sensory impairment, physical injury or illness, or psychological or social dysfunction. Occupational therapy utilizes therapeutic goal-directed activities to evaluate, prevent, or correct physical or emotional dysfunction or to maximize function in the life of the individual. Such activities are applied in the treatment of patients on an individual basis, in groups, or through social systems, by means of direct or monitored treatment or consultation.
Utah Utah Code Ann. §58-42a-102	"Occupational therapy" means the use of purposeful activity or occupational therapy interventions to develop or restore the highest possible level of independence of an individual who is limited by a physical injury or illness, a dysfunctional condition, a cognitive impairment, a psychosocial dysfunction, a mental illness, a developmental or learning disability, or an adverse environmental condition. "Occupational therapy services" include: (a) assessing, treating, educating, or consulting with an individual, family, or other persons; (b) developing, improving, or restoring an individual's daily living skills, work readiness, work performance, play skills, or leisure capacities, or enhancing an individual's educational performance skills; (c) developing, improving, or restoring an individual's sensory-motor, oral-motor, perceptual, or neuromuscular functioning, or the individual's range of motion; (d) developing, improving, or restoring the individual's emotional, motivational, cognitive, or psychosocial components of performance; (e) assessing the need for and recommending, developing, adapting, designing, or fabricating splints or assistive technology devices for individuals; (f) training individuals in the use of rehabilitative or assistive technology devices such as selected orthotic or prosthetic devices; (g) applying physical agent modalities as an adjunct to or in preparation for purposeful activity; (h) applying the use of ergonomic principles; and (i) adapting or modifying environments and processes to enhance or promote the functional performance, health, and wellness of individuals. "Practice of occupational therapy" means rendering or offering to render occupational therapy services to individuals, groups, agencies, organizations, industries, or the public.
Vermont Vt. Stat. Ann. §3351	"Occupational therapy" means the use of purposeful activity to maximize functional independence, prevent and remediate disability, and maintain the health of individuals who are limited by physical injury or illness, a cognitive impairment, psychosocial dysfunction, a mental illness, developmental or learning disabilities, or an adverse environmental condition. The practice of occupational therapy encompasses evaluation and testing, treatment, and consultation. Occupational therapists use skilled observation or administer and interpret standardized or nonstandardized tests and measurements to identify the need for occupational therapy services. Occupational therapists assess the need for and use of: the design, development, adaptation, or application of assistive technology devices; the design, fabrication, and application of rehabilitative technology such as selected orthotic devices; training in the use of assistive technology or orthotic and prosthetic devices; the application of therapeutic agents as an adjunct to, or in preparation for, purposeful activities; ergonomic principles; and the adaptation of environments and processes to enhance functional performance or the promotion of health and wellness. Occupational therapy services include: developing daily living skills; work readiness or work performance; play skills or leisure capacity; enhancing educational performance skills; assisting in the development of sensory-motor, perceptual or neuromuscular functioning, or range of motion; assisting in the development of emotional, motivational, cognitive, or psychosocial components of performance; or assisting individuals with eating/swallowing disorders. Occupational therapy services are provided individually, in groups, or through social systems, and may be carried out in consultation with the patient's family or other person interested in his or her welfare.
Virginia Va. Code Ann. §54.1-2900	"Practice of occupational therapy" means the evaluation, analysis, assessment, and delivery of education and training in activities of daily living (ADL); the design, fabrication, and application of orthoses (splints); guidance in the selection and use of adaptive equipment; therapeutic activities to enhance functional performance; prevocational evaluation and training; and consultation concerning the adaptation of physical environments for individuals who have disabilities.
Washington Wash. Rev. Code §8.59.020	"Occupational therapy" is the scientifically based use of purposeful activity with individuals who are limited by physical injury or illness, psychosocial dysfunction, developmental or learning disabilities, or the aging process in order to maximize independence, prevent disability, and maintain health. The practice encompasses evaluation, treatment, and consultation. Specific occupational therapy services include but are not limited to: Using specifically designed activities and exercises to enhance neurodevelopmental, cognitive, perceptual motor, sensory integrative, and psychomotor functioning; administering and interpreting tests such as manual muscle and sensory integration; teaching daily living skills; developing prevocational skills and play and avocational capabilities; designing, fabricating, or applying selected orthotic and prosthetic devices or selected adaptive equipment; and adapting environments for the handicapped. These services are provided individually, in groups, or through social systems.

State/Citation	Scope of Practice Language
West Virginia W. Va. Code §30-28-3	"Occupational therapy" means the evaluation, treatment and aid in diagnosis of problems interfering with functional performance in persons impaired by physical illness or injury, emotional disorder, congenital or developmental disability, or the aging process in order to achieve optimum functioning and for prevention and health maintenance. Specific occupational therapy services include, but are not limited to, activities of daily living (ADL); the design, fabrication and application of splints; sensorimotor activities; the use of specifically designed crafts; guidance in the selection and use of adaptive equipment; therapeutic activities to enhance functional performance; prevocational evaluation and training; and consultation concerning the adaption of physical environments for the handicapped. These services are provided to individuals or groups through medical, health, educational and social systems and for the maintenance of health through these systems.
Wisconsin Wis. Stat. §448.01	Occupational therapy means the use of purposeful activity with persons who are limited by physical injury or illness, psychosocial dysfunction, developmental or learning disability or the aging process, in order to maximize independent function, prevent further disability and achieve and maintain health and productivity, and encompasses evaluation, treatment and consultation services that are provided to a person or a group of persons.
Wyoming Wyo. Stat. §33-40-102	"Occupational therapy" is the use of purposeful activity with individuals who are limited by physical injury or illness, psychosocial dysfunction, developmental or learning disabilities or the aging process in order to maximize independence, prevent disability and maintain health. The practice encompasses evaluation, treatment and consultation. Specific occupational therapy services include but are not limited to the following services provided individually, in groups or through social systems: (A) Teaching daily living skills; (B) Developing perceptual-motor skills and sensory integrative functioning; (C) Developing play skills and prevocational and leisure capacities; (D) Assessing the need for designing, fabricating, training in the use of or applying selected orthotic devices or selective adaptive equipment; (E) Assessing the need for and training in the use of prosthetic devices; (F) Using specifically designed crafts and exercises to enhance functional performance; (G) Administering and interpreting tests such as manual muscle and range of motion; and (H) Adapting environments for the handicapped.

Chapter 3

State Regulation of Occupational Therapy Assistants

Thirty-nine states, the District of Columbia and Puerto Rico license occupational therapy assistants; 3 states have certification laws; 3 states have registration laws; and 1 state and Guam have trademark laws. Colorado, Hawaii, and Virginia do not regulate occupational therapy assistants. In New York, the State Board of Occupational Therapy, which licenses occupational therapists, does not license OTAs. The New York State Department of Education (NYSDE), the state agency with authority over occupational therapy practitioners, does not require that occupational therapy assistants pass the entry-level certification examination. However, the NYSDE does provide an agency "certification" for occupational therapy assistants. New York is the only state that has two different types of regulation for the two levels of the profession.

Regulation Procedures and Requirements

1. In order to practice in a state that has licensure, certification, or registration, you must be issued a license, certificate, or registration. It is your responsibility to contact the state agency, or board/council and request an application at least 6 to 8 weeks prior to your employment start date. Be sure to consult with your facility and state agency office to ensure that you meet any additional requirements for practice.
2. Consult your state regulatory agency/board for guidance in the following areas:
   - For persons who will be practicing in states that license or certify OTAs, you must
     - Contact the state regulatory board/council and request an application and a copy of the state occupational therapy laws and regulations; and
     - Submit the completed application, and/or letters of reference, and fees to the board/council. Be sure

to retain copies of your completed application packet including copies of your canceled checks/money order receipts for fees paid.
   - For persons who will be practicing in states that have registration or trademark laws, you must
     - Contact the appropriate state agency and facility and inquire about requirements for practice and request a copy of the state occupational therapy laws and regulations; and
     - Read and understand the regulations for Medicare, Medicaid, and other third-party payers.
   - For persons who will be practicing in states that are regulated but do not have a statutory scope of practice for occupational therapy, you should
     - Read and understand your facility's practice policies and the regulations for Medicare, Medicaid, and other third-party payers; and
     - Consult appropriate AOTA official documents for guidance in practice.
   - *Prior* to your first day working as an OTA, you should have
     - Received a license, certificate, or registration authorized by the board/council and provide a copy or the original to your supervisor to show that you have complied with the state requirements;
     - Read and understand the state OT laws and regulations; and
     - Read and understand the regulations for Medicare, Medicaid, and other third-party payers.

Note. If you are employed by a contract agency company that has initiated your application to practice in a state, it is ultimately your responsibility to follow through with the state board or agency to ensure that your application information is complete so that the board can render a decision on your eligibility to practice.

Scope of Practice

State regulation of occupational therapy practitioners is usually administered by an appointed regulatory board, council, or state agency. The regulatory bodies have statutory authority to define the scope of practice in state occupational therapy laws and regulations and also to establish policies that may impact the practice of occupational therapy. When a question arises regarding the interpretation of state occupational therapy laws and regulations, it is recommended that you *send a written request to the board and seek written clarification*. Most state boards use the services of the Office of the Attorney General to assist in responding to scope of practice issues. You should contact the board for copies of state occupational therapy laws and regulations so that you can be an informed practitioner. Remember, once you receive a license, certificate or registration to practice occupational therapy from a state regulatory board, it is presumed that you understand the laws and regulations governing the practice of occupational therapy in that state.

Continuing Education Requirements

Some states require completion of continuing education requirements for renewal of a license, certificate, or registration to practice. Contact the state regulatory board, and be sure to understand the dates and procedures for renewal. If you practice in more than one state, you should comply with the requirements of each state. An important caveat—states renew thousands of practitioners on similar renewal cycles. It is your responsibility to be proactive in this process and understand that mistakes can occur. For your records, maintain copies of all continuing education documentation and follow up with the board staff periodically for a status of your renewal application. If you wait to the last minute to complete the renewal requirements, you may run the risk of not receiving an updated license, certificate, or registration in a timely manner. This could jeopardize your employment status.

Supervision Requirements

Another facet of the jurisdiction of state regulatory boards is establishing requirements for occupational therapy assistant supervision. In the process of drafting regulations on this issue, most state regulatory boards consult with the AOTA State Policy and Practice Departments and refer to the AOTA documents, *Occupational Therapy Roles, Guide for Supervision of Occupational Therapy Personnel in the Delivery of Occupational Therapy Services,* and the *Model State Regulation for Supervision of Occupational Therapy Assistant and Aides* to develop specific parameters for supervision, documentation, cosignature and frequency and type/level of supervision.

Occupational therapy assistants should know

- State occupational therapy supervision and reimbursement requirements and
- If these requirements differ, an occupational therapy assistant should comply with the more restrictive requirements.

Occupational therapy assistants should

- Refer to state occupational therapy laws and regulations for guidance on documentation and types/levels of supervision required and
- Contact the state regulatory board if you are unsure of these requirements.

Disciplinary Procedures

Refer to specific occupational therapy laws and regulations for each state by contacting your state regulatory board. Some states have enhanced this section with the adoption of the AOTA *Occupational Therapy Code of Ethics*. Under certain circumstances, both AOTA and NBCOT may conduct investigations of alleged unethical/unprofessional conduct respectively subject to membership in AOTA or certification by NBCOT.

Special Note

- Consult your facility administrators to ascertain whether there are additional facility requirements/policies with which you must comply, and if you practice in a state that does not regulate the area of supervision, rely on your facility for direction and remind your facility of AOTA's official documents on this subject.
- Any person who practices occupational therapy in a regulated jurisdiction is subject to the laws and regulations of that jurisdiction and may be liable for violations to those laws and regulations.

DEFINITIONS OF TYPES OF REGULATION FOR OCCUPATIONAL THERAPY

Type of Regulation	Description	Requirements for Practice*	Oversight Agency
Licensure/Practice Act	Provides highest level of public protection by prohibiting unlicensed individuals from practicing occupational therapy or referring to themselves as occupational therapists/ occupational therapy assistants. Licensure laws reserve a certain scope of practice for those who are issued a license.	Mandates entry-level competence.	State Health Department delegates authority to an occupational therapy board or advisory board, consisting of occupational therapy practitioners, consumers, and/or other health professionals.
Mandatory Certification* [Certification as granted by the occupational therapy regulatory board or advisory board/council. To be distinguished from certification granted to individuals passing the National Board for Certification in Occupational Therapy (NBCOT) exam.]	Protects the public by prohibiting non-certified individuals from referring to themselves as occupational therapists/ occupational therapy assistants. Unlike licensure, individuals under certain circumstances can practice if they do not refer to their services as occupational therapy. Certification laws may provide for definition of occupational therapy.	Mandates entry-level competency.	Government agency maintains registry of individuals who successfully complete eligibility requirements.
Mandatory Registration*	Protects the public by prohibiting non-registered individuals from referring to themselves as occupational therapists/ occupational therapy assistants, although they can practice if they do not refer to their services as occupational therapy. Registration laws may provide for definition of occupational therapy.	Competency standards may be required by the government agency maintaining the register.	Government agency maintains registry of individuals who successfully complete eligibility requirements.
Voluntary Certification or Registration	Voluntary certification or registration do not protect either the title or the practice. The state does not have the legal authority to prohibit a non-certified or non-registered person from practicing occupational therapy unless that person has violated certain standards of care.	There are usually no state requirements for practice; however, the practitioner's professional association may advise on entry level competency. Practitioners are subject to the entry-level competency requirements for reimbursement by third-party insurers, private insurers, and Medicare.	Other than the state's constitutional authority to govern health, safety, and welfare, there are usually no express requirements for the governance of the profession.
Title Control (sometimes called a Trademark Act)	Prohibits non-NBCOT-certified individuals from referring to themselves as occupational therapists/occupational therapy assistants, although they can practice under certain circumstances, if they do not refer to their services as occupational therapy.	Mandates entry-level competency.	Government agency maintains registry of individuals who successfully complete eligibility requirements.

*The terms *registration* and *certification* are often used interchangeably. Therefore, it is important to understand the provisions and protections of each type or regulation rather than assuming certain provisions are automatically included.

The Occupational Therapy Assistant: Resources for Practice and Education

Jurisdictions Regulating Occupational Therapy Assistants

Jurisdictions With Licensure Law

1990	Alabama		1983	North Dakota
1987	Alaska		1976	Ohio
1989	Arizona		1984	Oklahoma
1977	Arkansas		1977	Oregon
1978	Connecticut		1982	Pennsylvania
1985	Delaware		1968	Puerto Rico
1978	District of Columbia		1997	Rhode Island
1975	Florida		1977	South Carolina
1976	Georgia		1986	South Dakota
1998	Guam		1983	Tennessee
1987	Idaho		1983	Texas
1983	Illinois		1977	Utah
1980	Iowa		2002	Vermont
2002	Kansas		1984	Washington
1986	Kentucky		1978	West Virginia
1979	Louisiana		2000	Wisconsin
1984	Maine		1991	Wyoming
1977	Maryland			
1983	Massachusetts		**States With Registration Law**	
2000	Minnesota		1988	Michigan
1988	Mississippi			
1997	Missouri		**States With Certification Law**	
1985	Montana		2000	California
1984	Nebraska		1989	Indiana
1991	Nevada			
1977	New Hampshire		**States That Do Not Regulate OTAs**	
1993	New Jersey		Colorado	
1983	New Mexico		Hawaii	
1984	North Carolina		Virginia	
			New York (see below)	

46 jurisdictions license occupational therapy assistants
1 state registers occupational therapy assistants
2 states certify occupational therapy assistants
———
Total: **49** **Jurisdictions Regulate Occupational Therapy Assistants**

3 states regulate occupational therapists and do not regulate occupational therapy assistants: **Colorado, Hawaii,** and **Virginia.**

1 state licenses occupational therapists and does not license occupational therapy assistants: **New York** (OTAs are certified by the New York State Department of Education).

Occupational Therapy Regulatory Body Contact List

ALABAMA
Ann Cosby, Executive Director
Alabama State Board of Occupational Therapy
64 N. Union Street, Suite 734
Montgomery, AL 36130
(334) 353-4466
(334) 353-4465 (fax)
email: acosby@asbot.state.al.us

ALASKA
Ruth Bluhm, Licensing Examiner
State of Alaska
Department of Commerce and Economic Development
Division of Occupational Licensing
State Occupational Therapy and Physical Therapy Board
PO Box 110806
Juneau, AK 99811-0806
(907) 465-3811
(907) 465-2974 (fax)

ARIZONA
Ed Logan, Executive Director
Arizona Board of Occupational Therapy Examiners
1400 W. Washington Street, Suite 240
Phoenix, AZ 85007-2931
(602) 542-6784
(602) 542-5469 (fax)
email: azot@primenet.com

ARKANSAS
Valerie Morgan
Medical Board Licensing Coordinator
Arkansas State Medical Board
2100 Riverfront Drive, Suite 200
Little Rock, AR 72202-1793
(501) 296-1802
(501) 296-1805 (fax)

CALIFORNIA (Trademark Law)
Occupational Therapy Association of California
4600 Northgate Boulevard, Suite 135
Sacramento, CA 95834
(916) 567-7000

COLORADO (Trademark Law)
Linda Graham or Jennifer Whitford
Occupational Therapy Association of Colorado
809 N. Cascade Avenue, Suite C
Colorado Springs, CO 80903
(719) 635-2190
(719) 635-1017 (fax)
email: otac99@hotmail.com

CONNECTICUT
Norma Shea or Richard Ouellet
Department of Public Health, Occupational Therapy Licensure
410 Capitol Avenue, Mail Stop #12APP
PO Box 340308
Hartford, CT 06134-0308
(860) 509-7561
(860) 509-8457 (fax)

DELAWARE
Dana Spruill, Administrative Assistant
Delaware State Board of Occupational Therapy
Division of Professional Regulation
Cannon Building, Suite 203
861 Silver Lake Boulevard
Dover, DE 19904
(302) 739-4522, ext. 205
(302) 739-2711 (fax)

DISTRICT OF COLUMBIA
Graphelia Ramseur
DC Board of Occupational Therapy
Department of Health
Office of Professional Licensing
825 N. Capitol Street NE, Suite 2224
Washington, D.C. 20002
(202) 442-9200
(202) 442-9430 (fax)

FLORIDA
Deborah Boutwell, PRS-II
Florida Department of Health
Board of Occupational Therapy Practice
2020 Capital Circle, SE
BIN #C05
Tallahassee, FL 32399-3255
(850) 488-0595
(850) 414-6860 (fax)
email: Deb-Boutwell@doh.state.fl.us

GEORGIA
Sandra Marshall
Georgia Board of Occupational Therapy
Examining Board Division
237 Coliseum Drive
Macon, GA 31217-3858
(912) 207-1620
(912) 207-1633

HAWAII
Lee Ann Teshima, Executive Officer
Occupational Therapy Program
Professional and Vocational Licensing Division
Commerce and Consumer Affairs Department
PO Box 3469
Honolulu, HI 96801
(808) 586-3000 Applications/registration
(808) 586-2694 Specific questions
(808) 586-2689 (fax)

IDAHO
Eileen Wilson, Office Specialist II
Idaho State Board of Medicine
PO Box 83720
280 N. 8th Street, Suite 202
Boise, ID 83720-0058
(208) 334-2822
(208) 334-2801 (fax)

ILLINOIS
Jennifer Witts Allen
Department of Professional Regulation
320 W. Washington Street, 3rd Floor
Springfield, IL 62786
(217) 782-8556
(217) 782-7645 (fax)

INDIANA
Maryann Seyfried, Director of Operations
Kimberly Tarnacki, Deputy Director of Health Professions
Bureau
Health Professions Bureau
402 W. Washington Street, Room 041
Indianapolis, IN 46204
(317) 232-2960
(317) 233-4236 (fax)

IOWA
Judy Manning, Board Administrator
Professional Licensure Office
Physical Therapy and Occupational Therapy Board
of Examiners
Lucas State Office Building
Des Moines, IA 50319-0075
(515) 281-7074

KANSAS
Rhonda Bohannon, Office Assistant
KS State Board of Healing Arts
235 South Topeka Boulevard
Topeka, KS 66603-3068
(785) 296-7413
(785) 296-0852 (fax)

KENTUCKY
Karen Gardenshire, Board Administrator
Kentucky Occupational Therapy Board
PO Box 456
Frankfort, KY 40602-0456
(502) 564-3296
(502) 564-4818 (fax)

LOUISIANA
Carol Duchmann
Louisiana State Board of Medical Examiners
630 Camp Street
New Orleans, LA 70130-0250
(504) 524-6763
(504) 568-8893 (fax)

MAINE
Diane Staples, Board Clerk
Department of Professional and Financial Regulation
Board of Occupational Therapy Practice, State House
Station #35
Augusta, ME 04333
(207) 624-8626
(207) 582-5415 (fax)

MARYLAND
Donna Ashman
Metro Executive Office Building
State Board of Occupational Therapy, 3rd Floor, Room 314
4201 Patterson Avenue
Baltimore, MD 21215-2299
(410) 764-4728
(410) 764-5987 (fax)

MASSACHUSETTS

Kimberly Hamel, Administrative Assistant
Board of Allied Health Professions
Division of Registration
239 Causeway Street
Boston, MA 02114
(617) 727-3071
(617) 727-2197 (fax)

MICHIGAN

Patricia Lewis
State of Michigan
Bureau of Health Services
PO Box 30670
Lansing, MI 48909-7518
(517) 335-0918 Applications/registration
(517) 373-8102 Specific questions

MINNESOTA

Cleone Griep
Minnesota Department of Health
121 E. 7th Place
PO Box 64975
St. Paul, MN 55164-0975
(651) 282-5624 (OT/OTA Registration—Mark Meath)

MISSISSIPPI

Stephen Quilter, Health Program Specialist
Professional Licensure
Mississippi State Department of Health
500 B East Woodrow Wilson Boulevard
Jackson, MS 39216
(601) 987-4153

MISSOURI

Desmond Peters, Executive Director
Missouri Board of Occupational Therapy
Box 1335
Jefferson City, MO 65102
(573) 751-0877

MONTANA

Helena Lee
Department of Commerce, Montana Board of
Occupational Therapy
111 N. Jackson, PO Box 200513
Helena, MT 59620-0513
(406) 444-3091

NEBRASKA

Brad Rohr
Division of Professional Licensing
Rehabilitation and Community Services Section
Health and Human Services
PO Box 95007
Lincoln, NE 68509-5007
(402) 471-0547 (Diane)
(402) 471-4908 (Delores)
(402) 471-0383 (fax)

NEVADA

Lorraine Pokorski, Executive Secretary
State of Nevada, Board of Occupational Therapy
PO Box 70220
Reno, NV 89570-0220
(775) 857-1700
(775) 857-2121 (fax)

NEW HAMPSHIRE

Veronique Soucy, Administrative Assistant
New Hampshire Board of Allied Health Professions,
Occupational Therapy Licensure
2 Industrial Park Drive
Concord, NH 03301
(603) 271-8389
(603) 271-6702 (fax)

NEW JERSEY

Laura Anderson, Executive Director
Advisory Council of Occupational Therapy
PO Box 45037
Newark, NJ 07101
(973) 504-6570
(973) 648-3536 (fax)

NEW MEXICO

J. J. Walker
New Mexico Board of Occupational Therapy Practice
2055 South Pacheco, Suite 400
PO Box 25101
Santa Fe, NM 87505
(505) 476-7117
(505) 476-7095 (fax)

NEW YORK

Ronnie Hausheer, Executive Secretary
New York State Board of Occupational Therapy
Room 3013 CEC
Empire State Plaza
Albany, NY 12230
(518) 473-0221
(518) 474-3817 (call for application)

NORTH CAROLINA

Theresa Kay, Administrative Assistant
North Carolina Board of Occupational Therapy
PO Box 2280
Raleigh, NC 27602
(919) 832-1380
(919) 833-1059 (fax)

NORTH DAKOTA

Ken Tupa, Executive Secretary
Kristin Narum, Executive Secretary
North Dakota State Board of Occupational Therapy
Practice
PO Box 4005
2900 E. Broadway #5
Bismark, ND 58502
(701) 250-0847 (phone & fax)

OHIO

Carl G. Williams, Executive Director
Ohio OT, PT, and AT Board
77 South High Street, 16th Floor
Columbus, OH 43266-0317
(614) 466-3774
(614) 644-8112 (fax)

OKLAHOMA

Kathy Plant, Executive Secretary
Board of Medical Licensure and Supervision
PO Box 18256
Oklahoma City, OK 73154
(405) 848-6841
(405) 848-8240 (fax)

OREGON

Peggy Smith
Oregon Occupational Therapy Licensing Board
800 NE Oregon #21, Suite 407
Portland, OR 97232
(503) 731-4048
(503) 731-4207 (fax)

PENNSYLVANIA

Clara Flinchum, Board Administrator
State Board of Occupational Therapy, Education,
and Licensure
Box 2649
Harrisburg, PA 17105-2649
(717) 783-1389
(717) 787-7769 (fax)

PUERTO RICO

Beverly Davila, Executive Director
Department of Health, Office of Regulations and
Certification of Health Professions
Call Box 10200
San Juan, PR 00908
(787) 725-8121
(787) 725-7903 (fax)

RHODE ISLAND

Donna Dickerman
Division of Professional Regulation
3 Capitol Hill, Room 104
Providence, RI 02908-5097
(401) 222-2827, ext. 106

SOUTH CAROLINA

Brenda M. Owens, Administrator
South Carolina Board of Occupational Therapy
110 Centerview Drive
Columbia, SC 29210
(803) 896-4683
(803) 896-4719 (fax)

SOUTH DAKOTA

Mitzi Turley
South Dakota Board of Medical and Osteopathic
Examiners
1323 S. Minnesota Avenue
Sioux Falls, SD 57105
(605) 336-1965

TENNESSEE

Virginia Jenkins
Lee Phelps
Tennessee Board of Occupational Therapy and Physical
Therapy Examiners
425 5th Avenue N., Cordell Building, First Floor
Nashville, TN 37247-1010
(615) 532-5135
(615) 532-5164 (fax)

TEXAS

Alicia Dimmik Essary, Coordinator of Occupational
Therapy Programs
Jennifer Jean Jones, Executive Assistant
Executive Council of Physical Therapy and Occupational
Therapy Examiners
Texas Board of Occupational Therapy Examiners
333 Guadalupe, Suite 2-510
Austin, TX 78701-3942
(512) 305-6900
(512) 305-6951 (fax)

UTAH

Karen McCall, Board Secretary
Division of Occupational and Professional Licensing
160 East 300 S.
PO Box 146741
Salt Lake City, UT 84114-6741
(801) 530-6632
(801) 530-6511 (fax)

VERMONT

Diane Lafaille, Staff Assistant
Secretary of State's Office
109 State Street
Montpelier, VT 05609-1106
(802) 828-2390
(802) 828-2496 (fax)

VIRGINIA

Cookie Ergens
Virginia Board of Medicine
6606 W. Broad Street, 4th Floor
Richmond, VA 23230-1717
(804) 662-7664

WASHINGTON

Carol Neva, Program Manager
Department of Health, Occupational Therapy Board
PO Box 47868
Olympia, WA 98504-7868
(360) 236-4872
(360) 753-0657 (fax)

WEST VIRGINIA

Cathy Whalen
West Virginia Board of Occupational Therapy
119 S. Price Street
Kingwood, WV 26537
(304) 329-0480
Mon–Thurs 8am–3pm/Calls answered 9am–noon

WISCONSIN

Tammy Buckingham
State of Wisconsin Department of Regulation and
Licensing
PO Box 8935
Madison, WI 53708-8935
(608) 266-2112
(608) 266-1396

WYOMING

Vickie L. Spires
Occupational Licensing Officer
Wyoming Board of Occupational Therapy
1116 Logan Avenue
Cheyenne, WY 82002
(307) 432-0488
(307) 432-0492(fax)

State	Permits/Licenses/Documents Issued	Number of Permits/ Licenses/Documents Board May Issue Number of Renewals Fees	Eligibility Criteria	Limitations
Alabama	Limited: Limited permit issued to persons pursuing license.	Limited: 1, no renewal OT: Limited Permit: $45 OTA: Limited Permit: $35	Limited: Applicant must have completed educational and fieldwork requirements.	Limited: Must practice under supervision of OT with current license. Valid until the date on which the results of the next qualifying exam have been made public. May not be renewed if the applicant has failed the exam.
Alaska	Temporary: Temporary permit issued to new applicants for licensure.	Temporary: 1 OT/OTA: Temporary Permit $50	Temporary: Applicant must have completed educational requirements. Foreign-trained applicants must have completed supervised fieldwork and meet the requirements of the Immigration and Nationality Act.	Temporary: Valid for 8 months or until the results of the first exam for which the applicant is scheduled are published, whichever occurs first. If the applicant fails to take the first exam for which the applicant is scheduled, the applicant's temporary permit lapses on the day of the exam. Permit valid until the results of the first exam for which the applicant is scheduled as published following the completion of the required internship.
	Limited: A limited permit is issued to a person to practice OT in the state as a visiting, nonresident OT or OTA.	Limited: 3 per lifetime. OT/OTA: Limited Permit $50	Limited: Applicant may have not been previously denied licensure in the state. The applicant must be licensed to practice in another state. Applicant must provide proof that they will not practice in the state for more than 120 days per year. Applicant must pay all fees.	Limited: May not receive more than 3 limited permits to practice OT during the person's lifetime.
Arizona	Limited: Board may grant limited permit to a person who has not taken the exam.	Limited: 1, 1 renewal OT/OTA: Application: $100 Permit: $30 Renewal: $35	Limited: Completed academic and fieldwork requirements. Foreign-trained applicants must have completed academic and fieldwork requirements and must submit proof of acceptance to take the licensure exam.	Limited: Must practice under direct supervision of licensed OT. A limited permit is valid for 4 months and becomes void if a person fails the exam.
Arkansas	Temporary: Board authorized to issue limited license to applicants who have not taken the exam.	Temporary: 1, with 1 renewal OT/OTA: License fee (includes fee for temporary license): $75 Renewal: $15	Temporary: Applicants must have the completed education and experience requirements and are required to be licensed to obtain employment as an OT.	Temporary: Valid until the date on which the results of the next qualifying exam have been made public. Temporary license may be renewed only once if the applicant has not passed the exam or if the applicant has failed to take the qualifying exam, unless that failure is justified by good cause acceptable at the discretion of the secretary of the board.
California	N/A	N/A	N/A	N/A
Colorado	N/A	N/A	N/A	N/A
Connecticut	Limited: The Commissioner is authorized to issue limited permit to graduates that have not taken licensure exam.	Limited: 1, no renewal OT/OTA: Permit: $25	Limited: Applicants must meet educational and field experience requirements and have not yet taken the exam.	Limited: Effective until the results of the exam next following the issuance of the permit are announced. Permittee is authorized to practice OT under the direct supervision of a licensed OT. May only practice in public, voluntary, or proprietary facility.

(Continued)

State	Permits/Licenses/Documents Issued	Number of Permits/Licenses/Documents Board May Issue Number of Renewals Fees	Eligibility Criteria	Limitations
Delaware	Temporary: Board may issue a temporary license to an applicant who has applied for licensure and is eligible to take the exam.	Temporary: 1, with 1 renewal **OT/OTA:** Application: $10 Temporary License: $30 Renewal: Prorated.	Temporary: Must have applied for licensure and be eligible to take the exam.	Temporary: Only available to person during first application for licensure. Must practice under the direct supervision of licensed OT.
District of Columbia	Limited: Limited permit authorized for applicants that have completed educational and experience requirements.	Limited: 1, with 1 renewal **OT/OTA:** Limited Permit: $155	Limited: Completed educational and experience requirements.	Limited: Must practice under the supervision of an OTR. The limited permit can be renewed only once until the date on which the results of the next qualifying exam have been made public.
Florida	Temporary: Temporary permit may be issued to applicants qualified to be licensed by endorsement until the next board meeting at which license applications are to be considered.	Temporary: 1 temporary permit by endorsement may be issued to an applicant, and it is not renewable. **OT/OTA:** Application: $100 Temporary Permit: $35	Temporary: Board may issue temporary permit to applicants qualified to be licensed by endorsement.	Temporary: The board may issue the applicant a temporary permit to practice OT until the next board meeting at which license applications are to be considered, but not for a longer period of time. Only 1 temporary permit by endorsement must be issued to an applicant, and it is not renewable.
	The Board may issue a temporary permit to an applicant that has not taken the exam.	1, no renewal** ** However, applicants enrolled in a full-time advanced master's OT education program who have completed all requirements for licensure except exam must, upon written request, be granted a temporary permit valid for 6 months even if that period extends beyond the next exam, provided the applicant has not failed the exam. This permit will remain valid only while the applicant remains a full-time student and, upon written request, must be renewed once for an additional 6 months. **OT/OTA:** Application: $100 Temporary Permit: $35	Applicants must meet all of the other requirements for licensure and applied for the next scheduled exam.	Must practice under the supervision of a licensed OT until notification of the results of the exam. An individual who has passed the exam may continue to practice OT under her or his temporary permit until the next meeting of the board. An individual who has failed the exam may not continue to practice OT under her or his temporary permit, and the permit will be revoked upon notification to the board of the exam results and the subsequent, immediate notification by the board to the applicant of the revocation.
Georgia	Limited: Board authorized to issue limited permit to persons who have completed education and experience requirements. Board authorized to issue a limited permit to persons who have successfully completed a certification exam approved by the board.	Limited: 1, no renewal **OT:** Application and License (includes limited permit): $60 **OTA:** Application and License (includes limited permit): $50	Limited: Completed education and experience requirements. Board authorized to issue a limited permit to persons who have successfully completed a certification exam approved by the board.	Limited: Allowed to practice under the supervision of licensed OT. Valid until the date on which the results of the next qualifying exam have been made public. Permits issued to persons who have completed a certification exam allow a person to practice OT for a period not to exceed 90 days under the supervision of an OT who holds a current license in the state.

State	Permits/Licenses/Documents Issued	Number of Permits/ Licenses/Documents Board May Issue / Number of Renewals / Fees	Eligibility Criteria	Limitations
Hawaii	N/A	N/A	N/A	N/A
Idaho	Limited: Limited permit may be granted to a person who has completed education and experience requirements.	Limited: 1, with 1 renewal. **OT/OTA:** Application (includes limited permit): $25 Renewal: $25	Limited: Completed education and experience requirements.	Limited: Allows person to practice OT in association with a licensed OT. Permit valid until the person is issued a license or until the results of the exam taken are available to the board.
Illinois	The Department may issue a Letter of Authorization that allows an applicant to practice without a license for 6 months.	1 letter issued, no renewal** **(1) If the date on which a person can take the next available exam authorized by the Department extends beyond 6 months from the date the person completes the OT program, the Department will extend the exemption until the results of that exam become available to the Department; or (2) If the Department is unable to complete its evaluation and processing of a person's application for a license within 6 months after the date on which the application is submitted to the Department in proper form, the Department will extend the exemption until the Department has completed its evaluation and processing of the application.	Person must complete application and be exam eligible.	If the applicant fails the exam, that person must stop working until the applicant is licensed to practice.
Indiana	Temporary: Temporary permit may be issued to applicants who have completed education requirements are exam eligible.	**OT/OTA:** Letter of Authorization: $25 Temporary: 1, no renewal** **OT/OTA:** Application: $30 Temporary Permit: $10 Renewal: $10 **Temporary permits of applicants who fail to appear for the scheduled exam will be invalidated. If the applicant shows good cause why they missed the exam, the committee may allow the applicant to submit a new application. The applicant may make up to 2 applications.	Temporary: Temporary permits may be issued to applicants who have completed education requirements and are exam eligible.	Temporary: A temporary permit expires the date the committee disapproves the person's certificate application. Permittees must practice under the supervision of an IN–certified OT.

(Continued)

State	Permits/Licenses/Documents Issued	Number of Permits/Licenses/Documents Board May Issue / Number of Renewals / Fees	Eligibility Criteria	Limitations
Iowa	Limited: Board may grant limited permit to persons who have completed education and experience requirements.	Limited: 1, no renewal OT/OTA: Limited Permit: $25	Limited: Completed education and experience requirements.	Limited: Person allowed to practice OT under the supervision of a licensed OT. Valid until the date on which the results of the next qualifying exam have been made public. The limited permit may not be renewed if the applicant failed the exam.
Kansas	Temporary: Board may issue temporary registration to qualified applicants.	Temporary: 1, no renewal. OT/OTA: Application: $60 Temporary Registration: $25	Temporary: Person must complete application, meet all requirements for registration except exam, and pay applicable fees.	Temporary: The registration expires 1 year from the date of issue or on the date that the board approves the application for registration.
Kentucky	Temporary: Board may issue temporary permit to a person who has completed education and experience requirements.	Temporary: 1, no renewal OT: License (Includes Temporary Permit): $50 OTA: License (Includes Temporary Permit): $35	Temporary: Completed education and experience requirements and applied for licensure.	Temporary: Allows the applicant to practice OT under the supervision of a licensed OT. Permit valid until the applicant is issued or denied a license. A permit may not extend for more than 60 days following the second application offered after the applicant has applied to take the exam.
Louisiana	Temporary: Board may issue a temporary license to persons who have completed academic supervised work requirements	Temporary: 1, with 1 renewal OT: Temporary License: $25 OTA: Temporary License: $17 Renewal: $25	Temporary: Completed academic supervised work experience requirements and are waiting exam.	Temporary: The temporary license is valid until the date on which the results of the qualifying exam have been known and acted upon by the board. The temporary license is renewable once, if the applicant has not passed the exam or if the applicant has failed to take the qualifying exam. Exceptions to the one extension rule can be given at the discretion of the board based upon an appeal identifying extenuating circumstances.
Maine	Temporary: Board may grant a temporary license to applicants who have completed the education and Level II fieldwork requirements and are eligible to take the exam.	Temporary: 1, with 1 renewal OT: Temporary License: $25 Renewal: $25 OTA: Temporary License: $20 Renewal: $25	Temporary: Completed the education and Level II fieldwork requirements and are eligible to take the exam. Foreign-trained applicants must receive approval to sit for the exam from NBCOT to be eligible for a temporary license.	Temporary: Allows the holder of the license to practice under the supervision of a licensed OT. Valid until the results are made available to the board. The temporary license of a person who has failed the exam may be renewed 1 time at the discretion of the board. If the person did not take the first available exam, the person must submit a letter to the board explaining the circumstances. At its discretion, the board may renew the person's temporary license to allow the person to sit for the next scheduled exam.
Maryland	Temporary: Board may issue a temporary license to an applicant that has met the education and experience requirements.	Temporary: 2, with no renewal OT/OTA: Application (Includes First Temporary License): $100 Second Temporary License: $50	Temporary: Meets education and experience requirements.	Temporary: A temporary license issued to an OT authorizes the holder to practice OT in association with an OT who is authorized to practice. A temporary license issued to an OTA authorizes the holder to practice limited OT only under the supervision of an OT who is authorized to practice in this state. A temporary license expires on the date when the results of the first exam that the holder was eligible to take are made public. The board may not issue more than 2 temporary licenses to an individual. The board may not renew a temporary license.
Massachusetts	Temporary: Board may issue temporary license to an individual whose application has been approved.	Temporary: 1, with 2 renewals. OT/OTA: Temporary License: $35 Renewal: $10	Temporary: Applicant who is awaiting passing exam.	Temporary: A temporary license holder is required to practice under the supervision of a supervisor in that discipline. The supervisor must co-sign all documentation until the applicant receives an unrestricted license. After the application is filed with the board, the applicant is required to take the next scheduled exam. A passing exam score will result in the issuance of an unrestricted license. Upon the receipt of the license, an applicant may practice without supervision. If the applicant fails the exam, they must stop practice immediately. When the board has approved reapplication for licensure, the applicant will be issued a second temporary license.

State	Permits/Licenses/Documents Issued	Number of Permits/ Licenses/Documents Board May Issue Number of Renewals Fees	Eligibility Criteria	Limitations
Michigan	N/A	N/A	N/A	N/A
Minnesota	Temporary: Commissioner may issue temporary registration to qualified applicants.	Temporary: 1, with 1 renewal **OT/OTA:** Temporary Registration: $50 Renewal: $50	Temporary: An applicant must have applied for registration and awaiting exam results.	Temporary: Applicants who have graduated from an accredited education program and have not passed the exam must practice under the supervision of a registered OT. The temporary registration expires 10 weeks following the exam date or until the board issues or denies registration, whichever comes first.
			An applicant who submits application materials and evidence of unrestricted credential in another state or NBCOT certification may receive a temporary registration. Applicants must submit an affidavit stating that they are not the subject of a pending investigation or disciplinary action.	A temporary registration issued to an applicant credentialed by NBCOT or another jurisdiction expires 90 days after it is issued.
Mississippi	Limited: Board may issue limited permit to applicant who has completed the education and experience requirements.	Limited: 1, with 1 renewal. **OT:** Application: $100 Limited Permit: $150 Renewal: $150 **OTA:** Application: $100 Limited Permit: $100 Renewal: $100	Limited: Completed education and experience requirements.	Limited: The limited permit allows an applicant to practice OT under the supervision of a licensed OT. The permit is valid until the date on which the results of the next qualifying exam have been made public. The limited permit may be renewed once if the applicant failed the exam.
Missouri	Limited: The division may issue a limited permit to an applicant that is eligible to take the exam.	Limited: 1, with 1 renewal **OT/OTA:** Application (includes Limited Permit): $50 Renewal: No charge	Limited: Submission of application and proof of eligibility to sit for the first available exam.	Limited: An applicant must practice under supervision of licensed OT. The permit is valid up to but not to exceed the time the results of the second available exam are released. Limited permits for successful exam candidates are valid for an additional 60 days.
Montana	Temporary: The board may issue a temporary practice permit to a person licensed in another state that has licensing standards substantially equivalent to those of this state if the board determines that there is no reason to deny the license under the laws of this state governing the profession or occupation.	Temporary: 1, no renewal **OT/OTA:** Temporary permit: $10	Temporary: The board may issue a temporary practice permit to a person licensed in another state that has licensing standards substantially equivalent to those of this state if the board determines that there is no reason to deny the license under the laws of this state governing the profession or occupation. The person may practice under the permit until a license is granted or until a notice of proposal to deny a license is issued. The permit may not be issued until the board receives verification from the state or states in which the person is licensed that the person is currently licensed and is not subject to pending charges or final disciplinary action for unprofessional conduct or impairment.	Temporary: The permit is valid until the person either fails the first license exam for which the person is eligible following issuance of the permit or passes the exam and is granted a license. Applicants who have previously taken the exam and failed are not eligible for a temporary practice permit. Temporary practice permit holders must work under the routine supervision of a certified OTA or a licensed OT.

(Continued)

State	Permits/Licenses/Documents Issued	Number of Permits/Licenses/Documents Board May Issue / Number of Renewals / Fees	Eligibility Criteria	Limitations
Montana (*cont.*)			A board may issue a temporary practice permit to a person seeking licensure in this state who has met all licensure requirements other than passage of the licensing exam. The permit is valid until the person either fails the first license exam for which the person is eligible following issuance of the permit or passes the exam and is granted a license.	
Nebraska	Temporary: The board may issue a temporary permit to any person who has applied to take the exam and has completed the education and experience requirements.	Temporary: 1, no renewal **OT/OTA:** Temporary permit: $25	Temporary: Applied to take exam and completed education and experience requirements.	Temporary: Must practice in association with a licensed OT. Valid until the date on which the results of the next licensure exam are available to the Department. Temporary permit may not be renewed if the applicant has failed the exam. Permit may be extended at the discretion of the board with the approval of the Department. Temporary permit may not be extended beyond 1 year.
Nevada	Temporary: Board may issue temporary license if the applicant is of good moral character and has completed education and experience requirements.	Temporary: 1, with 1 renewal **OT:** Temporary License: $250 Renewal: $100 **OTA:** Temporary License: $175 Renewal: $75	Temporary: Board may issue temporary license if the applicant is of good moral character and has completed education and experience requirements.	Temporary: Person may practice OT under the general supervision of licensed OT. The permit is valid for 6 months or until the person to whom it is issued otherwise obtains a license, whichever occurs first. The board may renew a temporary license no more than once.
New Hampshire	Interim: The governing boards of the Allied Health Professions may issue interim licenses to applicants who are qualified.	Interim: 1, no renewal. **OT/OTA:** Application (includes interim license): $60 Renewal: $35	Interim: Interim licenses are available to (1) a student awaiting results of an exam; (2) applicants licensed in other states who are waiting a final governing board decision.	Interim: Interim licenses valid for 9 months and may not be renewed.
New Jersey	Temporary: The Director of the Division of Consumer Affairs in the Department of Law and Public Safety may issue temporary license to applicants that have submitted application/fee and meet education and fieldwork requirements.	Temporary: 1, 1 renewal if exam is failed. **OT/OTA:** Application: $100 Temporary License: $50 Renewal: $50	Temporary: Director may issue temporary license to applicants that have submitted application/fee and meet education and fieldwork requirements.	Temporary: A temporary license is available to an applicant with his initial application for exam and he may practice only under the direct supervision of a licensed OT. A temporary license expires automatically upon the holder being notified of failure of the licensure exam. The temporary license may be renewed for an additional period until the results of the next licensure exam at which time it will automatically expire and must be surrendered to the Director.
New Mexico	Provisional: Provisional permit may be issued to a person who has completed the education and experience requirements.	Provisional: 1, no renewal **OT/OTA:** Temporary Permit: $25 Limited: 1, 1 renewal	Provisional: Provisional permit may be issued to a person who has completed the education and experience requirements.	Provisional: Allows person to practice OT under the supervision of a registered OT. The permit is valid until the date on which the results of the next qualifying exam have been made public. The permit may not be renewed if the applicant failed the exam.
New York	Limited: Limited permits may be issued to eligible applicants.	**OT:** Limited Permit: $70 Licensure: $270 **OTA:** No Provision	Limited: Limited permits may be issued to the following: (a) An OT who has graduated from an OT curriculum with a baccalaureate degree or certificate in OT which is substantially equivalent to a baccalaureate degree satisfactory to the board of OT and in accordance with the Commissioner's regulations; or	Limited: A permittee may practice OT only under the supervision of a licensed OT or a licensed physician and may practice only in a public, voluntary, or proprietary hospital, health care agency or in a preschool or an elementary or secondary school for the purpose of providing OT as a related service for a handicapped child. A limited permit is valid for 1 year. It may be renewed once for a period not to exceed 1 additional year, at the discretion of the Department, upon the submission of an explanation satisfactory to the Department for an applicant's failure

State	Permits/Licenses/Documents Issued	Number of Permits/ Licenses/Documents Board May Issue / Number of Renewals / Fees	Eligibility Criteria	Limitations
New York (*cont.*)			(b) A foreign OT who is in this country on a non-immigration visa for the continuation of OT study, pursuant to the exchange student program of the U.S. Department of State.	to become licensed within the original 1-year period. A limited permit becomes null and void if and when the holder fails to pass a licensing exam.
North Carolina	Provisional: The board may grant a provisional license to any individual who has successfully completed the educational and fieldwork experience requirements and has made application to take the exam.	Provisional: 1, no renewal **OT/OTA:** Provisional License: $35	Provisional: The board may grant a provisional license to any individual who has successfully completed the educational and fieldwork experience requirements and has made application to take the exam.	Provisional: A provisional license allows the individual to practice as an OT or OTA under the supervision of a licensed OT. A provisional license may not be issued to applicant who has failed the exam in this North Carolina or another jurisdiction. Provisional license is valid for 9 months.
North Dakota	Limited: The board may grant a limited permit to a person who has completed the education and experience requirements.	Limited: 1, with 1 renewal **OT:** Limited Permit: $40 **OTA:** Limited Permit: $30	Limited: The board may grant a limited permit to a person who has completed the education and experience requirements.	Limited: A limited permit allows the person to practice OT under supervision of a North Dakota-licensed OT. A limited permit is valid until the results of the exam are available to the board and the board decides to issue or deny a license to a person. The holder of a limited permit must take the next available exam. The permit expires if the holder fails to take the next available exam. A limited permit may be renewed one time if the person has failed the exam or, with good cause as determined by the board, failed to take the next exam.
Ohio	Limited: The OT may issue a limited permit to an applicant that is of good moral character and completes the fieldwork and education requirements.	Limited: 1, no renewal **OT/OTA:** Limited Permit: $50	Limited: The board may issue a limited permit to an applicant that is of good moral character and completes the fieldwork and education requirements.	Limited: The limited permit allows the person to practice as an OT or OTA under the supervision of a licensed OT and is valid until the date on which the results of the next qualifying exam are made public. The limited permit may not be renewed if the applicant has failed the exam. A limited permit may not be granted to any applicant who failed the qualifying exam prior to making application for a limited permit. The section may grant waivers of the limited permit requirements or extensions of time within which to fulfill the requirements. Waivers of the limited permit requirements may be granted by the section for any permit not to exceed the second test date results.
Oklahoma	Temporary Letter: The board may issue an informal letter that allows the applicant to practice under the on-site supervision of a licensed OT.	Temporary Letter: 1, no renewal** **OT/OTA:** Temporary Letter Fee: $100 **Upon failure of the exam for licensure by the applicant, the applicant can still function as a graduate OT/OTA student and take the exam the next time it is given.	An applicant who meets the academic, clinical, and educational requirements for licensure as an OT or OTA may practice under the on-site supervision of a licensed OT in the status of a graduate OT student or graduate OTA until the next meeting of the Oklahoma State Board of Medical Licensure and Supervision. The status is communicated to the applicant in the form of an informal letter.	The letter is valid until next board meeting. The progress to licensure of each applicant in the temporary status is evaluated at each meeting.

(Continued)

State	Permits/Licenses/Documents Issued	Number of Permits/ Licenses/Documents Board May Issue / Number of Renewals / Fees	Eligibility Criteria	Limitations
Oregon	Limited: Students who have successfully completed the educational and fieldwork requirements and students who have taken the certification exam, but do not yet have their test results, may apply for a limited permit to practice OT under at least routine supervision.	Limited: 1, no renewal** **OT/OTA:** Limited Permit: $25 **The board may grant an extension of a limited permit to persons who, because of extenuating circumstances, are unable to take the scheduled certification exam. Request must be made in writing to the board.	Limited: Students who have successfully completed the educational and fieldwork requirements and students who have taken the certification exam, but do not yet have their test results, may apply for a limited permit to practice OT under at least routine supervision. Applicants must submit application/fee, official transcript/proof of meeting education requirement, and show evidence of being approved to take the next certification exam.	Limited: An Oregon-licensed OT must sign the limited permit application verifying a supervisory role to the applicant. A limited permit may not be issued to applicants who have taken and failed the certification exam, and limited permits may not be renewed. A person who fails the exam must immediately surrender the limited permit upon receipt of exam scores.
Pennsylvania	Temporary: The board may grant a temporary license to an applicant who has completed the education and experience requirements and is eligible to take the exam. The board may issue a temporary license to an applicant that has failed the exam and has applied for reexam. The board may issue a temporary license to an OT or OTA who is qualified to practice in another state or is AOTCB certified as long as services are provided no longer than 6 consecutive months in a calendar year.	Temporary: 1, no renewal **OT/OTA:** Temporary permit: $20	Temporary: The board may grant a temporary license to an applicant who has completed the education and experience requirements and is eligible to take the exam. The board may issue a temporary license to an applicant that has failed the exam and has applied for reexam. The temporary license expires automatically upon receipt by that person of notice of failure of the reexam and that the person is not be eligible for a temporary license for a period of 1 year from the date of the reexam. A temporary license may be granted to a person engaged in the performance of occupational therapy services who is a nonresident and not licensed under this act, provided the services of the licensee are performed for not longer than a 6-consecutive-month period in a calendar year and are performed in association with an occupational therapist licensed under this act and that one of the following exists: (1) The person is licensed under the laws of a state, District of Columbia, or territory of the United States which has licensure requirements substantially equal to the requirements of the statute. (2) The person has met the requirements for certification, as an occupational therapist registered (OTR) or a certified occupational therapy assistant (COTA), established by the American Occupational Therapy Association.	Temporary: The issuance by the board of a temporary license authorizes the practice of OT or providing services only as an assistant under the direct supervision of a licensed OT. The temporary license expires automatically upon the failure of the applicant to take the licensure exam, except for an appropriate excuse approved by the board. The temporary license expires automatically upon receipt by the applicant of notice of failure of reexam, and the applicant may not be eligible for another temporary license for a period of 1 year from the date of the notice. Even after 1 year from the date of notice of failure of reexam, the applicant may not be issued another temporary license, except at the discretion of the board.

State	Permits/Licenses/Documents Issued	Number of Permits/ Licenses/Documents Board May Issue Number of Renewals Fees	Eligibility Criteria	Limitations
Puerto Rico	Provisional: The board must issue a provisional license to practice to a person requesting for the first time to be admitted to the exam.	Provisional: 1, with 3 renewals **OT:** Provisional License: $35 Renewal: $20 **OTA:** Provisional License: $25 Renewal: $20	Provisional: The board must issue a provisional license to practice to a person, practicing under the supervision of a licensed OT, requesting for the first time to be admitted to the exam.	Provisional: The provisional license is canceled 1 year after its issuance. The provisional license may be renewed 3 times. To be entitled to the renewals, the applicant must take the exam at least once a year in consecutive terms. Before a renewal is granted, a candidate must demonstrate that he has received or is receiving additional training or pursuing further studies in the field of OT. The board may also waive the requirement that the applicant take the exam in consecutive terms.
Rhode Island	Graduate Status: A graduate from an approved OT school who has filed a completed application for licensure may, upon receiving a receipt from the division, perform as an OT or OTA.	Graduate Status: Renewal not applicable **OT/OTA:** No fee.	Graduate Status: A graduate an approved OT school who has filed a completed application for licensure may, upon receiving a receipt from the division, perform as an OT or OTA, under the supervision of an OT licensed in this state, only until the next scheduled exam.	Graduate Status: Must perform under the supervision of a licensed OT. If an applicant fails to take the next succeeding exam without due cause or fails to pass the exam and received a license, the graduate status privileges automatically cease. During the interim period (between time of application and exam) an individual must identify himself or herself only as a "graduate occupational therapist" or "graduate occupational therapy assistant."
South Carolina	Temporary: A temporary license may be granted to a person who has completed an educational program approved by ACOTE or other AOTA-endorsed accrediting body for OT and who has applied to take the next scheduled board-approved certification exam following graduation or who has taken the exam and has not received the exam results. The board may issue a temporary license to a licensee whose OT or OTA license has been inactive or lapsed for 3 years or more and who has applied to reactivate the license.	Temporary (for new applicants): 1, with 1 renewal **OT:** Application fee (includes temporary license): $135 **OTA:** Application fee (includes temporary license): $115 Temporary (license has been inactive or lapsed for 3 years or more): 1, with no renewal **OT:** Application fee (includes temporary license): $135 **OTA:** Application fee (includes temporary license): $115 Limited: 1, with 1 renewal	Temporary: A temporary license may be granted to a person who has completed an educational program approved by ACOTE or other AOTA-endorsed accrediting body for OT and who has applied to take the next scheduled board-approved certification exam following graduation or who has taken the exam and has not received the exam results. The board may issue a temporary license to a licensee whose OT or OTA license has been inactive or lapsed for 3 years or more and who has applied to reactivate the license.	Temporary: A temporary license authorizes the temporary licensee to practice OT under the direct supervision of a licensed OT, and the temporary license is valid until the date on which the results of the next qualifying exam are received by the board. The applicant must submit to the board a completed supervisory form for each place of employment. Temporary licenses may be renewed once in the discretion of the board, if good cause is demonstrated. The temporary license is valid for 1 year from the date of issue, may not be renewed, and authorizes the temporary licensee to work under the on-site supervision of an OT licensed in this State in order to obtain the minimum number of contact hours required to reactivate the license.
South Dakota	Limited: The board may grant a limited permit to any person who has completed the education and experience requirements.	**OT/OTA:** Limited Permit: $25	Limited: Must have completed education and experience requirements. Must demonstrate evidence that applicant may sit for the exam. Must include statement including name and address of person or institution employing the applicant during the time of limited license.	Limited: The permit allows the person to practice OT under supervision of in consultation with a licensed OT. Permit is valid until the person is issued a license or until the results of the exam taken are available to the board. The permit may be renewed once if the person failed the exam.

(Continued)

State	Permits/Licenses/Documents Issued	Number of Permits/Licenses/Documents Board May Issue / Number of Renewals / Fees	Eligibility Criteria	Limitations
Tennessee	Limited: A limited permit may be issued to an applicant who has successfully completed the educational and experience requirements and is scheduled for the initial exam.	Limited: 1, with 1 renewal. **OT:** Application (includes permit): $235 Renewal: $185 **OTA:** Application (includes permit): $160 Renewal: $130	Limited: A limited permit may be issued to an applicant who has successfully completed the educational and experience requirements and is scheduled for the initial exam.	Limited: The permit allows the applicant to practice OT in association with a licensed OT. If the applicant fails the exam, the permit is valid until the results of the exam are available to the committee. The permit of an applicant who fails the initial exam and is scheduled for the next exam may be renewed once. If the applicant passes the exam, the permit is valid until the board grants the certificate.
Texas	Temporary: The board may issue temporary licenses. There two types of temporary licenses in Texas:			
	(1) Temporary License Pending Examination	(1) Temporary License Pending Examination 1**, no renewal ** The Application Review Committee may allow a second temporary license to an individual who failed to take the exam for which he or she was registered, if there are documented extraordinary circumstances that prevented the individual from taking the Examination. **OT** (Temporary License): Application: $10 License Fee: $90 Temporary to Regular: $60 **OTA** (Temporary License): Application: $10 License Fee: $65 Temporary to Regular: $45	(1) Temporary License Pending Examination—The applicant meets all the qualifications for a license except taking the first available exam after completion of all educational requirements.	(1) Temporary License Pending Examination—Continuing supervision by a licensed OTR or LOT is required while holding this type of license. The temporary license expires upon notification to the board of failure to pass the exam and must be returned to the board. No second temporary licenses are issued after failure of the exam.
	(2) Temporary Extended License	(2) Temporary Extended License 1, no renewal **OT** (Temporary Extended License): Application: $10 License Fee: $115 Temporary to Regular: $60 **OTA** (Temporary Extended License): Application: $10 License Fee: $90 Temporary to Regular: $45	(2) Temporary Extended License—The applicant has passed the Examination and has not been employed as an OTR, LOT, COTA, or LOTA for 5 years or more from the receipt date of current, complete application for licensure with TBOTE.	(2) Temporary Extended License—A temporary license is issued for a maximum of 12 months, during which time the exam must be taken. The temporary license will be canceled if the applicant fails the exam and must be returned to the board. The continuing supervision by a licensed OTR or LOT is required, and the licensee must complete additional hours of continuing education within a specified period of time as determined by the Coordinator of the Occupational Therapy Program.

State	Permits/Licenses/Documents Issued	Number of Permits/ Licenses/Documents Board May Issue / Number of Renewals / Fees	Eligibility Criteria	Limitations
Texas (*cont.*)	Provisional: If an applicant for a regular license is from another state, foreign country, or the federal government, non-licensing state and is unable to provide complete documentation that he or she meets the qualification for a regular license, the board may issue a provisional license.	Provisional: 1, no renewal **OT** (Provisional): Application: $15 License Fee: $35 Temporary to Regular: $60 **OTA** (Provisional): Application: $15 License Fee: $25 Temporary to Regular: $45	Provisional: The applicant must provide satisfactory interim documentation, including evidence of having passed the exam.	Provisional: The provisional license will be valid for not more than 120 days. Upon receipt of full documentation the board may issue a regular license. The applicant must be sponsored by and practice with a person licensed by the board. An applicant may be excused from this requirement if it constitutes a hardship to the applicant. A request for hardship exemption must be submitted in writing to the board.
Utah	Temporary: The division may issue a temporary license to a person who has met all license requirements except the passing of an examination.	Temporary: 1, no renewal **OT/OTA:** Temporary License Application: (includes temporary license and license once exam is passed): $110	Temporary: An applicant for temporary licensure must: (1) submit an application for temporary license which includes a verification that the applicant has registered to take the next available Occupational Therapy Certification Examination required to become certified by the American Occupational Therapy Certification Board; (2) pay the required temporary license application fee; and (3) submit a "supervision" affidavit.	Temporary: The licensee must take the next available examination. The temporary license automatically expires upon release of official examination results if the applicant fails the examination. An OT or OTA who is issued a temporary license must practice OT under the general supervision of a licensed OT. A temporary license is valid for 10 months.
Vermont	Temporary: The Director of the Office of Professional Regulation may issue a temporary certificate to a qualified applicant.	Temporary: 1, with no renewal **OT/OTA:** Application (includes certification): $100 Temporary Certificate: $50	Temporary: An applicant must have completed the education and clinical supervised experience requirements. They must submit verification of employment.	Temporary: Valid for 60 days after exam.
Virginia	No temporary or limited permits/licenses or documents issued. **	No provision. No fee.	** A person who has graduated from an accredited education program can practice under the supervision of licensed OT for 1 year or until he has taken and received the examination results, whichever comes first.	No provision.
Washington	Limited: A limited permit may be granted to persons who have completed the education and experience requirements for licensure.	Limited: 1, with 1 extension. **OT/OTA:** Application and Initial License Fee: $125 Limited Permit: $40	Limited: A limited permit may be granted to persons who have completed the education and experience requirements for licensure.	Limited: The limited permit allows the applicant to practice in association with an OT. The limited permit is valid until the results of the next examination have been made public. One extension of this permit may be granted if the applicant has failed the examination, but during this period the person shall be under the direct supervision of an OT.
	**Temporary Permit: An applicant who is currently licensed in another jurisdiction is entitled to a temporary permit that allows the person to practice until the licensure process is completed.	Temporary: 1, with no renewal. **OT/OTA:** Application and Initial License Fee: $125 Limited Permit: $40	Temporary: An applicant who is currently licensed in another jurisdiction is entitled to a temporary permit that allows the person to practice until the licensure process is completed.	Temporary: The temporary permit expires upon issuance of a license by the board, initiation of an investigation by the board, or 90 days. ** Staff report temporary permits are rarely issued. In most cases they are issued to practitioners so that they may practice while completing a state-required AIDS education course.

(Continued)

State	Permits/Licenses/Documents Issued	Number of Permits/ Licenses/Documents Board May Issue / Number of Renewals / Fees	Eligibility Criteria	Limitations
West Virginia	Limited: The board must issue a limited permit to an applicant that has completed the education and experience requirements.	Limited: 1, with no renewal **OT:** Application Packet: $15 Initial License Fee: $190 Limited Permit Fee: $140 (will be applied to permanent license fee) **OTA:** Application Packet: $15 Initial License: $140 Limited Permit Fee: $90 (will be applied to permanent license fee)	Limited: The board must issue a limited permit to an applicant that has completed the education and experience requirements.	Limited: The limited permit allows a person to practice under the direct supervision of a licensed OT. The permit is valid until the date on which the results of the next qualifying examination have been made public. The limited permit may not be renewed if the applicant failed the exam.
Wisconsin	Temporary: An applicant for certification may apply to the board for a temporary certificate.	Temporary: 1, no renewal. **OT/OTA:** Application: $41 Temporary Certificate: $10	Temporary: The applicant must be a graduate of an approved school and scheduled to take the exam or awaiting results.	Temporary: Practice during the period of the temporary certificate must be in consultation, at least monthly, with an OT. The OT must endorse the activities of the person holding the certificate on a monthly basis. OTAs must practice under the supervision of an OT. The temporary certificate expires on the date the applicant is notified that he or she has failed the exam or the date the board grants or denies an applicant permanent certification. A temporary certificate expires on the first day of the next exam if the applicants failed to take the exam. A temporary certificate may not be renewed.

Wyoming	Limited: A limited permit may be granted to allow a person to practice under the general supervision of a registered OT.
	
	Temporary: An applicant who is currently licensed to practice in another jurisdiction and meets the requirements for licensure by endorsement may obtain a temporary license while the application is being processed by the board.
		Limited: 1, with 1 renewal
		
		OT:
		Application: $125
		License
		  Before Feb 1: $105
		  On or After Feb 1: $50
		Limited Permit: $55
		
		OTA:
		Application: $125
		License:
		  Before Feb 1: $50
		  On or After Feb 1: $25
		Limited Permit: $25
		
		OT:
		Application: $125
		License
		  Before Feb 1: $105
		  On or After Feb 1: $50
		Temporary License: $55
		
		OTA:
		Application: $125
		License:
		  Before Feb 1: $50
		  On or After Feb 1: $25
		Temporary License: $25
			Limited: A limited permit may be granted to allow a person to practice under the general supervision of a registered OT. A limited permit may be granted to a person who has completed the educational and experience requirements and is seeking licensure. A limited permit may also be granted to a licensee who has inactive status for more than 5 years or who has failed to renew a license for more than 5 years.
			
			Temporary: An applicant who is currently licensed to practice in another jurisdiction and meets the requirements for licensure by endorsement may obtain a temporary license while the application is being processed by the board. The applicant must submit the application, fee, temporary license fee, and a copy of the current license held in another jurisdiction.
				Limited: The permit expires 6 months after issuance when the person is issued a license.
				
				Temporary: The temporary license is in effect until the board issues a permanent license. A temporary license expires 90 days from the date of issuance.

State	Application Fee	License/Certification/ Registration Fees	Renewal Fees	Miscellaneous
Alabama	**OT** Initial Application: $30 Reciprocity: N/A	**OT** Initial License: $60 Certification: N/A Registration: N/A Duplicate: $0 Endorsement: N/A Reinstatement: N/A Reinstatement of Revoked (or Suspended): N/A	**OT** Renewal: $90 Temp/Limited Permit License (Renewal): N/A	**OT** Limited Permit: $45 Verification: $0 Late: N/A
	OTA Initial Application: $30 Reciprocity: N/A	**OTA** Initial License: $40 Certification: N/A Registration: N/A Duplicate: $0 Endorsement: N/A Reinstatement: N/A Reinstatement of Revoked (or Suspended): N/A	**OTA** Renewal: $65 Temp/Limited Permit License (Renewal): N/A	**OTA** Limited Permit: $35 Verification: $0 Late: N/A
Alaska	**OT** Initial Application: $50 Reciprocity: N/A	**OT** Initial License: $180 Certification: N/A Registration: N/A Duplicate: $5 Endorsement: N/A Reinstatement: N/A Reinstatement of Revoked (or Suspended): N/A	**OT** Renewal: $180 (biennial) Temp/Limited Permit License (Renewal): N/A	**OT** Temporary Permit: $50 Limited Permit: $50 Verification: $20 Late: N/A Wall Certificate Fee: $20
	OTA Initial Application: $50 Reciprocity: N/A	**OTA** Initial License: $130 Certification: N/A Registration: N/A Duplicate: $5 Endorsement: N/A Reinstatement: N/A Reinstatement of Revoked (or Suspended): N/A	**OTA** Renewal: $130 (biennial) Temp/Limited Permit License (Renewal): N/A	**OTA** Temporary Permit: $50 Limited Permit: $50 Verification: $20 Late: N/A Wall Certificate Fee: $20
Arizona	**OT** Initial Application: $100 Reciprocity: N/A	**OT** Initial License: $135 Certification: N/A Registration: N/A Duplicate: $10 Endorsement: N/A Reinstatement: $75 Reinstatement of Revoked (or Suspended): N/A	**OT** Renewal: $135 Temp/Limited Permit License (Renewal): N/A	**OT** Temp/Limited Permit or License: $35 (Will be credited toward initial application fee upon full licensure) Verification: N/A Late: N/A Inactive Status Renewal Fee: $25
	OTA Initial Application: $100 Reciprocity: N/A	**OTA** Initial License: $70 Certification: N/A Registration: N/A Duplicate: $10 Endorsement: N/A Reinstatement: $75 Reinstatement of Revoked (or Suspended): N/A	**OTA** Renewal: $70 Temp/Limited Permit License (Renewal): N/A	**OTA** Temp/Limited Permit License: $35 (Will be credited toward initial application fee upon full licensure) Verification: N/A Late: N/A Inactive Status Renewal Fee: $15

(Continued)

State	Application Fee	License/Certification/Registration Fees	Renewal Fees	Miscellaneous
Arkansas	**OT** Initial Application: $50 Reciprocity: $50 Application for License by Waiver of Exam: $50	**OT** Initial License: N/A (Included with initial application) Certification: N/A Registration: N/A Duplicate: N/A Endorsement: N/A Reinstatement: All delinquent fees plus $10 per year for all years delinquent. Reinstatement of Revoked (or Suspended): N/A	**OT** Renewal: $25 Temp/Limited Permit License (Renewal): N/A	**OT** Temp/Limited Permit License: $25 Verification: N/A Late: N/A
	OTA Initial Application: $25 Reciprocity: $25 Application for License by Waiver of Exam: $25	**OTA** Initial License: N/A Certification: N/A Registration: N/A Duplicate: N/A Endorsement: N/A Reinstatement: All delinquent fees plus $10 per year for all years delinquent. Reinstatement of Revoked (or Suspended): N/A	**OTA** Renewal: $25 Temp/Limited Permit License (Renewal): N/A	**OTA** Temp/Limited Permit License: $25 Verification: N/A Late: N/A
California	N/A	N/A	N/A	N/A
Colorado	N/A	N/A	N/A	N/A
Connecticut	**OT** Initial Application: N/A Reciprocity: N/A	**OT** Initial License: $100 Certification: N/A Registration: N/A Duplicate: N/A Endorsement: N/A Reinstatement: N/A Reinstatement of Revoked (or Suspended): N/A	**OT** Renewal: $100 (biennial) Temp/Limited Permit License (Renewal): N/A	**OT** Temp/Limited Permit License: $25 Verification: N/A Late: $50
	OTA Initial Application: N/A Reciprocity: N/A	**OTA** Initial License: $100 Certification: N/A Registration: N/A Duplicate: N/A Endorsement: N/A Reinstatement: N/A Reinstatement of Revoked (or Suspended): N/A	**OTA** Renewal: $100 (biennial) Temp/Limited Permit License (Renewal): N/A	**OTA** Temp/Limited Permit License: $25 Verification: N/A Late: $50
Delaware	**OT** Initial Application: $10 Reciprocity: N/A	**OT** Initial License: $105 Certification: N/A Registration: N/A Duplicate: N/A Endorsement: N/A Reinstatement: Renewal + Late Fee Reinstatement of Revoked (or Suspended): N/A	**OT** Renewal: $108 Temp/Limited Permit License (Renewal): N/A	**OT** Temporary License: $30 (plus $10 application fee) Verification: $10 Late Renewal: $54
	OTA Initial Application: $10 Reciprocity: N/A	**OTA** Initial License: $40 Certification: N/A Registration: N/A Duplicate: N/A Endorsement: N/A Reinstatement: Renewal + Late Fee Reinstatement of Revoked (or Suspended): N/A	**OTA** Renewal: $40 Temp/Limited Permit License (Renewal): N/A	**OTA** Temporary License: $30 (plus $10 application fee) Verification: $10 Late Renewal: $54

State	Application Fee	License/Certification/ Registration Fees	Renewal Fees	Miscellaneous
District of Columbia	**OT** Initial Application: $50 Reciprocity: N/A	**OT** Initial License: $105 Certification: N/A Registration: N/A Duplicate: N/A Endorsement: N/A Reinstatement: N/A Reinstatement of Revoked (or Suspended): N/A	**OT** Renewal: $105 (2 years) Temp/Limited Permit License (Renewal): N/A	**OT** Limited Permit: $155 Verification: N/A Late Renewal: $25
	OTA Initial Application: $50 Reciprocity: N/A	**OTA** Initial License: $105 Certification: N/A Registration: N/A Duplicate: N/A Endorsement: N/A Reinstatement: N/A Reinstatement of Revoked (or Suspended): N/A	**OTA** Renewal: $105 (2 years) Temp/Limited Permit License (Renewal): N/A	**OTA** Limited Permit: $155 Verification: N/A Late Renewal: $25
Florida	**OT** Initial Application: $100 Reciprocity: N/A	**OT** Initial License: $50 Certification: N/A Registration: N/A Duplicate: $25 Endorsement: N/A Reinstatement: N/A Reinstatement of Revoked (or Suspended): N/A	**OT** Renewal: $50 (biennial, due by January 31) Temp/Limited Permit License (Renewal): N/A	**OT** Temp/Limited Permit License: $35 Verification: N/A Late: N/A
	OTA Initial Application: $100 Reciprocity: N/A	**OTA** Initial License: $50 Certification: N/A Registration: N/A Duplicate: $25 Endorsement: N/A Reinstatement: N/A Reinstatement of Revoked (or Suspended): N/A	**OTA** Renewal: $50 Temp/Limited Permit License (Renewal): N/A	**OTA** Temp/Limited Permit License: $35 Verification: N/A Late: N/A
Georgia	**OT** Initial Application: N/A Reciprocity: N/A	**OT** Initial License: $60 (includes application and limited permit) Certification: N/A Registration: N/A Duplicate: $15 Endorsement: N/A Reinstatement: $100 Reinstatement of Revoked (or Suspended): N/A	**OT** Renewal: $60 Temp/Limited Permit License (Renewal): N/A	**OT** Temp/Limited Permit License: Included in initial license fee. Verification: $15 Late Renewal: $75 Wall License: $15 I.D. Card: $10
	OTA Initial Application: N/A Reciprocity: N/A	**OTA** Initial License: $50 (includes application and limited permit) Certification: N/A Registration: N/A Duplicate: $15 Endorsement: N/A Reinstatement: $80 Reinstatement of Revoked (or Suspended): N/A	**OTA** Renewal: $40 Temp/Limited Permit License (Renewal): N/A	**OTA** Temp/Limited Permit License: Included in initial license fee Verification: $15 Late Renewal: $60 Wall License: $15 I.D. Card: $10

(Continued)

State	Application Fee	License/Certification/Registration Fees	Renewal Fees	Miscellaneous
Hawaii	**OT** Initial Application: N/A Reciprocity: N/A	**OT** Initial License: N/A Certification: N/A Registration: (1) Based on NBCOT Certificate Issued during odd-numbered year: $85 Issued during even-numbered year: $68 (2) Temporary Registration for State of Hawaii Department of Health Employees: $85 (3) Reclassification—if filing from temporary status to registration based on NBCOT status: $10 Duplicate: N/A Endorsement: N/A Reinstatement: N/A Reinstatement of Revoked (or Suspended): N/A	**OT** Renewal: N/A Temp/Limited Permit License (Renewal): N/A	**OT** Temp/Limited Permit License: N/A Verification: N/A Late: N/A
	OTA Initial Application: N/A Reciprocity: N/A	**OTA** Initial License: N/A Certification: N/A Registration: N/A Duplicate: N/A Endorsement: N/A Reinstatement: N/A Reinstatement of Revoked (or Suspended): N/A	**OTA** Renewal: N/A Temp/Limited Permit License (Renewal): N/A	**OTA** Temp/Limited Permit License: N/A Verification: N/A Late: N/A
Idaho	**OT** Initial Application: N/A Reciprocity: N/A	**OT** Initial License: $110 Certification: N/A Registration: N/A Duplicate: N/A Endorsement: N/A Reinstatement: $35 (plus lapsed license fees) Reinstatement of Revoked (or Suspended): N/A	**OT** Renewal: $65 Temp/Limited Permit License (Renewal): N/A	**OT** Limited Permit: $25 Verification: N/A Late: N/A Inactive License: $45
	OTA Initial Application: N/A Reciprocity: N/A	**OTA** Initial License: $80 Certification: N/A Registration: N/A Duplicate: N/A Endorsement: N/A Reinstatement: $35 (plus lapsed license fees) Reinstatement of Revoked (or Suspended): N/A	**OTA** Renewal: $45 Temp/Limited Permit License (Renewal): N/A	**OTA** Limited Permit: $25 Verification: N/A Late: N/A Inactive License: $45
Illinois	**OT** Initial Application: $25 Reciprocity: N/A	**OT** Initial License: N/A (included with application) Certification: N/A Registration: N/A Duplicate: $20 Endorsement: $50 Reinstatement: N/A Reinstatement of Revoked (or Suspended): N/A	**OT** Renewal: $20 Temp/Limited Permit License (Renewal): N/A	**OT** Letter of Temporary Authorization: $25 Verification: $20 Late: N/A Reactivation of Inactive License: $20 Restoration of License (Other Than Inactive): $10 plus all lapsed renewal fees Wall Certificate: Cost of producing the certificate

State	Application Fee	License/Certification/ Registration Fees	Renewal Fees	Miscellaneous
Illinois (*cont.*)	**OTA** Initial Application: $25 Reciprocity: N/A	**OTA** Initial License: N/A (included with application) Certification: N/A Registration: N/A Duplicate: $20 Endorsement: $50 Reinstatement: N/A Reinstatement of Revoked (or Suspended): N/A	**OTA** Renewal: $10 Temp/Limited Permit License (Renewal): N/A	**OTA** Letter of Temporary Authorization: $25 Verification: $20 Late: N/A Reactivation of Inactive License: $10 Restoration of License (Other Than Inactive): $10 plus all lapsed renewal fees Wall Certificate: Cost of producing the certificate
Indiana	**OT** Initial Application: N/A Reciprocity: N/A	**OT** Initial License: N/A Certification: $30 Registration: N/A Duplicate: N/A Endorsement: N/A Reinstatement: N/A Reinstatement of Revoked (or Suspended): N/A	**OT** Renewal: $20 (every 2 years, due by December 31 of even-numbered years) Temp/Limited Permit License (Renewal): N/A	**OT** Temp/Limited Permit or License: $10 Verification: $10 Late Renewal (up to 3 years): $10, plus all past due and current renewal fees
	OTA Initial Application: N/A Reciprocity: N/A	**OTA** Initial License: N/A Certification: $30 Registration: N/A Duplicate: N/A Endorsement: N/A Reinstatement: N/A Reinstatement of Revoked (or Suspended): N/A	**OTA** Renewal: $20 (every 2 years, due by December 31 of even-numbered years) Temp/Limited Permit License (Renewal): N/A	**OTA** Temp/Limited Permit or License: $10 Verification: $10 Late Renewal (up to 3 years): $10, plus all past due and current renewal fees
Iowa	**OT** Initial Application: $100 (includes license) Reciprocity: N/A	**OT** Initial License: N/A Certification: N/A Registration: N/A Duplicate: $10 Endorsement: N/A Reinstatement: $100 Reinstatement of Revoked (or Suspended): N/A	**OT** Renewal: $55 (biennial) Temp/Limited Permit License (Renewal): N/A	**OT** Limited Permit: $25 Verification: N/A Late Renewal: $55 Failure to Complete CE Requirements: $50 Failure to Complete CE Report During Renewal Period: $50 Failure to Report Change of Address Within 30 Days: $10 Failure to Report Change of Name Within 30 Days: $10
	OTA Initial Application: $90 (includes initial license) Reciprocity: N/A	**OTA** Initial License: N/A Certification: N/A Registration: N/A Duplicate: $10 Endorsement: N/A Reinstatement: $100 Reinstatement of Revoked (or Suspended): N/A	**OTA** Renewal: $45 (biennial) Temp/Limited Permit License (Renewal): N/A	**OTA** Limited Permit: $25 Verification: N/A Late Renewal: $45 Failure to Complete CE Requirements: $50 Failure to Complete CE Report During Renewal Period: $50 Failure to Report Change of Address Within 30 Days: $10 Failure to Report Change of Name Within 30 Days: $10

(Continued)

State	Application Fee	License/Certification/ Registration Fees	Renewal Fees	Miscellaneous
Kansas	**OT** Initial Application (Includes Initial Registration): $40 Reciprocity: N/A	**OT** Initial License: N/A Certification: N/A Registration: N/A Duplicate: N/A Endorsement: N/A Reinstatement: $40 Reinstatement of Revoked (or Suspended): N/A	**OT** Renewal: $30 Temp/Limited Permit License (Renewal): N/A	**OT** Temporary Registration: $15 Verification: N/A Late Registration Renewal Fee: $35 Certified Copy of Registration: $15
	OTA Initial Application (Includes Initial Registration): $40 Reciprocity: N/A	**OTA** Initial License: N/A Certification: N/A Registration: N/A Duplicate: N/A Endorsement: N/A Reinstatement: $40 Reinstatement of Revoked (or Suspended): N/A	**OTA** Renewal: $30 Temp/Limited Permit License (Renewal): N/A	**OTA** Temporary Registration: $15 Verification: N/A Late Registration Renewal Fee: $35 Certified Copy of Registration: $15
Kentucky	**OT** Initial Application: N/A Reciprocity: N/A	**OT** Initial License: $50 Certification: N/A Registration: N/A Duplicate: $10 Endorsement: N/A Reinstatement: $75 Reinstatement of Revoked (or Suspended): N/A	**OT** Renewal: $50 Temp/Limited Permit License (Renewal): N/A	**OT** Temp Permit: Included with initial license Verification: N/A Late Renewal Fee: $75
	OTA Initial Application: N/A Reciprocity: N/A	**OTA** Initial License: $35 Certification: N/A Registration: N/A Duplicate: $10 Endorsement: N/A Reinstatement: $75 Reinstatement of Revoked (or Suspended): N/A	**OTA** Renewal: $35 Temp/Limited Permit License (Renewal): N/A	**OTA** Temp/Limited Permit License: Included with initial license Verification: N/A Late Renewal Fee: $75
Louisiana	**OT** Initial Application: $55 Reciprocity: $80	**OT** Initial License: Included with application Certification: N/A Registration: N/A Duplicate: $10 Endorsement: N/A Reinstatement: $35 Reinstatement of Revoked (or Suspended): N/A	**OT** Renewal: $25 Temp/Limited Permit License (Renewal): N/A	**OT** Temporary Permit: $25 Verification: N/A Late Renewal: $35
	OTA Initial Application: $35 Reciprocity: $55	**OTA** Initial License: Included with application Certification: N/A Registration: N/A Duplicate: $10 Endorsement: N/A Reinstatement: $35 Reinstatement of Revoked (or Suspended): N/A	**OTA** Renewal: $25 Temp/Limited Permit License (Renewal): N/A	**OTA** Temporary Permit: $25 Verification: N/A Late Renewal: $35

State	Application Fee	License/Certification/ Registration Fees	Renewal Fees	Miscellaneous
Maine	**OT** Initial Application: $60 Reciprocity: N/A	**OT** Initial License: $80 Certification: N/A Registration: N/A Duplicate: $5 Endorsement: N/A Reinstatement: N/A Reinstatement of Revoked (or Suspended): N/A	**OT** Renewal: $80 Temp/Limited Permit License (Renewal): $25	**OT** Temp/Limited Permit License: $25 Verification: N/A Late: N/A
	OTA Initial Application: $60 Reciprocity: N/A	**OTA** Initial License: $70 Certification: N/A Registration: N/A Duplicate: $5 Endorsement: N/A Reinstatement: N/A Reinstatement of Revoked (or Suspended): N/A	**OTA** Renewal: $25 Temp/Limited Permit License (Renewal): $20	**OTA** Temp/Limited Permit License: $20 Verification: N/A Late: N/A
Maryland	**OT** Initial Application: $100 (includes temporary license) Reciprocity: N/A	**OT** Initial License: Certification: Registration: Duplicate: $50 Endorsement: Reinstatement: $300 Reinstatement of Revoked (or Suspended):	**OT** Renewal: $160 Temp/Limited Permit License (Renewal): $50 (for 6 months or until results of exam)	**OT** Temp/Limited Permit License: Included with application Verification: $20 Late Renewal: $25 (within 20 days from renewal deadline)
	OTA Initial Application: $100 (includes temporary license) Reciprocity: N/A	**OTA** Initial License: Certification: Registration: Duplicate: $50 Endorsement: Reinstatement: $300 Reinstatement of Revoked (or Suspended):	**OTA** Renewal: $110 Temp/Limited Permit License (Renewal): $50 (for 6 months or until results of exam)	**OTA** Temp/Limited Permit License: Included with application Verification: $20 Late Renewal: $25 (within 20 days from renewal deadline)
Massachu-setts	**OT** Initial Application: $25 Reciprocity: N/A	**OT** Initial License: Included with application Certification: N/A Registration: N/A Duplicate: $11 Endorsement: N/A Reinstatement: N/A Reinstatement of Revoked (or Suspended): N/A	**OT** Renewal: $25 (every 2 years, by January 31 of even years) Temporary License (Renewal): $10	**OT** Temporary License: $10 (plus application fee) Verification: $10 Late Renewal: $25 Lost Certificate: $18
	OTA Initial Application: $25 Reciprocity: N/A	**OTA** Initial License: N/A Certification: N/A Registration: N/A Duplicate: $11 Endorsement: N/A Reinstatement: N/A Reinstatement of Revoked (or Suspended): N/A	**OTA** Renewal: $25 (every 2 years, by January 31 of even years) Temporary License (Renewal): $10	**OTA** Temporary License: $10 (plus application fee) Verification: $10 Late Renewal: $25 Lost Certificate: $18

(Continued)

State	Application Fee	License/Certification/ Registration Fees	Renewal Fees	Miscellaneous
Michigan	**OT** Initial Application: $80 Reciprocity: N/A	**OT** Initial License: N/A Certification: N/A Registration: Included with application Duplicate: N/A Endorsement: $80 Reinstatement: N/A Reinstatement of Revoked (or Suspended): N/A	**OT** Renewal: $100 (2 years) Temp/Limited Permit License (Renewal): N/A	**OT** Temp/Limited Permit License: N/A Verification: N/A Late: N/A
	OTA Initial Application: $80 Reciprocity: N/A	**OTA** Initial License: N/A Certification: N/A Registration: Included with application Duplicate: N/A Endorsement: $80 Reinstatement: N/A Reinstatement of Revoked (or Suspended): N/A	**OTA** Renewal: $100 (2 years) Temp/Limited Permit License (Renewal): N/A	**OTA** Temp/Limited Permit License: N/A Verification: N/A Late: N/A
Minnesota	**OT** Initial Application: N/A Reciprocity: N/A	**OT** Initial License: N/A Certification: N/A Registration: $180 Duplicate: N/A Endorsement: N/A Reinstatement: N/A Reinstatement of Revoked (or Suspended): N/A	**OT** Renewal: $180 Temp/Limited Permit License (Renewal): N/A Provisional Registration Renewal Fee: $90	**OT** Temporary Registration: $50 Initial Provisional Registration Fee: $647 Limited Registration: $96 Verification to Institutions: $10 Late Renewal: $25 Fee for Course Approval After Lapse of Registration: $96 Certification to Other States: $25 Surcharge (due upon application and registration renewal): $62
	OTA Initial Application: N/A Reciprocity: N/A **Surcharge**: For 5 years after June 17, 1996, all registrants must pay a surcharge fee in addition to other applicable fees	**OTA** Initial License: N/A Certification: N/A Registration: $150 Duplicate: N/A Endorsement: N/A Reinstatement: N/A Reinstatement of Revoked (or Suspended): N/A	**OTA** Renewal: $100 Temp/Limited Permit License (Renewal): N/A Provisional Registration Renewal Fee: $50	**OTA** Temporary Registration: $50 Initial Provisional Registration Fee: $647 Limited Registration: $96 Verification to institutions: $10 Late Renewal: $25 Fee for Course Approval After Lapse of Registration: $96 Certification to Other States: $25 Surcharge (due upon application and registration renewal) $36

State	Application Fee	License/Certification/ Registration Fees	Renewal Fees	Miscellaneous
Mississippi	**OT** Initial Application: $100 Reciprocity: N/A	**OT** Initial License: $150 Certification: N/A Registration: N/A Duplicate: N/A Endorsement: N/A Reinstatement: N/A Reinstatement of Revoked (or Suspended): N/A	**OT** Renewal: $150 Limited Permit (Renewal): $150	**OT** Limited Permit: $150 Verification: $25 Late Renewal: $125 Inactive License: $50 ID Card Replacement: $10 Certificate Replacement: $25 Duplicate Certificate: $25
	OTA Initial Application: $100 Reciprocity: N/A	**OTA** Initial License: $100 Certification: N/A Registration: N/A Duplicate: N/A Endorsement: N/A Reinstatement: N/A Reinstatement of Revoked (or Suspended): N/A	**OTA** Renewal: $150 Limited Permit (Renewal): $100	**OTA** Limited Permit: $100 Verification: $25 Late Renewal: $125 Inactive License: $50 ID Card Replacement: $10 Certificate Replacement: $25 Duplicate Certificate: $25
Missouri	**OT** Initial Application: $150 Reciprocity: N/A	**OT** Initial License: Included with application Certification: N/A Registration: Duplicate: $10 Endorsement: N/A Reinstatement: N/A Reinstatement of Revoked (or Suspended): N/A	**OT** Renewal: $150 (2 years) Limited Permit (Renewal): $0	**OT** Limited Permit: $50 Verification: $10 Late Renewal Fee: $50 Inactive License: $30 Replacement Wall-Hanging Fee: $15
	OTA Initial Application: $100 Reciprocity: N/A	**OTA** Initial License: Included with application Certification: N/A Registration: N/A Duplicate: $10 Endorsement: N/A Reinstatement: N/A Reinstatement of Revoked (or Suspended): N/A	**OTA** Renewal: $100 (2 years) Limited Permit (Renewal): $0	**OTA** Limited Permit: $50 Verification: $10 Late Renewal Fee: $50 Inactive License: $25 Replacement Wall-Hanging Fee: $15
Montana	**OT** Initial Application: $20 Reciprocity: N/A	**OT** Initial License: $20 Certification: N/A Registration: N/A Duplicate: $10 Endorsement: N/A Reinstatement: N/A Reinstatement of Revoked (or Suspended): N/A	**OT** Renewal: $20 Temp/Limited Permit License (Renewal): N/A	**OT** Temporary Permit: $10 Verification: $10 Late renewal: $20 Inactive Fee Renewal: $10
	OTA Initial Application: $20 Reciprocity: N/A	**OTA** Initial License: $20 Certification: N/A Registration: N/A Duplicate: $10 Endorsement: N/A Reinstatement: N/A Reinstatement of Revoked (or Suspended): N/A	**OTA** Renewal: $20 Temp/Limited Permit License (Renewal): N/A	**OTA** Temporary Permit: $10 Verification: $10 Late Renewal: $20 Inactive Fee Renewal: $10

(Continued)

State	Application Fee	License/Certification/Registration Fees	Renewal Fees	Miscellaneous
Nebraska	**OT** Initial Application: $200 + $1 license assistance fee per year for each year remaining during the current biennial renewal process Reciprocity: N/A	**OT** Initial License: Included with application Certification: N/A Registration: N/A Duplicate: $10 Endorsement: $25 Reinstatement: $10 Reinstatement of Revoked (or Suspended): N/A	**OT** Renewal: $150 + $2 license assistance fee Temp/Limited Permit License (Renewal): N/A	**OT** Temporary Permit: $25 Verification: $5 Late Renewal: $25 Inactive status: $35 If rejected, applicant is entitled to refund of fee, except for $25 administrative fee
	OTA Initial Application: $175 + $1 license assistance fee per year for each year remaining during the current biennial renewal process Reciprocity: N/A	**OTA** Initial License: Included with application Certification: N/A Registration: N/A Duplicate: $10 Endorsement: $25 Reinstatement: $10 Reinstatement of Revoked (or Suspended): N/A	**OTA** Renewal: $125 + $2 license assistance fee Temp/Limited Permit License (Renewal): N/A	**OTA** Temporary Permit: $25 Verification: $5 Late Renewal: $25 Inactive Status: $35 If rejected, applicant is entitled to refund of fee, except for $25 administrative fee
Nevada	**OT** Initial Application: $250 Reciprocity: N/A	**OT** Initial License: $150 Certification: N/A Registration: N/A Duplicate: $50 Endorsement: N/A Reinstatement: $350 Reinstatement of Revoked (or Suspended): N/A	**OT** Renewal: $175 Temporary License (Renewal): $100	**OT** Application for Temporary License: $100 Verification: Late Renewal: $290 Inactive License: $150 Reinstatement of Inactive License: $100
	OTA Initial Application: $75 Reciprocity: N/A	**OTA** Initial License: $100 Certification: N/A Registration: N/A Duplicate: $50 Endorsement: N/A Reinstatement: $250 Reinstatement of Revoked (or Suspended): N/A	**OTA** Renewal: $125 Temporary License (Renewal): $75	**OTA** Application for Temporary License: $75 Verification: Late Renewal: $230 Inactive License: $100 Reinstatement of Inactive License: $90
New Hampshire	**OT** Initial Application (Includes License and Interim License): $60 Reciprocity: N/A	**OT** Initial License: Included with application Certification: N/A Registration: N/A Duplicate: $2 Endorsement: N/A Reinstatement: N/A Reinstatement of Revoked (or Suspended): N/A	**OT** Renewal: $100 (biennial) Temp/Limited Permit License (Renewal): N/A	**OT** Interim License: Included with application Verification: $10 Late Renewal: $200
	OTA Initial Application (Includes License and Interim License): $60 Reciprocity: N/A	**OTA** Initial License: Included with application Certification: N/A Registration: N/A Duplicate: $2 Endorsement: N/A Reinstatement: N/A Reinstatement of Revoked (or Suspended): N/A	**OTA** Renewal: Temp/Limited Permit License (Renewal): N/A	**OTA** Interim License: Included with application Verification: $10 Late Renewal: $200

State	Application Fee	License/Certification/Registration Fees	Renewal Fees	Miscellaneous

New Jersey	**OT**
	Initial Application: $100
	Reciprocity: N/A
		OT
		Initial License:
		  $160 (first year of biennial process)
		  $80 (second year of biennial process
		Certification: N/A
		Registration: N/A
		
		Duplicate: N/A
		Endorsement: N/A
		Reinstatement: $80 (over 60 days late)
		Reinstatement of Revoked (or Suspended): N/A
			OT
			Renewal: $160
			
			Temporary License (Renewal): $50
				OT
				Temporary License: $50
				
				Verification: N/A
				Late Renewal: $40
				Duplicate Wall Certificate: $40
				Registration Fee: $25 (biennial)

	OTA
	Initial Application: $100
	Reciprocity: N/A
		OTA
		Initial License:
		  $100 (first year of biennial process)
		  $50 (second year of biennial process)
		Certification: N/A
		Registration: N/A
		
		Duplicate: N/A
		Endorsement: N/A
		Reinstatement: $80 (over 60 days late)
		Reinstatement of Revoked (or Suspended): N/A
			OTA
			Renewal: $100
			
			Temporary License (Renewal): $50
				OTA
				Temporary License: $50
				
				Verification: N/A
				Late Renewal: $40
				Duplicate Wall Certificate: $40
				Registration Fee: $25

New Mexico	**OT** Application Information Packet: $10 Reciprocity: N/A	**OT** Initial License: $100 If received between April 1 and July 31: $50 Certification: N/A Registration: N/A Duplicate: $10 Endorsement: N/A Reinstatement: N/A Reinstatement of Revoked (or Suspended): N/A	**OT** Renewal: $60 Temp/Limited Permit License (Renewal): N/A	**OT** Provisional Permit: $25 Jurisprudence Examination: $10 Verification: $20 Late: 3 months: $30 3-6 months: $50 6-12 months: $75 Over 12 months: $100 Each year after, up to 5 years: $100
	OTA Application Information Packet: $10 Reciprocity: N/A	**OTA** Initial License: $100 If received between April 1 and July 31: $50 Certification: N/A Registration: N/A Duplicate: $10 Endorsement: N/A Reinstatement: N/A Reinstatement of Revoked (or Suspended): N/A	**OTA** Renewal: $40 Temp/Limited Permit License (Renewal): N/A	**OTA** Provisional Permit: $25 Jurisprudence Examination: $10 Verification: $20 Late: 3 months: $30 3-6 months: $50 6-12 months: $75 Over 12 months: $100 Each year after, up to 5 years: $100

(Continued)

State	Application Fee	License/Certification/Registration Fees	Renewal Fees	Miscellaneous

New York	**OT**
	Initial Application: N/A
	Reciprocity: N/A
		OT
		Initial License: $270
		Certification: N/A
		Registration: N/A
		
		Duplicate: N/A
		Endorsement: N/A
		Reinstatement: N/A
		Reinstatement of Revoked (or Suspended): N/A
			OT
			Renewal: $155 (triennial)
			
			Temp/Limited Permit
			License (Renewal): N/A
				OT
				Limited Permit: $70
				
				Verification:
				   $20 verification of credentials for other states
				   $10 employer or insurance company
				   $10 letter of good standing
				Late Renewal: $10 per month late
				Parchment Certificate: $10

	OTA
	Initial Application: N/A
	Reciprocity: N/A
		OTA
		Initial License: N/A
		Certification: N/A
		Registration: $95
		
		Duplicate: N/A
		Endorsement: N/A
		Reinstatement: N/A
		Reinstatement of Revoked (or Suspended): N/A
			OTA
			Renewal: $50 (triennial)
			
			Temp/Limited Permit
			License (Renewal): N/A
				OTA
				Limited Permit: N/A
				
				Verification:
				   $20 verification of credentials for other states
				   $10 employer or insurance company
				   $10 letter of good standing
				Late Renewal: $10 per month late
				Parchment Certificate: $10

North Carolina	**OT** Initial Application (for Regular or Provisional License): $10 Reciprocity: N/A	**OT** Initial License: $100 Certification: N/A Registration: N/A Duplicate: N/A Endorsement: N/A Reinstatement: N/A Reinstatement of Revoked (or Suspended): N/A	**OT** Renewal: $50 Temp/Limited Permit License (Renewal): N/A	**OT** Provisional License: $35 Verification: N/A Late Renewal: $50
	OTA Initial Application (for Regular or Provisional License): $10 Reciprocity: N/A	**OTA** Initial License: $100 Certification: N/A Registration: N/A Duplicate: N/A Endorsement: N/A Reinstatement: N/A Reinstatement of Revoked (or Suspended): N/A	**OTA** Renewal: $50 Temp/Limited Permit License (Renewal): N/A	**OTA** Provisional License: $35 Verification: N/A Late Renewal: $50
North Dakota	**OT** Initial Application: N/A Reciprocity: N/A	**OT** Initial License: $40 Certification: N/A Registration: N/A Duplicate: N/A Endorsement: N/A Reinstatement: N/A Reinstatement of Revoked (or Suspended): N/A	**OT** Renewal: Renewal and late fees are based on an assessment of the previous year's expenses, divided by the number of total licensed therapist and assistants. The renewal fee may not exceed the initial license fee. Temp/Limited Permit License (Renewal): N/A	**OT** Limited Permit (Includes License): $40 Verification: N/A Late: Renewal and late fees are based on an assessment of the previous year's expenses, divided by the number of total licensed therapist and assistants. The renewal fee may not exceed the initial license fee. Therapists who initially become licensed after April 1 of any year are exempt from the renewal fee for 1 year.

State	Application Fee	License/Certification/ Registration Fees	Renewal Fees	Miscellaneous
North Dakota *(cont.)*	**OTA** Initial Application: $50 Reciprocity: N/A	**OTA** Initial License: $55 Certification: N/A Registration: N/A Duplicate: N/A Endorsement: N/A Reinstatement: N/A Reinstatement of Revoked (or Suspended): N/A	**OTA** Renewal: Renewal and late fees are based on an assessment of the previous year's expenses, divided by the number of total licensed therapist and assistants. The renewal fee may not exceed the initial license fee. Temp/Limited Permit License (Renewal): N/A	**OTA** Limited Permit (Includes License): $30 Verification: N/A Late: Renewal and late fees are based on an assessment of the previous year's expenses, divided by the number of total licensed therapist and assistants. The renewal fee may not exceed the initial license fee. Therapists who initially become licensed after April 1 of any year are exempt from the renewal fee for 1 year.
Ohio	**OT** Initial Application: $100 Reciprocity: N/A	**OT** Initial License: Included with license Certification: N/A Registration: N/A Duplicate: N/A Endorsement: N/A Reinstatement: N/A Reinstatement of Revoked (or Suspended): N/A	**OT** Renewal: $80 (biennial) Temp/Limited Permit License (Renewal): N/A	**OT** Limited Permit: $50 Verification: $15 Late: Wallet Card: $10 Wall Certificate: $5
	OTA Initial Application: $100 Reciprocity: N/A	**OTA** Initial License: Included with license Certification: N/A Registration: N/A Duplicate: N/A Endorsement: N/A Reinstatement: N/A Reinstatement of Revoked (or Suspended): N/A	**OTA** Renewal: $80 (biennial) Temp/Limited Permit License (Renewal): N/A	**OTA** Limited Permit: $50 Verification: $15 Late: Wallet Card: $10 Wall Certificate: $5
Oklahoma	**OT** Application Processing Fee: $50 Application Reprocessing Fee: $25 Reciprocity: N/A	**OT** Initial License: $50 Certification: N/A Registration: N/A Duplicate: $50 Endorsement: N/A Reinstatement: N/A Reinstatement of Revoked (or Suspended): N/A	**OT** Renewal: Application Processing Fee: $55 Annual Renewal Fee: $20 Temp/Limited Permit License (Renewal): N/A	**OT** Temporary Status Letter: $100 Verification: $20 Late Renewal (after October 31): $20
	OTA Application Processing Fee: $50 Application Reprocessing Fee: $25 Reciprocity: N/A	**OTA** Initial License: $50 Certification: N/A Registration: N/A Duplicate: $50 Endorsement: N/A Reinstatement: N/A Reinstatement of Revoked (or Suspended): N/A	**OTA** Renewal: Application Processing Fee: $55 Annual Renewal Fee: $20 Temp/Limited Permit License (Renewal): N/A	**OTA** Temporary Status Letter: $100 Verification: $20 Late Renewal (after October 31): $20
Oregon	**OT** Initial Application: N/A Reciprocity: N/A	**OT** Initial License: $75 Certification: N/A Registration: N/A Duplicate: N/A Endorsement: N/A Reinstatement: N/A Reinstatement of Revoked (or Suspended): N/A	**OT** Renewal: $85 (due before June 1 of each year) Temp/Limited Permit License (Renewal): N/A	**OT** Limited Permit: $25 Verification: N/A Late Renewal: $50

(Continued)

State	Application Fee	License/Certification/Registration Fees	Renewal Fees	Miscellaneous
Oregon (cont.)	**OTA** Initial Application: N/A Reciprocity: N/A	**OTA** Initial License: $60 Certification: N/A Registration: N/A Duplicate: N/A Endorsement: N/A Reinstatement: N/A Reinstatement of Revoked (or Suspended): N/A	**OTA** Renewal: $70 (due before June 1 of each year) Temp/Limited Permit License (Renewal): N/A	**OTA** Limited Permit: $25 Verification: N/A Late Renewal: $50
Pennsylvania	**OT** Initial Application (Includes License): $30 Reciprocity: N/A	**OT** Initial License: N/A Certification: N/A Registration: N/A Duplicate: N/A Endorsement: N/A Reinstatement: N/A Reinstatement of Revoked (or Suspended): N/A	**OT** Renewal: $55 Temp/Limited Permit License (Renewal): N/A	**OT** Temporary License: $20 Verification: N/A Late: N/A
	OTA Initial Application (Includes License): $30 Reciprocity: N/A	**OTA** Initial License: N/A Certification: N/A Registration: N/A Duplicate: N/A Endorsement: N/A Reinstatement: N/A Reinstatement of Revoked (or Suspended): N/A	**OTA** Renewal: $45 Temp/Limited Permit License (Renewal): N/A	**OTA** Temporary License: $20 Verification: N/A Late: N/A
Puerto Rico	**OT** Initial Application: N/A Reciprocity: N/A	**OT** Initial License: $15 Certification: N/A Registration: N/A Duplicate: N/A Endorsement: N/A Reinstatement: N/A Reinstatement of Revoked (or Suspended): N/A	**OT** Renewal: $20 Provisional License (Renewal): $20	**OT** Provisional License: $10 Verification: N/A Late: N/A
	OTA Initial Application: N/A Reciprocity: N/A	**OTA** Initial License: $15 Certification: N/A Registration: N/A Duplicate: N/A Endorsement: N/A Reinstatement: N/A Reinstatement of Revoked (or Suspended): N/A	**OTA** Renewal: $20 Provisional License (Renewal): $20	**OTA** Provisional License: $10 Verification: N/A Late: N/A
Rhode Island	**OT** Initial Application: $50 Reciprocity: N/A	**OT** Initial License: Included with application Certification: N/A Registration: N/A Duplicate: N/A Endorsement: N/A Reinstatement: N/A Reinstatement of Revoked (or Suspended): N/A	**OT** Renewal: $50 Temp/Limited Permit License (Renewal): N/A	**OT** Graduate Status: $0 Verification: N/A Late Renewal: $25

State	Application Fee	License/Certification/ Registration Fees	Renewal Fees	Miscellaneous
Rhode Island (*cont.*)	**OTA** Initial Application: $50 Reciprocity: N/A	**OTA** Initial License: Included with application Certification: N/A Registration: N/A Duplicate: N/A Endorsement: N/A Reinstatement: N/A Reinstatement of Revoked (or Suspended): N/A	**OTA** Renewal: $50 Temp/Limited Permit License (Renewal): N/A	**OTA** Graduate Status: $0 Verification: N/A Late Renewal: $25
South Carolina	**OT** Initial Application: $135 Reciprocity: N/A	**OT** Initial License: Included with application Certification: N/A Registration: N/A Duplicate: $5 Endorsement: N/A Reinstatement: $10 per year delinquent up to a maximum of 3 years Reinstatement of Revoked (or Suspended): N/A	**OT** Renewal: $50 Temp/Limited Permit License (Renewal): N/A	**OT** Temporary License: Included with application fee. Verification: $15 Late Renewal: $10 Duplicate ID Card: $2
	OTA Initial Application: $115 Reciprocity:	**OTA** Initial License: Included with application Certification: N/A Registration: N/A Duplicate: $5 Endorsement: N/A Reinstatement: $10 per year delinquent up to a maximum of 3 years Reinstatement of Revoked (or Suspended): N/A	**OTA** Renewal: $45 Temp/Limited Permit License (Renewal): N/A	**OTA** Temporary License: Included with application fee. Verification: $15 Late Renewal: $10 Duplicate ID Card: $2
South Dakota	**OT** Initial Application: N/A Reciprocity: $50	**OT** Initial License: $50 Certification: N/A Registration: N/A Duplicate: N/A Endorsement: $50 Reinstatement: N/A Reinstatement of Revoked (or Suspended): N/A	**OT** Renewal: $50 (by January 1 of each year) Temp/Limited Permit License (Renewal): N/A	**OT** Limited Permit: $25 Verification: N/A Late Renewal: $25
	OTA Initial Application: Reciprocity: $50	**OTA** Initial License: $50 Certification: N/A Registration: N/A Duplicate: N/A Endorsement: $50 Reinstatement: N/A Reinstatement of Revoked (or Suspended): N/A	**OTA** Renewal: $50 (by January 1 of each year) Temp/Limited Permit License (Renewal): N/A	**OTA** Limited Permit: $25 Verification: N/A Late Renewal: $25
Tennessee	**OT** Initial Application: $50 Reciprocity: N/A	**OT** Initial License: $150 Certification: N/A Registration: N/A Duplicate: $25 Endorsement: N/A Reinstatement: N/A Reinstatement of Revoked (or Suspended):	**OT** Renewal: $150 (biennial) Limited Permit (renewal): $185	**OT** Limited Permit: $25 State Regulatory Fee: $10 (biennial) Verification: $25 Late Renewal: $15 Certificate Fee: $75 Registration Fee: $75 (One time fee paid by initial certificate holders for issuance of certificate of registration)

(Continued)

State	Application Fee	License/Certification/ Registration Fees	Renewal Fees	Miscellaneous
Tennessee (*cont.*)	**OTA** Initial Application: $30 Reciprocity: N/A	**OTA** Initial License: $120 Certification: N/A Registration: N/A Duplicate: $25 Endorsement: Reinstatement: Reinstatement of Revoked (or Suspended):	**OTA** Renewal: $120 (biennial) Limited Permit (Renewal): $130	**OTA** Limited Permit: $25 State Regulatory Fee: $10 (biennial) Verification: $25 Late Renewal: $15 Certificate Fee: $75 Registration Fee: $75 (One time fee paid by initial certificate holders for issuance of certificate of registration)
Texas	**OT** Initial Application: Provisional Application: $15 Temporary Application: $10 Extended Temporary Application: $10 Regular Application: $10 Reciprocity: N/A	**OT** License: Provisional: $35 Regular (to Birth Month): $50 Certification: N/A Registration: N/A Duplicate: License: $25 Renewal Certificate/Wallet Card: $25 Endorsement: N/A Reinstatement: N/A Reinstatement of Revoked (or Suspended): $50	**OT** Renewal: $100 Temp/Limited Permit License (Renewal): N/A Inactive/Retiree: $0	**OT** Temporary: $90 Extended Temporary: $115 Temporary/Provisional to Regular (to Birth Month): $60 Active to Inactive/Retiree Status: $25 Inactive to Active Status: $175 Inactive to Retiree Status: $0 Verification: $40 Late Renewal Fees: Regular License (A) Late 90 days or less—Regular fee plus late fee which is equal to ½ of the certification exam fee (B) Late more than 90 days but less than 1 year—Regular fee plus late fee which is equal to the certification examination fee Inactive License: (A) Late 90 days or less—$12 (B) Late more than 90 days but less than 1 year—$25
	OTA Initial Application: Provisional Application: $15 Temporary Application: $10 Extended Temporary Application: $10 Regular Application: $10 Reciprocity: N/A	**OTA** License: Provisional: $25 Regular (to Birth Month): $35 Certification: N/A Registration: N/A Duplicate: License: $25 Renewal Certificate/Wallet Card: $25 Endorsement: N/A Reinstatement: N/A Reinstatement of Revoked (or Suspended): $50	**OTA** Renewal: $75 Temp/Limited Permit License (Renewal): N/A Inactive/Retiree: $0	**OTA** Temporary: $65 Extended Temporary: $90 Temporary/Provisional to Regular (to Birth Month): $35 Active to Inactive/Retiree Status: $25 Inactive to Active Status: $125 Inactive to Retiree Status: $0 Verification: $40 Late Renewal Fees: Regular License (A) Late 90 days or less—Regular fee plus late fee which is equal to ½ of the certification exam fee (B) Late more than 90 days but less than 1 year—Regular fee plus late fee which is equal to the certification examination fee Inactive License: (A) Late 90 days or less—$12 (B) Late more than 90 days but less than 1 year—$25

State	Application Fee	License/Certification/Registration Fees	Renewal Fees	Miscellaneous
Utah	**OT** Initial Application: $60 Reciprocity: N/A	**OT** Initial License: Included with application Certification: N/A Registration: N/A Duplicate: $10 Endorsement: N/A Reinstatement: $50 Reinstatement of Revoked (or Suspended): N/A	**OT** Renewal: $35 (by May 31 of odd years) Temp/Limited Permit License (Renewal): N/A	**OT** Temporary License: $110 (includes $60 application fee) Verification: N/A Late Renewal: $20 Inactive Fee: $50 Reactivation Fee: $50
	OTA Initial Application: $60 Reciprocity: N/A	**OTA** Initial License: Included with application Certification: N/A Registration: N/A Duplicate: $10 Endorsement: N/A Reinstatement: $50 Reinstatement of Revoked (or Suspended): N/A	**OTA** Renewal: $35 (by May 31 of odd years) Temp/Limited Permit License (Renewal): N/A	**OTA** Temporary License: $110 (includes $60 application fee) Verification: N/A Late Renewal: $20 Inactive Fee: $50 Reactivation Fee: $50
Vermont	**OT** Initial Application: N/A Reciprocity: N/A	**OT** Initial License: N/A Certification: $100 Registration: N/A Duplicate: N/A Endorsement: N/A Reinstatement: N/A Reinstatement of Revoked (or Suspended): N/A	**OT** Renewal: $200 Temp/Limited Permit License (Renewal): N/A	**OT** Temp Certificate: $50 (Plus certification application fee) Verification: N/A Late: N/A
	OTA Initial Application: N/A Reciprocity: N/A	**OTA** Initial License: N/A Certification: $100 Registration: N/A Duplicate: N/A Endorsement: N/A Reinstatement: N/A Reinstatement of Revoked (or Suspended): N/A	**OTA** Renewal: $200 Temp/Limited Permit License (Renewal): N/A	**OTA** Temp Certificate: $50 (Plus certification application fee) Verification: N/A Late: N/A
Virginia (Does not regulate OTAs)	**OT** Initial Application: N/A Reciprocity: N/A	**OT** Initial License: $100 Certification: N/A Registration: N/A Duplicate: N/A Endorsement: N/A Reinstatement: $150 Reinstatement of Revoked (or Suspended): $500	**OT** Renewal: $85 (due in the birth month of licensed therapist each even-numbered year) Temp/Limited Permit License (Renewal): N/A	**OT** Temp/Limited Permit License: N/A Verification: $10 Late: N/A
	OTA Initial Application: N/A Reciprocity: N/A	**OTA** Initial License: N/A Certification: N/A Registration: N/A Duplicate: N/A Endorsement: N/A Reinstatement: N/A Reinstatement of Revoked (or Suspended): N/A	**OTA** Renewal: N/A Temp/Limited Permit License (Renewal): N/A	**OTA** Temp/Limited Permit License: N/A Verification: N/A Late: N/A

(Continued)

State	Application Fee	License/Certification/ Registration Fees	Renewal Fees	Miscellaneous
Washington	**OT** Initial Application: N/A Reciprocity: N/A	**OT** Initial License: $125 Certification: N/A Registration: N/A Duplicate: $15 Endorsement: N/A Reinstatement: N/A Reinstatement of Revoked (or Suspended): N/A	**OT** Renewal: $95 Temp/Limited Permit License (Renewal): N/A	**OT** Temp/Limited Permit License: $40 Verification: $25 Late Renewal: $50 Expired License Reissuance: $50 Inactive License: $5 Expired Inactive License Reissuance: $5
	OTA Initial Application: N/A Reciprocity: N/A	**OTA** Initial License: $125 Certification: N/A Registration: N/A Duplicate: $15 Endorsement: N/A Reinstatement: N/A Reinstatement of Revoked (or Suspended): N/A	**OTA** Renewal: $70 Temp/Limited Permit License (Renewal): N/A	**OTA** Temp/Limited Permit License: $40 Verification: $25 Late Renewal: $50 Inactive License: $5 Expired License Reissuance: $40
West Virginia	**OT** Initial Application: $15 Reciprocity: N/A	**OT** Initial License: $190 Certification: N/A Registration: N/A Duplicate: N/A Endorsement: N/A Reinstatement: N/A Reinstatement of Revoked (or Suspended): N/A	**OT** Renewal: $60 Temp/Limited Permit License (Renewal): N/A	**OT** Temp/Limited Permit License: $140 (will be applied to permanent license fee) Verification: N/A Late Renewal: $50
	OTA Initial Application: $15 Reciprocity: N/A	**OTA** Initial License: $140 Certification: N/A Registration: N/A Duplicate: N/A Endorsement: N/A Reinstatement: N/A Reinstatement of Revoked (or Suspended): N/A	**OTA** Renewal: $50 Temp/Limited Permit License (Renewal): N/A	**OTA** Temp/Limited Permit License: $90 (will be applied to permanent license fee) Verification: N/A Late Renewal: $50
Wisconsin	**OT** Initial Application: N/A Reciprocity: $41	**OT** Initial License: N/A Certification: $41 Registration: N/A Duplicate: $10 Endorsement: $10 Reinstatement: N/A Reinstatement of Revoked (or Suspended): N/A	**OT** Renewal: $42 (November 1 of each odd-numbered year) Temp/Limited Permit License (Renewal): N/A	**OT** Temporary Certificate: $10 Verification: N/A Late: N/A
	OTA Initial Application: N/A Reciprocity: $41	**OTA** Initial License: N/A Certification: $41 Registration: N/A Duplicate: $10 Endorsement: $10 Reinstatement: N/A Reinstatement of Revoked (or Suspended):	**OTA** Renewal: $42 (November 1 of each odd-numbered year) Temp/Limited Permit License (Renewal): N/A	**OTA** Temporary Certificate: $10 N/A Verification: N/A Late: N/A

State	Application Fee	License/Certification/ Registration Fees	Renewal Fees	Miscellaneous
Wyoming	**OT** Initial Application: $125 Reciprocity: N/A	**OT** Initial License: Before February 1: $105 On or After February 1: $50 Certification: N/A Registration: N/A Duplicate: $10 Endorsement: N/A Reinstatement: N/A Reinstatement of Revoked (or Suspended): N/A	**OT** Renewal: $125 Temp/Limited Permit License (Renewal): N/A	**OT** Temporary License: $55 Limited Permit: $55 Verification: $10 Late Renewal: $40 Reactivation: $25
	OTA Initial Application: $125 Reciprocity: N/A	**OTA** Initial License: Before February 1: $50 On or After February 1: $25 Certification: N/A Registration: N/A Duplicate: $10 Endorsement: N/A Reinstatement: N/A Reinstatement of Revoked (or Suspended): N/A	**OTA** Renewal: $75 Temp/Limited Permit icense (Renewal): N/A	**OTA** Temp License: $25 Limited Permit: $25 Verification: $10 Late Renewal: $40 Reactivation: $25

PART II

Supervision, Roles, and Responsibilities

The question of supervision of occupational therapy assistants has been debated since 1958, when the Representative Assembly of the American Occupational Therapy Association (AOTA) first authorized the training of occupational therapy assistants. As the regulations have changed over the past few years, supervision has become an even larger issue. Occupational therapists and occupational therapy assistants must make informed decisions about supervision with input from many entities. This section contains resources that will help occupational therapy practitioners make well-informed and appropriate decisions about supervision based on a variety of factors.

Supervision is a process in which two or more people participate in a joint effort to establish, maintain, and elevate a level of performance. Supervision, which enhances both the occupational therapist and the occupational therapy assistant, must be a collaborative effort for it to be successful. The process of determining what roles and responsibilities to delegate is difficult. The most important component of this process is good communication.

Delegation is entrusting another, assigning responsibility or authority, or empowering another to act. When occupational therapists make choices about what to delegate to occupational therapy assistants, three considerations are used in the decision-making process: (1) the legal obligation of occupational therapists and occupational therapy assistants to follow the requirements of the regulatory body in the state in which the practice occurs, (2) the often-overlooked affective or emotional components, and (3) the knowledge and skills that both therapists and assistants possess.

First, to make the most informed decision, occupational therapists must have a thorough understanding of the knowledge and skills of the occupational therapy assistant in the current practice setting and within the state regulatory requirements. To fully understand the knowledge and skills that need to be considered in the practice area, the occupational therapist and the occupational therapy assistant must look at the diversity and complexity of the client population and the specific occupational therapy requirements for the practice setting. Second, the occupational therapist must examine the biases, both positive and negative, that might influence the delegation process. Empowering others and entrusting them with duties requires effective communication and affects how they function as a team.

Finally, one must consider the service competency—not only the years of experience but also the skill set—of the occupational therapist and the occupational therapy assistant within that setting and with the specific populations. When entering a new practice environment or developing new skills, the therapist and the assistant must consider the complexity of the treatment when looking at supervision requirements.

Defining, determining, and documenting service competency often are discussed in state regulations. However, many practice acts don't define these or give direction. *Competency* is the ability to apply skills and knowledge effectively. A competency describes the cluster of related knowledge, skills, and attributes expressed as behavior that contributes to successful performance, can be measured against well-accepted standards, and can be improved through training and development. This is a complex issue and has many implications for the supervisory process.

To help resolve these issues, the following resources are included in this section:

- Chapter 4: AOTA Guidelines for Supervision, Roles, and Responsibilities During the Delivery of Occupational Therapy
- Chapter 5: Sample Supervision Matrix
- Chapter 6: Model State Regulation for Supervision of Occupational Therapy Assistants and Aides
- Chapter 7: State Occupational Therapy Assistant Supervision Requirements
- Chapter 8: A Guide for Managers and Supervisors to Develop a System for Assessment of Competencies

- Chapter 9: AOTA Standards for Continuing Competence
- Chapter 10: Model Continuing Competence Guidelines for Occupational Therapists and Occupational Therapy Assistants: A Resource for State Regulatory Boards
- Chapter 11: Competency Checklists
- Chapter 12: Sample State Occupational Therapy Supervision Logs
- Chapter 13: Forging OTA–OT Partnerships That Work
- Chapter 14: Medicare Supervision Requirements for Reimbursement
- Chapter 15: HIPAA Guidelines for Fieldwork.

Chapter 4

AOTA Guidelines for Supervision, Roles, and Responsibilities During the Delivery of Occupational Therapy

This document contains four sections that direct the delivery of occupational therapy services: guidelines for the supervision of occupational therapy personnel,[1] supervision of occupational therapists and occupational therapy assistants, roles and responsibilities of occupational therapists and occupational therapy assistants during the delivery of occupational therapy services, and supervision of occupational therapy aides.

Guidelines for the Supervision of Occupational Therapy Personnel

These guidelines provide a definition of supervision and outline parameters to be used by occupational therapy personnel regarding effective supervision as it relates to the delivery of occupational therapy services. These supervision guidelines are to assist occupational therapy personnel in the appropriate and effective provision of occupational therapy services. The guidelines themselves cannot be interpreted to constitute a standard of supervision in any particular locality. All personnel are expected to meet applicable state and federal regulations, adhere to relevant workplace policies and the *Occupational Therapy Code of Ethics* (American Occupational Therapy Association [AOTA], 2000), and participate in ongoing professional development activities to maintain continuing competency.

In these guidelines, *supervision* is viewed as a cooperative process in which two or more people participate in a joint effort to establish, maintain, and/or elevate a level of competence and performance. Supervision is based on mutual understanding between the supervisor and the supervisee about each other's competence, experience, education, and credentials. It fosters growth and development, promotes effective utilization of resources, encourages cre-

ativity and innovation, and provides education and support to achieve a goal (AOTA, 1999a). Within the scope of occupational therapy practice, supervision is a process aimed at ensuring the safe and effective delivery of occupational therapy services and fostering professional competence and development.

Supervision of Occupational Therapists and Occupational Therapy Assistants

Occupational Therapists

Based on their education and training, occupational therapists, after initial certification, are autonomous practitioners who are able to deliver occupational therapy services independently. The occupational therapist is responsible for all aspects of occupational therapy service delivery and is accountable for the safety and effectiveness of the occupational therapy service delivery process. Occupational therapists are encouraged to seek supervision and mentoring to develop best practice approaches and promote professional growth.

Occupational Therapy Assistants

Based on their education and training, occupational therapy assistants must receive supervision from an occupational therapist to deliver occupational therapy services. The occupational therapy assistant delivers occupational therapy services under the supervision of and in partnership with the occupational therapist. The occupational therapist and the occupational therapy assistant are responsible for collaboratively developing a plan for supervision.

General Principles

1. Supervision involves guidance and oversight related to the delivery of occupational therapy services and the facilitation of professional growth and competence. It is the responsibility of the occupational therapist and the occupational therapy assistant to seek the appropriate

---

[1]Occupational therapy personnel include occupational therapists, occupational therapy assistants, and occupational therapy aides (AOTA, 1999a).

quality and frequency of supervision to ensure safe and effective occupational therapy service delivery.

2. To ensure safe and effective occupational therapy services, it is the responsibility of the occupational therapist and occupational therapy assistant to recognize when supervision is needed and to seek supervision that supports current and advancing levels of competence.

3. The specific frequency, methods, and content of supervision may vary by practice setting and are dependent upon the
   a. Complexity of client needs,
   b. Number and diversity of clients,
   c. Skills of the occupational therapist and the occupational therapy assistant,
   d. Type of practice setting,
   e. Requirements of the practice setting, and
   f. Other regulatory requirements.

4. Supervision that is more frequent than the minimum level required by the practice setting or regulatory agencies may be necessary when
   a. The needs of the client and the occupational therapy process are complex and changing,
   b. The practice setting provides occupational therapy services to a large number of clients with diverse needs, or
   c. The occupational therapist and occupational therapy assistant determine that additional supervision is necessary to ensure safe and effective delivery of occupational therapy services.

5. A variety of types and methods of supervision should be used. Methods may include direct face-to-face contact and indirect contact. Examples of methods or types of supervision that involve direct face-to-face contact include observation, modeling, co-treatment, discussions, teaching, and instruction. Examples of methods or types of supervision that involve indirect contact include phone conversations, written correspondence, and electronic exchanges.

6. Occupational therapists and occupational therapy assistants must abide by agency and state requirements regarding the documentation of a supervision plan and supervision contacts. Documentation may include the
   a. Frequency of supervisory contact,
   b. Method(s) or type(s) of supervision,
   c. Content areas addressed,
   d. Evidence to support areas and levels of competency, and
   e. Names and credentials of the persons participating in the supervisory process.

7. Supervision related to professional growth, such as leadership and advocacy development, may differ from that

needed to provide occupational therapy services. The person providing this supervision, as well as the frequency, method, and content of supervision, should be responsive to the supervisee's advancing levels of professional growth.

Supervision Outside the Delivery of Occupational Therapy Services

The education and expertise of occupational therapists and occupational therapy assistants prepare them for employment in arenas other than those related to the delivery of occupational therapy. In these other arenas, supervision may be provided by non–occupational therapy professionals.

1. The guidelines of the setting, regulatory agencies, and funding agencies direct the supervision requirements.

2. The occupational therapist and occupational therapy assistant should obtain and use credentials or job titles commensurate with their roles in these other employment arenas.

3. The following are used to determine whether the services provided are related to the delivery of occupational therapy:
   a. State practice acts
   b. Regulatory agency standards and rules
   c. The domain of occupational therapy practice
   d. The written and verbal agreement among the occupational therapist, the occupational therapy assistant, the client, and the agency or payer about the services provided.

Roles and Responsibilities of Occupational Therapists and Occupational Therapy Assistants During the Delivery of Occupational Therapy Services

General Statement

The focus of occupational therapy is to facilitate the engagement of the client in occupations that support participation in daily life situations in context or contexts. Occupational therapy addresses the needs and goals of the client related to areas of occupation, performance skills, performance patterns, occupational context, activity demands, and client factors.

1. The occupational therapist is responsible for all aspects of occupational therapy service delivery and is accountable for the safety and effectiveness of the occupational therapy service delivery process. The occupational therapy service delivery process involves evaluation, intervention planning, intervention implementation, intervention review, and outcome evaluation.

2. The occupational therapist must be directly involved in the delivery of services during the initial evaluation and regularly throughout the course of intervention and outcome evaluation.

3. The occupational therapy assistant delivers occupational therapy services under the supervision of and in partnership with the occupational therapist.

4. It is the responsibility of the occupational therapist to determine when to delegate responsibilities to other occupational therapy personnel. It is the responsibility of the occupational therapy personnel who perform the delegated responsibilities to demonstrate service competency.

5. The occupational therapist and the occupational therapy assistant demonstrate and document service competency for clinical reasoning and judgment during the service delivery process as well as for the performance of specific techniques, assessments, and intervention methods used.

6. When delegating aspects of occupational therapy services, the occupational therapist considers the following factors:
   a. The complexity of the client's condition and needs
   b. The knowledge, skill, and competence of the occupational therapy practitioner
   c. The nature and complexity of the intervention
   d. The needs and requirements of the practice setting.

Roles and Responsibilities

Regardless of the setting in which occupational therapy services are delivered, the occupational therapist and the occupational therapy assistant assume the following generic responsibilities during evaluation, intervention, and outcomes evaluation.

Evaluation

1. The occupational therapist directs the evaluation process.

2. The occupational therapist is responsible for directing all aspects of the initial contact during the occupational therapy evaluation, including
   a. Determining the need for service,
   b. Defining the problems within the domain of occupational therapy that need to be addressed,
   c. Determining the client's goals and priorities,
   d. Establishing intervention priorities,
   e. Determining specific further assessment needs, and
   f. Determining specific assessment tasks that can be delegated to the occupational therapy assistant.

3. The occupational therapist initiates and directs the evaluation, interprets the data, and develops the intervention plan.

4. The occupational therapy assistant contributes to the evaluation process by implementing delegated assessments and by providing verbal and written reports of observations and client capacities to the occupational therapist.

5. The occupational therapist interprets the information provided by the occupational therapy assistant and integrates that information into the evaluation and decision-making process.

Intervention Planning

1. The occupational therapist has overall responsibility for the development of the occupational therapy intervention plan.

2. The occupational therapist and the occupational therapy assistant collaborate with the client to develop the plan.

3. The occupational therapy assistant is responsible for being knowledgeable about evaluation results and for providing input into the intervention plan, based on client needs and priorities.

Intervention Implementation

1. The occupational therapist has overall responsibility for implementing the intervention.

2. When delegating aspects of the occupational therapy intervention to the occupational therapy assistant, the occupational therapist is responsible for providing appropriate supervision.

3. The occupational therapy assistant is responsible for being knowledgeable about the client's occupational therapy goals.

4. The occupational therapy assistant selects, implements, and makes modifications to therapeutic activities and interventions that are consistent with demonstrated competency levels, client goals, and the requirements of the practice setting.

Intervention Review

1. The occupational therapist is responsible for determining the need for continuing, modifying, or discontinuing occupational therapy services.

2. The occupational therapy assistant contributes to this process by exchanging information with and providing documentation to the occupational therapist about the client's responses to and communications during intervention.

Outcome Evaluation

1. The occupational therapist is responsible for selecting, measuring, and interpreting outcomes that are related to the client's ability to engage in occupations.

2. The occupational therapy assistant is responsible for being knowledgeable about the client's targeted occupational therapy outcomes and for providing information and documentation related to outcome achievement.

3. The occupational therapy assistant may implement outcome measurements and provide needed client discharge resources.

Supervision of Occupational Therapy Aides[2]

An aide, as used in occupational therapy practice, is an individual who provides supportive services to the occupational therapist and the occupational therapy assistant. Aides are not primary service providers of occupational therapy in any practice setting. Therefore, aides do not provide skilled occupational therapy services. An aide is trained by an occupational therapist or an occupational therapy assistant to perform specifically delegated tasks. The occupational therapist is responsible for the overall use and actions of the aide. An aide first must demonstrate competency to be able to perform the assigned, delegated client and non-client tasks.

1. The occupational therapist must oversee the development, documentation, and implementation of a plan to supervise and routinely assess the ability of the occupational therapy aide to carry out non-client- and client-related tasks. The occupational therapy assistant may contribute to the development and documentation of this plan.
2. The occupational therapy assistant can supervise the aide.
3. Non-client-related tasks include clerical and maintenance activities and preparation of the work area or equipment.
4. Client-related tasks are routine tasks during which the aide may interact with the client but does not act as a primary service provider of occupational therapy services. The following factors must be present when an occupational therapist or occupational therapy assistant delegates a selected client-related task to the aide:
   a. The outcome anticipated for the delegated task is predictable.
   b. The situation of the client and the environment is stable and will not require that judgment, interpretations, or adaptations be made by the aide.
   c. The client has demonstrated some previous performance ability in executing the task.
   d. The task routine and process have been clearly established.
5. When performing delegated client-related tasks, the supervisor must ensure that the aide
   a. Is trained and able to demonstrate competency in carrying out the selected task and using equipment, if appropriate;

b. Has been instructed on how to specifically carry out the delegated task with the specific client; and
   c. Knows the precautions, signs, and symptoms for the particular client that would indicate the need to seek assistance from the occupational therapist or occupational therapy assistant.
6. The supervision of the aide needs to be documented. Documentation includes information about frequency and methods of supervision used, the content of supervision, and the names and credentials of all persons participating in the supervisory process.

Summary

These guidelines about supervision, roles, and responsibilities are to assist in the appropriate utilization of occupational therapy personnel and in the appropriate and effective provision of occupational therapy services. All personnel are expected to meet applicable state and federal regulations, adhere to relevant workplace policies and the *Occupational Therapy Code of Ethics* (AOTA, 2000), and participate in ongoing professional development activities to maintain continuing competency.

References

American Occupational Therapy Association. (1999a). Guide for supervision of occupational therapy personnel in the delivery of occupational therapy services. *American Journal of Occupational Therapy, 53,* 592–594 [correction, *54*(2): 235].

American Occupational Therapy Association. (1999b). Guidelines for the use of aides in occupational therapy practice. *American Journal of Occupational Therapy, 53,* 595–597 [correction, *54*(2): 235].

American Occupational Therapy Association. (2000). Occupational therapy code of ethics. *American Journal of Occupational Therapy, 54,* 614–616.

Additional Reading

American Occupational Therapy Association. (1998). Standards of practice for occupational therapy. *American Journal of Occupational Therapy, 52,* 866–869.

American Occupational Therapy Association. (2002a). Parameters for appropriate supervision of the occupational therapy assistant. *OT Practice, 7*(15), 9.

American Occupational Therapy Association. (2002b). Roles and responsibilities of the occupational therapist and the occupational therapy assistant during the delivery of occupational therapy services. *OT Practice, 7*(15), 9–10.

---

[2]Depending on the setting in which service is provided, *aides* may be referred to by various names. Examples include but are not limited to *rehabilitation aides, restorative aides, extenders, paraprofessionals,* and *rehab techs* (AOTA, 1999b).

Authors

THE COMMISSION ON PRACTICE
Sara Jane Brayman, PhD, OTR/L, FAOTA, Chairperson
Gloria Frolek Clark, MS, OTR/L, FAOTA
Janet V. DeLany, DEd, OTR/L
Eileen R. Garza, PhD, OTR, ATP
Mary V. Radomski, MA, OTR/L, FAOTA
Ruth Ramsey, MS, OTR/L
Carol Siebert, MS, OTR/L
Kristi Voelkerding, BS, COTA/L
Pataricia D. LaVesser, PhD, OTR/L, SIS Liaison
Lenna Aird, ASD Liaison
Deborah Lieberman, MHSA, OTR/L, FAOTA, AOTA
    Headquarters Liaison

for

THE COMMISSION ON PRACTICE
Sara Jane Brayman, PhD, OTR/L, FAOTA, Chairperson

Adopted by the Representative Assembly 2004C24

This document replaces the following AOTA documents

- 1999 *Guidelines for Use of Aides in Occupational Therapy Practice* (previously published and copyrighted in 1999 by the *American Journal of Occupational Therapy, 53,* 595–597 [correction, *54*(2): 235]).

- 1999 *Guide for Supervision of Occupational Therapy Personnel in the Delivery of Occupational Therapy Services* (previously published and copyrighted in 1999 by the *American Journal of Occupational Therapy, 53,* 592–594 [correction, *54*(2):235].

- 2002 *Parameters for Appropriate Supervision of the Occupational Therapy Assistant* (previously published and copyrighted by *OT Practice, 7*(15), 9.

- 2002 *Roles and Responsibilities of the Occupational Therapist and the Occupational Therapy Assistant During the Delivery of Occupational Therapy Services* (previously published and copyrighted by *OT Practice, 7*(15), 9–10).

Originally published as American Occupational Therapy Association. (2004). AOTA guidelines for supervision, roles, and responsibilities during the delivery of occupational therapy. *American Journal of Occupational Therapy, 58,* 663–667.

Chapter 5

Sample Supervision Matrix

Directions for Use of the Supervision Matrix

To ensure safe, effective, and legal delivery of occupational therapy services, it is the responsibility of the occupational therapist and the occupational therapy assistant to recognize when supervision is needed and to seek supervision that supports current and advancing levels of competence. Utilizing this matrix will help ensure that the supervisory process meets these objectives and enhances the professional growth and competence of both the occupational therapist and the occupational therapy assistant.

Start at the beginning with regulation and scope of practice and proceed down the matrix addressing each of the areas. Once you have determined the needs of the environment and the skills of the occupational therapist and the occupational therapy assistant, you can then determine the level of supervision based on all of the above factors.

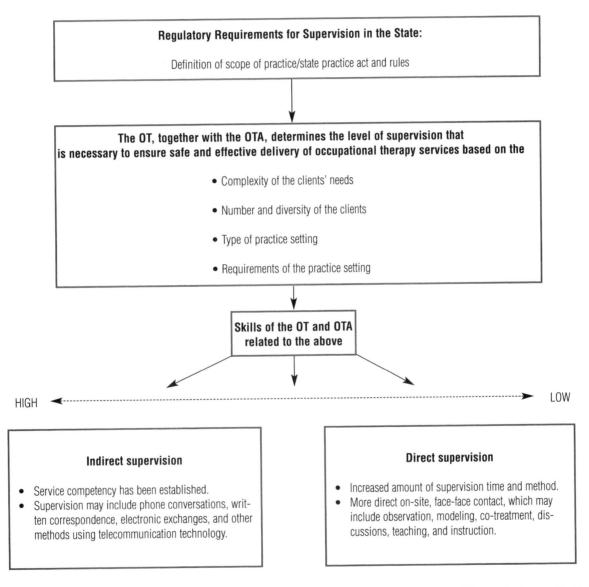

Regulatory Requirements for Supervision in the State:

Definition of scope of practice/state practice act and rules

The OT, together with the OTA, determines the level of supervision that is necessary to ensure safe and effective delivery of occupational therapy services based on the

- Complexity of the clients' needs
- Number and diversity of the clients
- Type of practice setting
- Requirements of the practice setting

Skills of the OT and OTA related to the above

HIGH ← - → LOW

Indirect supervision

- Service competency has been established.
- Supervision may include phone conversations, written correspondence, electronic exchanges, and other methods using telecommunication technology.

Direct supervision

- Increased amount of supervision time and method.
- More direct on-site, face-face contact, which may include observation, modeling, co-treatment, discussions, teaching, and instruction.

Based on the AOTA Documents Guidelines for Supervision, Roles, and Responsibilities During the Delivery of Occupational Therapy Services *and the* Model State Regulation for Supervision, Roles, and Responsibilities During the Delivery of Occupational Therapy Services.

Chapter 6

Model State Regulation for Supervision of Occupational Therapy Assistants and Aides

Purpose

The purpose of this Model State Regulation for Supervision of Occupational Therapy Personnel is to provide the template for use by state agencies and occupational therapy regulatory boards when drafting regulations to govern the clinical supervision of certain occupational therapists, occupational therapy assistants, and aides. The model is intended to help safeguard the public health, safety, and welfare by establishing minimal guidelines that are consistent with accepted standards and practice in the profession.

General Regulations

1. Definitions

A. In this chapter, the following terms have the meanings indicated.

1. "Board" means the _____ State "Board of Occupational Therapy Examiners."
2. "Licensed occupational therapist" means, unless the context requires otherwise, an occupational therapist who is licensed (certified or registered) by the Board and whose license (certificate or registration) is in good standing as determined by the Board.
3. "Licensed occupational therapy assistant" means, unless the context requires otherwise, an occupational therapy assistant who is licensed (certified or registered) by the state Board to assist in the practice of occupational therapy under the supervision of a licensed occupational therapist.
4. "Occupational therapy practitioner" is a generic term that refers to an occupational therapist or an occupational therapy assistant who is licensed (certified or registered) by the Board.
5. "Aide" means an individual who is not certified by a nationally recognized occupational therapy certifying body or licensed (certified or registered) by the Board as an occupational therapy practitioner and who provides supportive services to the occupational therapy practitioner as defined by Regulation 4 of this chapter.
6. "Supervision" means the periodic review and inspection of all aspects of occupational therapy services by the appropriate licensed (certified or registered) occupational therapy practitioner.
7. "Continuous supervision" applies to aides and means the occupational therapy supervisor is in sight of the aide who is performing delegated client-related tasks.
8. "Close supervision" means daily, direct contact at the site of work and applies only to occupational therapists with initial skill development proficiencies or occupational therapy assistants, as appropriate, for the delivery of occupational therapy services.
9. "Routine supervision" means direct contact at least every 2 weeks at the site of work, with interim supervision occurring by other methods, such as telephonic, electronic, or written communication and applies only to occupational therapy assistants.
10. "General supervision" means at least monthly direct contact, with interim supervision available as needed by other methods, and applies only to occupational therapists with increased skill development and mastery of basic role functions or occupational therapy assistants, as appropriate, for the delivery of occupational therapy services.
11. "Minimal supervision" means supervision provided on a less-than-monthly basis to occupational therapy assistants when performing non-clinical administrative responsibilities.
12. "Good standing" means the individual has not been convicted of a felony or a misdemeanor or disciplined by the recognized professional certifying or standards-setting body within 5 years prior to application or renewal of license.

2. Scope of Occupational Therapy Assistant's License (Certificate or Registration)

A. *In general*—Subject to subsection B of this section, an occupational therapy assistant's license (certificate or registration) authorizes the licensee to practice occupational therapy under the supervision of a licensed occupational therapist. In addition to the requirements set forth in Regulation 3 of this chapter, the level of supervision will depend upon the ability and established competency of the occupational therapy assistant to safely and effectively provide direct service that follows routine and accepted procedure under the supervision of the licensed occupational therapist.

B. *Supervision required*—A licensed (certified or registered) occupational therapy assistant may practice only under the supervision of an occupational therapist who is authorized to practice occupational therapy in this state.

3. Supervision Parameters

A. Supervision is a collaborative process that requires both the licensed (certified or registered) occupational therapist and the licensed (certified or registered) occupational therapy assistant to share responsibility. Appropriate supervision will include consideration given to factors such as level of skill, the establishment of service competency (the ability to use the identified intervention in a safe and effective manner), experience and work setting demands, as well as the complexity and stability of the client population to be treated.

B. Supervision is an interactive process that requires both the licensed (certified or registered) occupational therapist and the licensed (certified or registered) occupational therapy assistant or other supervisee to share responsibility for communication between the supervisor and the supervisee.

The licensed (certified or registered) occupational therapist should provide the supervision, and the supervisee should seek it. An outcome of appropriate supervision is to enhance and promote supervision quality occupational therapy services and the professional development of the individuals involved.

C. Supervision of occupational therapy services provided by a licensed (certified or registered) occupational therapy assistant shall be implemented as follows:

1. Entry-level occupational therapy assistants are persons working on initial skill development (less than 1 year of work experience) or who are entering new practice environments or developing new skills (1 or more years of experience) and shall require close supervision.

2. Intermediate-level occupational therapy assistants are persons working on increased skill development, mastery of basic role functions (minimum 1–3 years of experience or dependent on practice environment or previous experience) and shall require routine supervision.

3. Advanced-level occupational therapy assistants are persons refining specialized skills (more than 3 years work experience or the ability to understand complex issues affecting role functions) and shall require general supervision.

4. Licensed (certified or registered) occupational therapy assistants, regardless of their years of experience, may require closer supervision by the licensed (certified or registered) occupational therapist for interventions that are more complex or evaluative in nature and for areas in which service competencies have not been established.

5. Certain occupational therapy assistants may only require minimal supervision when performing non-clinical administrative responsibilities.

4. Scope of the Use of an Aide

A. *In general*—The licensed (certified or registered) occupational therapist is ultimately responsible and accountable for the use of aides. An aide provides supportive services to the occupational therapy practitioner which may include client-related and non-client-related duties and which do not require the knowledge, skills, or judgment of a licensed (certified or registered) occupational therapy practitioner. The occupational therapist or the occupational therapy assistant shall delegate to aides only specifically selected routine tasks for which the aide has been trained and is able to demonstrate competency. Appropriate delegation of specifically selected routine tasks and appropriate supervision by an occupational therapist or an occupational therapy assistant is essential when using aides.

B. A supervising licensed (certified or registered) occupational therapist or occupational therapy assistant working with an aide shall provide continuous supervision when the aide is performing delegated client-related tasks which are specifically selected routine aspects of the intervention session.

C. Selected non-client-related tasks that may be delegated to an aide include, but are not limited to, routine clerical and maintenance activities or preparation of a work area or equipment.

Adopted 2/8/99 by Representative Assembly mail ballot (1999M92)

Chapter 7

State Occupational Therapy Assistant Supervision Requirements

State	Citation	Legislative/Regulatory information
Alabama	**Statute:** AL code 1975, §34-39-3.6	*Occupational Therapy Assistant* A person licensed to assist in the practices of occupational therapy under the supervision of, or with the consultation of, a licensed occupational therapist whose license is in good standing.

	Regulation: Chapter 625 -X-8-.01	*Supervision of Licensed Occupational Therapy Assistants*
		 1. All occupational therapy assistants shall assist in the practice of occupational therapy only under the supervision of an occupational therapist.
		 2. Supervision of an occupational therapy assistant by an occupational therapist shall consist of at least 5% of work hours per month of one-to-one on-site supervision for each certified occupational therapy assistant with supervision including:
		   a. The monitoring of a patient's progress by the occupational therapist;
		   b. Evaluation of the treatment plan and determination of treatment termination by the occupational therapist.
		 3. The Occupational Therapist shall ensure that the occupational therapy assistant is assigned only those duties and responsibilities for which the assistant has been specifically educated and which the occupational therapy assistant is qualified to perform.
		 4. The provisions as enumerated in subsection (1), (2), and (3), shall apply to any individual holding a temporary permit as issued by the Board.

	625-X-8-.02	*Supervision of Therapists/Assistants With Limited Permits*
		 Any individual issued a limited permit under the provision of §34-39-11, shall be supervised in accordance with the requirements of 625-X-8-.01 as set here and above.
		   a. Supervision of limited permit holders shall consist of one-to-one on-site supervision a minimum of 50 percent of direct patient time by an occupational therapist who holds a current license in this state.
		   b. Supervision of limited permit holders who are in the reentry process, as stated in 625-X-3-.08, shall consist of 100%, in-sight supervision by an Alabama licensed occupational therapist with no less than five years continuous experience.

Alaska	**Statute:** §08.84.190	4. "Occupational therapy assistant" means a person who assists in the practice of occupational therapy under the supervision of an occupational therapist;

	Regulation: 12 AAC 54.810	*Supervision of Occupational Therapy Assistants*
		 a. An occupational therapy assistant shall work under the supervision of a licensed occupational therapist. To meet this supervision requirement,
		   1. At least once per month the occupational therapist supervising the licensed occupational therapy assistant shall be physically present while the occupational therapy assistant being supervised implements a treatment plan with a patient; and
		   2. The occupational therapist supervising the occupational therapy assistant shall be available for consultation with the occupational therapy assistant being supervised, through telephone consultations, written reports, or inperson conferences.
		 b. If the licensed occupational therapist agrees to supervise an occupational therapy assistant, the occupational therapist shall
		   1. Determine the frequency and manner of consultations, taking into consideration the treatment settings being used, patient rehabilitation status, and the competency of the occupational therapy assistant being supervised;
		   2. Fully document the supervision provided, including a record of all consultations provided, and maintain those records at the occupational therapy assistant's place of employment; and
		   3. Countersign the patient treatment record each time the occupational therapist supervising the occupational therapy assistant is physically present and directly supervises the treatment of a patient by the occupational therapy assistant being supervised.

	12 AAC 54.820	*Standards for Supervision* For the purposes of 12 AAC 54.600–12 AAC 54.820, "supervision" means the occupational therapist 1. Will be present whenever a patient is evaluated, a treatment program is established, or a treatment program is changed; and 2. Is present to personally review the diagnosis of the condition to be treated, authorize the procedure, and, before dismissal of the patient, evaluate the performance of the treatment given.

State	Citation	Legislative/Regulatory information
Arizona	**Statute:** §32-3401.3	"Direct Supervision" means that the supervising occupational therapist is on the premise at all times while a limited permittee is performing occupational therapy services or when an unlicensed person is performing authorized tasks.
	§32-3401.7	"Occupational therapy assistant" means a person who is licensed pursuant to this chapter, who is a graduate of an accredited occupational therapy education program or the equivalent, who assists in the practice of occupational therapy and who performs delegated procedures commensurate with his education and training.
	Regulation: R4-43-101.11	"Supervision" means a collaborative process for the responsible periodic review and inspection of all aspects of occupational therapy services. The following levels of supervision are minimal. An occupational therapist may assign an increased level of supervision if deemed necessary for the safety of a patient or client. The levels of supervision are: a. "Continuous supervision" means the supervising occupational therapist is in the immediate area of the occupational therapy aide performing supportive services. b. "Close supervision" means the supervising occupational therapist provides initial direction to the occupational therapy assistant and daily contact while on the premises. c. "Routine supervision" means the supervising occupational therapist has face-to-face contact with the occupational therapy assistant at least once every 15 calendar days on a per patient or client basis while on the premises, with the supervising occupational therapist available by telephone or by written communication. d. "General supervision" means the supervising occupational therapist has face-to-face contact with the occupational therapy assistant at least once every 30 calendar days on a per patient or client basis while on the premises, with the supervising occupational therapist available by telephone or by written communication. e. "Minimal supervision" means the supervising occupational therapist has face-to-face contact with the occupational therapy assistant at least once every 30 calendar days while on the premises.
	R4-43-401	*Supervision of Occupational Therapy Assistants* A. Only a licensed occupational therapist shall: 1. Prepare an initial treatment plan, initiate or re-evaluate a client or patient's treatment plan, or authorize in writing a change of a treatment plan; 2. Delegate duties to a licensed occupational therapy assistant, designate an assistant's duties, and assign a level of supervision; and 3. Authorize a patient discharge. B. A licensed occupational therapy assistant shall not: 1. Evaluate or develop a treatment plan independently; 2. Initiate a treatment plan before a client or patient is evaluated and a treatment plan is prepared by an occupational therapist; 3. Continue a treatment procedure appearing harmful to a patient or client until the procedure is reevaluated by an occupational therapist; or 4. Continue or discontinue occupational therapy services unless the treatment plan is approved or reapproved by a supervising occupational therapist. C. A supervising occupational therapist shall supervise a licensed occupational therapy assistant as follows: 1. Not less than routine supervision if the occupational therapy assistant has less than 12 months' work experience in a particular practice setting or with a particular skill. 2. Not less than general supervision if the occupational therapy assistant has more than 12 months but less than 24 months of experience in a particular practice setting or with a particular skill. 3. Not less than minimal supervision if an occupational therapy assistant has more than 24 months of experience in a particular practice setting or with a particular skill. 4. Increased level of supervision, if necessary, for the safety of a patient or client.
Arkansas	**Statute:** 17-88-102	3. "Occupational therapy assistant" means a person licensed to assist in the practice of occupational therapy under the frequent and regular supervision by or with consultation with an occupational therapist, whose license is in good standing. The definition of "frequent" and "regular" will be established by the Arkansas State Occupational Therapy Examining Committee
	Regulation: Regulation 6, 6.2, Arkansas State Occupational Therapy Licensing Act 381 of 1977.	*Frequent and Regular Supervision Defined* As specified in the Occupational Therapy Practice Act 17-88-102 (3), an "occupational therapy assistant" means a person licensed to assist in the practice of occupational therapy under the frequent and regular supervision by or in consultation with an occupational therapist whose license is in good standing. "Frequent" and "regular" are defined by the Arkansas State Occupational Therapy Examining Committee as consisting of the following elements: A. The supervising occupational therapist shall have a legal and ethical responsibility to provide supervision, and the supervisee shall have a legal and ethical responsibility to obtain supervision regarding the patients seen by the occupational therapy assistant. B. Supervision by the occupational therapist of the supervisee's occupational therapy services shall always be required, even when the supervisee is experienced and highly skilled in a particular area. C. Frequent/Regular Supervision of an occupational therapy assistant by the occupational therapist is as follows: 1. The supervising occupational therapist shall meet with the occupational therapy assistant for on-site, face to face supervision a minimum of one (1) hour per forty (40) occupational therapy work hours performed by the occupational therapy assistant, to review each patient's progress and objectives. 2. The supervising occupational therapist shall meet with each patient being treated by the occupational therapy assistant on a monthly basis, to review patient progress and objectives. D. The occupational therapists shall assign, and the occupational therapy assistant shall accept, only those duties and responsibilities for which the occupational therapy assistant has been specifically trained and is qualified to perform, pursuant to the judgment of the occupational therapist.

(Continued)

State	Citation	Legislative/Regulatory information
Arkansas (*cont.*)		1. Assessment/reassessment. Patient evaluation is the responsibility of the occupational therapist. The occupational therapy assistant may contribute to the evaluation process by gathering data, and reporting observations. The occupational therapy assistant may not evaluate independently or initiate treatment prior to the occupational therapist's evaluation.
		2. Treatment planning/Intervention. The occupational therapy assistant may contribute to treatment planning as directed by the occupational therapist. The occupational therapist shall advise the patient/client as to which level of practitioner will carry out the treatment plan.
		3. Discontinuation of intervention. The occupational therapy assistant may contribute to the discharge process as directed by the occupational therapist. The occupational therapist shall be responsible for the final evaluation session and discharge documentation.
		E. Before an occupational therapy assistant can assist in the practice of occupational therapy, he must file with the Board a signed, current statement of supervision of the licensed occupational therapist(s) who will supervise the occupational therapy assistant. Change in supervision shall require a new status report to be filed with the Board.
		F. In extenuating circumstances, when the occupational therapy assistant is without supervision, the occupational therapy assistant may carry out established programs for up to thirty calendar days while appropriate occupational therapy supervision is sought. It shall be the responsibility of the occupational therapy assistant to notify the Board of these circumstances.
		G. Failure to comply with the above will be considered unprofessional conduct and may result in punishment by the Board.
California	**Statute:** §2570.2	"Occupational therapy assistant" means an individual who is certified pursuant to the provisions of this chapter, who is in good standing as determined by the board, and based thereon, who is qualified to assist in the practice of occupational therapy under this chapter, and who works under the appropriate supervision of a licensed occupational therapist.
	§2570.3	j. "Supervision of an occupational therapy assistant" means that the responsible occupational therapist shall at all times be responsible for all occupational therapy services provided to the client. The occupational therapist who is responsible for appropriate supervision shall formulate and document in each client's record, with his or her signature, the goals and plan for that client, and shall make sure that the occupational therapy assistant assigned to that client functions under appropriate supervision. As part of the responsible occupational therapist's appropriate supervision, he or she shall conduct at least weekly review and inspection of all aspects of occupational therapy services by the occupational therapy assistant.
		1. The supervising occupational therapist has the continuing responsibility to follow the progress of each patient, provide direct care to the patient, and to assure that the occupational therapy assistant does not function autonomously.
		2. An occupational therapist shall not supervise more occupational therapy assistants, at any one time, than can be appropriately supervised in the opinion of the board. Two occupational therapy assistants shall be the maximum number of occupational therapy assistants supervised by an occupational therapist at any one time, but the board may permit the supervision of a greater number by an occupational therapist if, in the opinion of the board, there would be adequate supervision and the public's health and safety would be served. In no case shall the total number of occupational therapy assistants exceed twice the number of occupational therapists regularly employed by a facility at any one time.
	§2570.13	a. Consistent with this section, subdivisions (a), (b), and (c) of Section 2570.2, and accepted professional standards, the board shall adopt rules necessary to assure appropriate supervision of occupational therapy assistants and aides.
		b. A certified occupational therapy assistant may practice only under the supervision of an occupational therapist who is authorized to practice occupational therapy in this state.
		c. An aide providing delegated, client-related supportive services shall require continuous and direct supervision by an occupational therapist.
Colorado		No relevant statutes or regulations.
Connecticut	**Statute:** Chapter 376a, §20-74a	"Occupational therapy assistant" means a person licensed to practice occupational therapy as defined in this chapter and whose license is in good standing.
	Regulation:	No relevant regulations.
Delaware	**Statute:** Sec. 20-74a-3	"Occupational therapy assistant" shall mean a person licensed to assist in the practice of occupational therapy, under the supervision of an occupational therapist.
	Sec. 20-74a-8	"Supervision" shall mean the interactive process between the licensed occupational therapist and the occupational therapy assistant. It shall be more than a paper review or cosignature. The supervising occupational therapist is responsible for insuring the extent, kind and quality of the services rendered by the occupational therapy assistant.
	Regulation: 24 Del.C. §2007 (a) (1)	1.0 *Supervision/Consultation Requirements for Occupational Therapy Assistants*
		1.1 "Occupational therapy assistant" shall mean a person licensed to assist in the practice of occupational therapy under the supervision of an occupational therapist. "Under the supervision of an occupational therapist" means the interactive process between the licensed occupational therapist and the occupational therapy assistant. It shall be more than a paper review or co-signature. The supervising occupational therapist is responsible for insuring the extent, kind, and quality of the services rendered by the occupational therapy assistant. The phrase, "Under the supervision of an occupational therapist," as used in the definition of occupational therapist assistant includes, but is not limited to the following requirements:
		1.1.1 Communicating to the occupational therapy assistant the results of patient/client evaluation and discussing the goals and program plan for the patient/client;
		1.1.2 In accordance with supervision level and applicable health care, educational, professional and institutional regulations, reevaluating the patient/client, reviewing the documentation, modifying the program plan if necessary and co-signing the plan;
		1.1.3 Case management;

State	Citation	Legislative/Regulatory information

Delaware *(cont.)*

1.1.4 Determining program termination;

1.1.5 Providing information, instruction and assistance as needed;

1.1.6 Observing the occupational therapy assistant periodically; and

1.1.7 Preparing on a regular basis, but at least annually, a written appraisal of the occupational therapy assistant's performance and discussion of that appraisal with the assistant. The supervisor may assign to a competent occupational therapy assistant the administration of standardized tests, the performance of activities of daily living evaluations and other elements of patient/client evaluation and reevaluation that do not require the professional judgment and skill of an occupational therapist.

1.2 Supervision for Occupational Therapy Assistants is defined as follows:

1.2.1 Direct Supervision requires the supervising occupational therapist to be on the premises and immediately available to provide aid, direction, and instruction while treatment is performed in any setting including home care. Occupational therapy assistants with experience of less than one (1) full year are required to have direct supervision.

1.2.2 Routine Supervision requires direct contact at least every two (2) weeks at the site of work, with interim supervision occurring by other methods, such as telephonic or written communication.

1.2.3 General Supervision requires at least monthly direct contact, with supervision available as needed by other methods.

1.3 Minimum supervision requirements:

1.3.1 Occupational therapy assistants with experience of less than one (1) full year are required to have direct supervision. Occupational therapy assistants with experience greater than one (1) full year must be supervised under either direct, routine or general supervision based upon skill and experience in the field as determined by the supervising OT.

1.3.2 Supervising occupational therapists must have at least one (1) year clinical experience after they have received permanent licensure.

1.3.3 An occupational therapist may supervise up to three (3) occupational therapy assistants but never more than two (2) occupational therapy assistants who are under direct supervision at the same time.

1.3.4 Levels of supervision should be determined by the occupational therapist before the individuals enter into a supervisor/supervisee relationship. The chosen level of supervision should be reevaluated regularly for effectiveness.

1.3.5 The supervising occupational therapist, in collaboration with the occupational therapy assistant, shall maintain a written supervisory plan specifying the level of supervision and shall document the supervision of each occupational therapy assistant. Levels of supervision should be determined by the occupational therapist before the individuals enter into a supervisor/supervisee relationship. The chosen level of supervision should be reevaluated regularly for effectiveness. This plan shall be reviewed at least every six months or more frequently as demands of service changes.

1.3.6 A supervisor who is temporarily unable to provide supervision shall arrange for substitute supervision by an occupational therapist licensed by the Board with at least one (1) year of clinical experience, as defined above, to provide supervision as specified by Rule 1.0 of these rules and regulations.

District of Columbia

Statute: Title 3, §3-1201.02-9

B. An individual licensed as an occupational therapy assistant pursuant to this chapter may assist in the practice of occupational therapy under the supervision of or in consultation with a licensed occupational therapist.

Regulation: Chapter 636399

Direct supervision—Supervision in which an occupational therapist is available on the premises and within vocal communication either directly or by a communications device.

Occupational therapy assistant—A person licensed to practice as an occupational therapy assistant under the Act.

Florida

Statute: §468.203-6

"Occupational therapy assistant" means a person licensed to assist in the practice of occupational therapy, who works under the supervision of an occupational therapist, and whose license is in good standing.

§468.203-8

"Supervision" means responsible supervision and control, with the licensed occupational therapist providing both initial direction in developing a plan of treatment and periodic inspection of the actual implementation of the plan. Such plan of treatment shall not be altered by the supervised individual without prior consultation with, and the approval of, the supervising occupational therapist. The supervising occupational therapist need not always be physically present or on the premises when the assistant is performing services; however, except in cases of emergency, supervision shall require the availability of the supervising occupational therapist for consultation with and direction of the supervised individual.

Georgia

Statute: §43-28-3.7

"Occupational therapy assistant" means a person licensed to assist the occupational therapist in the practice of occupational therapy under the supervision of or with the consultation of the licensed occupational therapist and whose license is in good standing.

Regulation: §671-2-02

Supervision Defined
Supervision as used in the law shall mean personal involvement of the licensed occupational therapist in the supervisee's professional experience which includes evaluation of his or her performance. Further, supervision shall mean personal supervision with weekly verbal contact and consultation, monthly review of patient care documentation, and specific delineation of tasks and responsibilities by the licensed occupational therapist and shall include the responsibility for personally reviewing and interpreting the results of any habilitative or rehabilitative procedures conducted by the supervisee. It is the responsibility of the licensed occupational therapist to ensure that the supervisee does not perform duties for which he or she is not trained. C.O.T.A.s and limited permit holders must be supervised.

§671-2-.03

Direct Supervision Defined
Direct supervision as used in the Law shall mean daily on-site, close contact whereby the supervisor is able to respond quickly to the needs of the client or supervisee. It requires specific delineation of task and responsibilities by a licensed Occupational Therapist and shall include the responsibility of personally reviewing and interpreting the result of any habilitative or rehabilitative procedures conducted by the supervisee. It is the responsibility of the licensed occupational therapist to ensure that the supervisee does not perform duties for which he/she is not trained.

(Continued)

State	Citation	Legislative/Regulatory information
Guam	**Statute:** Chapter 12, Article 14, §121401	*Definitions* d. Occupational therapy assistant means a person licensed to assist in the practice of occupational therapy who works under the indirect supervision of an occupational therapist, or as otherwise determined by the supervising occupational therapist.
	§121410	*Scope of Practice: Occupational Therapy Assistant* The occupational therapy assistant works under the supervision of the occupational therapist. The amount, degree and pattern of supervision a practitioner requires varies depending on the employment setting, method of service provision, the practitioner's competence and the demands of service. The occupational therapist is responsible for the evaluation of the client or patient. The treatment plan may be developed by the occupational therapy assistant in collaboration with the occupational therapy assistant. Once the evaluation and treatment plans are established, the occupational therapy assistant may implement and modify various therapeutic interventions as permitted by the Board under the supervision of the occupational therapist.
	Regulation:	No relevant regulations.
Hawaii	**Statute:** §457G	"Direct supervision" means daily, direct contact at the site of work by a registered occupational therapist.
	Regulations:	No relevant regulations.
Idaho	**Statute:** 54-3702-7	"Occupational therapy assistant" means a person licensed to assist in the practice of occupational therapy, who works under the supervision of an occupational therapist.
	Regulation: 22.01.09.010.6	*Occupational Therapy Assistant* A person licensed to assist in the practice of Occupational Therapy, who works under the supervision of an Occupational Therapist. a. Occupational Therapy Assistant Supervision. The occupational therapist shall be responsible for the supervision of the occupational therapy assistant. The supervising and consulting therapist need not be physically present or on the premises at all times the occupational therapy assistant is performing the service. The mode and extent of the communication between the supervising or consulting occupational therapist and the occupational therapy assistant shall be determined by the competency of the assistant, the treatment setting and the diagnostic category of the client.
	22.01.09.010.0 8	*Graduate Occupational Therapy Assistant* A person who holds a certificate of graduation from an approved Occupational Therapy Assistant curriculum, has submitted a completed application for licensure by examination and is performing the duties of Occupational Therapy Assistant in association with and under the supervision of an Occupational Therapist and under the authority of a Limited Permit. a. Graduate OTA Supervision. Supervision of a "Graduate Occupational Therapy Assistant" shall require the supervising licensed occupational therapist to review and countersign all patient documentation.
Illinois	**Statute:** 225 ILCS 75/2	"Certified occupational therapy assistant" means a person licensed to assist in the practice of occupational therapy under the supervision of a registered occupational therapist, and to implement the occupational therapy treatment program as established by the registered occupational therapist. Such program may include training in activities of daily living, the use of therapeutic activity including task oriented activity to enhance functional performance, and guidance in the selection and use of adaptive equipment.

	Regulation:
	§1315.163
		Supervision of an Occupational Therapy Assistant
		a. A certified occupational therapy assistant shall practice only under the supervision of a registered occupational therapist. Supervision is a process in which 2 or more persons participate in a joint effort to establish, maintain and elevate a level of performance and shall include the following criteria:
		  1. To maintain high standards of practice based on professional principles, supervision shall connote the physical presence of the supervisors and the assistant at regularly scheduled supervision sessions.
		  2. Supervision shall be provided in varying patterns as determined by the demands of the areas of patient/client service and the competency of the individual assistant. Such supervision shall be structured according to the assistant's qualifications, position, level of preparation, depth of experience and the environment within which he/she functions.
		  3. The supervisors shall be responsible for the standard of work performed by the assistant and shall have knowledge of the patients/clients and the problems being discussed.
		  4. A minimum guideline of formal supervision is as follows:
		    A. The occupational therapy assistant who has less than one year of work experience or who is entering new practice environments or developing new skills shall receive a minimum of 5% on-site face-to-face supervision from a registered occupational therapist per month. On-site supervision consists of direct, face-to-face collaboration in which the supervisor must be on the premises. The remaining work hours must be supervised.
		    B. The occupational therapy assistant with more than one year of experience in his/her current practice shall have a minimum of 5% direct supervision from a registered occupational therapist per month. The 5% direct supervision shall consist of 2% direct, face-to-face collaboration. The remaining supervision shall be a combination of telephone or electronic communication or face-to-face consultation.
		b. Record Keeping. It is the responsibility of the occupational therapy assistant to maintain on file at the job site signed documentation reflecting supervision activities. This supervision documentation shall contain the following: date of supervision, means of communication, information discussed and the outcomes of the interaction. Both the supervising occupational therapist and the occupational therapy assistant must sign each entry.

The Occupational Therapy Assistant: Resources for Practice and Education

State	Citation	Legislative/Regulatory information
Indiana	**Statute:** IC 25-23.5-1-6	"Occupational therapy assistant" means a person who provides occupational therapy services under the supervision of an occupational therapist.
	Regulation: 844 IAC 10-5-5 844 IAC 10-5-6	*Supervision of Occupational Therapy Assistant* Under the supervision of an occupational therapist, an occupational therapy assistant may contribute to the evaluation process by performing objective tests. The occupational therapy assistant may also contribute to the development and implementation of the treatment plan and the monitoring and documentation of progress. The occupational therapy assistant may not independently develop the treatment plan and/or initiate treatment. Documentation. The occupational therapist shall countersign within seven (7) calendar days all documentation written by the occupational therapy assistant, which will become part of the patient's permanent record.
Iowa	**Statute:** §148B.2-4	"Occupational therapy assistant" means a person licensed under this chapter to assist in the practice of occupational therapy.

	§645-206.8 (272C)	*Supervision Requirements*
		1. Care rendered by unlicensed personnel shall not be documented or charged as occupational therapy unless direct in-sight supervision is provided by an OT or an OTA.
		2. A licensed OTA, OTA limited permit holder or OTA applicant working prior to licensure shall be supervised by a licensed occupational therapist. The supervisor shall:
		  a. Ensure that the OTA has a current occupational therapy license and that the OTA limited permit holder or applicant working prior to licensure has a copy of the letter from the board verifying that a current application is on file;
		  b. Provide direct on-site and in-sight supervision for a minimum of four hours per month;
		  c. Complete a patient evaluation prior to treatment by the licensed OTA, OTA limited permit holder, or the OTA applicant working prior to licensure. The time spent evaluating the patient by the supervising OT shall not be considered time spent supervising;
		  d. Complete a written treatment plan outlining which elements have been delegated to the licensed OTA, OTA limited permit holder, or OTA applicant working prior to licensure;
		  e. Monitor patient progress;
		  f. Complete an evaluation of the treatment plan and write a discharge plan; and
		  g. Assign to the licensed OTA, OTA limited permit holder, or OTA applicant only those duties and responsibilities for which the assistant, limited permit holder, or applicant has been specifically trained and is qualified to perform.
		3. Supervision of an OT limited permit holder or an OT applicant. An OT limited permit holder or an OT applicant working prior to licensure shall be supervised by a licensed OT. The supervisor shall:
		  a. Ensure that the OT limited permit holder or OT applicant working prior to licensure has a copy of the letter from the board verifying that a current application is on file;
		  b. Provide one-to-one supervision for a minimum of two hours per week.
		  The applicant who is practicing prior to licensure may perform the duties of the occupational therapist under the supervision of an Iowa-licensed occupational therapist, except for providing supervision to an occupational therapy assistant.
		4. Occupational therapist limited permit holders and occupational therapist applicants working prior to licensure may evaluate clients, plan treatment programs, and provide periodic reevaluations only under supervision of a licensed occupational therapist who shall bear full responsibility for care provided under the occupational therapist's supervision.

	§645-206.9 (147)	*Occupational Therapy Assistant Responsibilities* An occupational therapy assistant shall: 1. Follow the treatment plan written by the supervising occupational therapist outlining which elements have been delegated; 2. Maintain a plan of supervision; and 3. Maintain documentation of supervision on a daily basis that shall be available for review upon request of the board.
Kansas	**Statute:** Chapter 655402	e. "Occupational therapy assistant" means a person licensed to assist in the practice of occupational therapy under the supervision of an occupational therapist.
	Regulation: 100-54-9	*Occupational Therapy Assistants: Information to Board* Before an occupational therapist allows an occupational therapy assistant to work under the occupational therapist's direction, the occupational therapist shall inform the board of the following: a. The name of each occupational therapy assistant who intends to work under the direction of that occupational therapist; b. The occupational therapy assistant's place of employment; and c. The address of the employer.
Kentucky	**Statute:** §319A.010	4. "Occupational therapy assistant" means a person licensed to assist in the practice of occupational therapy under this chapter, who works under the supervision of an occupational therapist;

	Regulation: 201 KAR 28:130.1	*Supervision of Licensed Certified Occupational Therapy Assistants*
		1. COTA/Ls shall assist in the practice of occupational therapy only under the supervision of an OTR/L.
		2. Supervision by an OTR/L of a COTA/L shall consist of no less than three (3) direct contact hours per week of supervision for each occupational therapy assistant; the amount of supervision time shall be prorated for the part-time COTA/L. Supervision shall be an interactive process between the OTR/L and the COTA/L It shall be more than a paper review or cosignature.
		  a. Assessment/reassessment. Patient evaluation is the responsibility of the OTR/L. The COTA/L may contribute to the evaluation process by gathering data, administering structured tests, and reporting observations. The COTA/L may not evaluate independently or initiate treatment prior to the OTR/L's evaluation.
		  b. Treatment planning. The OTR/L shall take primary responsibility for the treatment planning. The COTA/L may contribute to the treatment planning as directed by the OTR/L.

(Continued)

State	Citation	Legislative/Regulatory information
Kentucky *(cont.)*		c. Intervention. The OTR/L shall be responsible for the outcome of the occupational therapy intervention and for assigning appropriate intervention components to the COTA/L.
		d. Discontinuation of intervention. The OTR/L shall be responsible for the outcome of occupational therapy. The COTA/L may contribute to the discontinuation of intervention as directed by the OTR/L.
		3. The OTR/L shall assign and the COTA/L shall accept only those duties and responsibilities for which the COTA/L has been specifically trained and which the COTA/L is qualified to perform.
		4. In extenuating circumstances, when the COTA/L is without supervision, the COTA/L may continue carrying out established programs for up to thirty (30) calendar days under agency supervision while appropriate occupational therapy supervision is sought. It shall be the responsibility of the COTA/L to notify the board of these circumstances and to submit, in writing, a plan for resolution of the situation.
Louisiana	**Statute:** LRS 37:3003	D. "Occupational therapy assistant" means a person who is certified as a certified occupational therapy assistant (COTA) by the American Occupational Therapy Association, Inc. (AOTA), and is licensed to assist in the practice of occupational therapy under the supervision of, and in activity programs with the consultation of, an occupational therapist licensed under this Act.
	Regulation: LAC 46 §1903	Occupational Therapy Assistant is a person who is certified as a certified occupational therapy assistant (COTA) by the American Occupational Therapy Association, Inc. (AOTA), and is licensed to assist in the practice of occupational therapy under the supervision of, and in activity programs with the consultation of, an occupational therapist licensed under this chapter.

	LAC 46 §4925	*Supervision of Occupational Therapy Assistant in Home Health Setting*
		A. An occupational therapy assistant may administer occupational therapy in the home health setting under the supervision of a licensed occupational therapist, without the necessity of the continuous physical presence of the supervision occupational therapist, provided that the following conditions and restrictions are strictly observed and complied with.
		  1. The occupational therapy assistant shall have had not less than two years experience in providing occupational therapy in a physical disability setting prior to assuming responsibility for the provision of occupational therapy in a home health environment.
		  2. Before the occupational therapy assistant undertakes to provide occupational therapy to or for a client in a home health setting, the licensed occupational therapist under whose supervision the occupational therapy assistant may provide services shall have conducted an assessment of the client and have established the goals and treatment plan for the client.
		  3. Each client in a home health setting to whom an occupational therapy assistant administers occupational therapy shall be visited jointly by the occupational therapy assistant and the supervision licensed occupational therapist not less than once every two weeks or every fifth treatment session.
		  4. All therapy administered by an occupational therapy assistant in a home health setting shall be promptly, accurately, and completely documented by the occupational therapy assistant and, within 72 hours of the completion of such documentation, countersigned by the supervision occupational therapist.
		B. The administration of occupational therapy in a home health setting by an occupational therapy assistant other than in accordance with the provisions of this section shall be deemed a violation of these rules, subjecting the occupational therapy assistant to suspension or revocation of licensure pursuant to § 4921.A.18.

Maine	**Statute:** §2272-5	*Certified Occupational Therapy Assistant* "Certified occupational therapy assistant" means an individual who has passed the certification examination of the National Board for Certification in Occupational Therapy for an occupational therapy assistant or who was certified as an occupational therapy assistant prior to June 1977 and who is licensed to practice occupational therapy under this chapter in the State under the supervision of an occupational therapist.
	§2272-14	*Supervision of COTA* "Supervision of COTA" means initial directions and periodic inspection of the service delivery and provision of relevant in-service training. The supervising licensed occupational therapist shall determine the frequency and nature of the supervision to be provided based on the clients' required level of care and the COTA's caseload, experience and competency.

	Regulation:
	02-477-5.1
		Role of the Occupational Therapy Assistant
		The occupational therapy assistant:
		  1. Is permitted to assist in the practice of occupational therapy only under the supervision of an occupational therapist;
		  2. Must exercise sound judgement and provide appropriate care in the performance of duties;
		  3. Must not initiate a treatment program until the client has been evaluated and treatment has been planned by the occupational therapist, and may not discharge the client from a treatment program without supervision from the occupational therapist;
		  4. Must not perform an evaluation, but is permitted to contribute to the evaluation process with the supervision of the occupational therapist;
		  5. Is permitted to participate in the screening process by collecting data, such as records, by general observation and/or by conducting a general interview, and communicate in writing or orally the information gathered to the occupational therapist;
		  6. Is permitted to track the need for reassessment, report changes in status that might warrant reassessment or referral, and administer the reassessment under the supervision of the occupational therapist; and
		  7. Must immediately discontinue any specific treatment procedure which appears harmful to the client and so notify the supervising occupational therapist.

	02-477-5.2	*Skill and Supervision Levels Applicable to Occupational Therapy Assistants and Temporary Occupational Therapists*
		Skill levels:
		  1. Entry Level—Working on initial skill development (0–1 year experience) or working in a new area of practice.
		  2. Intermediate level—Increased independence and mastery basic roles and functions. Demonstrates ability to respond to new situations based on previous experience (generally 1–5 years' experience).
		  3. Advanced level—Refinement of skills with the ability to understand complex issues and respond accordingly.

State	Citation	Legislative/Regulatory information

Maine
(*cont.*)

Supervision levels:

1. Direct Supervision—Daily, direct contact at the site of work with the supervisor physically present at all times within the facility when the supervisee renders care. This supervision may be recommended by the Board or chosen by the supervisor in specific circumstances.
2. Close Supervision—Daily, direct contact at the site of work. The occupational therapist provides direction in developing the plan of treatment and periodically inspects the actual implementation of the plan. This supervision is appropriate for the temporary and entry level occupational therapy assistants.
3. Routine Supervision—Requires direct contact at least every two weeks at the site of work, with interim supervision occurring by other methods, such as by telephone or written communication. This supervision is appropriate for a temporary occupational therapist or for an intermediate level occupational therapy assistant.
4. General Supervision—Initial direction and periodic review of the following: service delivery, update of treatment plans, and treatment outcomes. The supervisor need not at all times be present at the premises where the occupational therapy assistant is performing the professional services. However, not less than monthly direct contact must be provided, with supervision available as needed by other methods. This supervision is appropriate for an intermediate to advanced occupational therapy assistant.

02-477-5.3

Supervision of Occupational Therapy Assistants and Temporary Occupational Therapists

1. Supervision principles

   The occupational therapist has the ultimate responsibility for occupational therapy treatment outcomes. Supervision is a shared responsibility. The supervising occupational therapist has a legal and ethical responsibility to provide supervision, and the supervisee has a legal and ethical responsibility to obtain supervision. Supervision is required even when the supervisee is experienced and/or highly skilled in a particular area.

2. Supervision parameters

   The level of supervison required shall be determined by the skill level of the individual whose practice is being supervised.
   - Direct—Daily direct contact and supervisor present at all times within the facility when the supervisee renders care. Chosen in specific circumstances or by supervisor.
   - Close—Daily direct contact at the site of work, OT provides direction in developing the plan of Rx, and OT periodically inspects the actual implementation of the plan. Entry-level OTA or temporary OTA.
   - Routine—Direct contact at least once every two weeks at site of work and interim supervision by other methods, such as telephone or written communication. Temporary OT or Intermediate-level OTA.
   - General—Initial direction, periodic review and inspection of service delivery, update of treatment plans and treatment outcomes. Not less frequent that monthly direct contact Supervisor need not be present on the premises where OTA renders care for contact to qualify as "direct monthly." Intermediate-level OTA or Advanced-level OTA.

3. Supervision standards

   A. To maintain high standards of practice: "Supervision" connotes the physical presence of the supervisor and the supervisee at regularly scheduled one-to-one supervision sessions.

   B. Supervision is provided in varying patterns as determined by the demands of the areas of client service and the competency of the individual supervisee. Supervision is structured according to the supervisee's qualifications, position, level of preparation, depth of experience and the environment within which he/she functions.

   C. The supervisor is responsible for the standard of work performed by the supervisee and must have knowledge of the client and the problems being discussed.

   D. A minimum guideline of formal on-site face-to-face supervision is 2.5 percent (or 1 hour per 40 hours worked) of the supervisee's work hours. Supervision shall be provided a minimum of once a month. For the temporary and entry level occupational therapy assistant, a minimum guideline of formal on-site face-to-face supervision is 5 percent (or 2 hours per 40 hours worked).

4. Documentation of supervision

   A. Supervisor's Affidavit—The licensed occupational therapy assistant or temporary occupational therapy practitioner shall designate, on a Board approved form, the supervising occupational therapist and the facilities or settings within which the occupational therapy assistant or temporary occupational therapy practitioner shall work. A form shall be filed for each place of employment for the licensed occupational therapy assistant or temporary occupational therapy practitioner. In a setting where there is more than one occupational therapist delegating to a occupational therapy assistant or temporary occupational therapy practitioner, one occupational therapist shall be the designated supervisor who completes the affidavit form and ensures the requirements have been met.

   B. Change in Supervision—The Board shall be notified regarding changes in supervision for temporary licensees and occupational therapy assistants within fifteen (15) days of the change. Notification shall be in the form of a signed supervisor's affidavit form.

   C. Supervisor Absence—In extenuating circumstances, when the supervising occupational therapist is absent from the job, occupational therapy assistant or temporary occupational therapy practitioner is limited to carry out established programs under employer supervision for up to 15 calendar days while appropriate occupational therapy supervision is sought. The occupational therapist shall provide up-to-date treatment documentation prior to any planned absence.

   D. The documentation of supervision shall be available for inspection if requested by the Board. This supervision shall meet the minimum guidelines outlined in Section 2 of this chapter. This shall include dates, general content of supervision session, and time. This documentation shall be completed by the individual who has signed the affidavit to verify that the supervision has been provided.

(Continued)

Maryland

Statute:
§10-101

e. Direct supervision

"Direct supervision" means supervision provided on a face-to-face basis by a supervising therapist when delegated client-related tasks are performed.

h. Licensed occupational therapy assistant

"Licensed occupational therapy assistant" means, unless the context requires otherwise, an occupational therapy assistant who is licensed by the Board to practice limited occupational therapy.

m. Occupational therapy assistant

"Occupational therapy assistant" means an individual who practices limited occupational therapy.

q. On-site supervision

"On-site supervision" means supervision in which a supervisor is immediately available on a face-to-face basis when client procedures are performed or as otherwise necessary.

r. Periodic supervision

1. "Periodic supervision" means supervision by a licensed occupational therapist on a face-to-face basis, occurring the earlier of at least:
   i. Once every 10 therapy visits; or
   ii. Once every 30 calendar days.
2. "Periodic supervision" includes:
   i. Chart review; and
   ii. Meetings to discuss client treatment plans, client response, or observation of treatment.

s. Supervision

"Supervision" means aid, direction, and instruction provided by an occupational therapist to adequately ensure the safety and welfare of clients during the course of occupational therapy.

§10-310

Scope of Occupational Therapy Assistant License

a. In general—Subject to subsection (b) of this section, an occupational therapy assistant license authorizes the licensee to practice limited occupational therapy while the license is effective.

b. Supervision required—A licensed occupational therapy assistant may practice limited occupational therapy only under the supervision of an occupational therapist who is authorized to practice occupational therapy in this State.

Regulation:
10.46.01.5

"Direct supervision" means supervision provided on a face-to-face basis by a supervising therapist when delegated client-related tasks are performed.

10.46.01.10

"Occupational therapy assistant" means, unless the context requires otherwise, an occupational therapy assistant who is licensed by the Board to practice limited occupational therapy.

10.46.01.11

"On-site supervision" means supervision in which a supervisor is immediately available on a face-to-face basis when client procedures are performed or as otherwise necessary.

10.46.01.12

12. *Periodic Supervision*
   a. "Periodic supervision" means supervision by an occupational therapist on a face-to-face basis, for each client, occurring the earlier of at least:
      i. Once every 10 therapy visits; or
      ii. Once every 30 calendar days.
   b. "Periodic supervision" includes:
      i. Chart review; and
      ii. Meetings to discuss client treatment plans, client response, or observation of treatment.

10.46.01.15

"Supervision" means the giving, by an individual designated as supervisor, of aid, direction, and instruction that is adequate to ensure the safety and welfare of clients during the provision of occupational therapy.

10.46.01.03

Supervision Requirements

A. Occupational Therapist.

1. An occupational therapist shall exercise sound judgment and provide adequate care in the performance of duties as provided in nationally recognized standards of practice.
2. An occupational therapist shall document client information as follows:
   a. Evaluation;
   b. Treatment program;
   c. Progress reports;
   d. Reevaluations;
   e. Discharge summaries;
   f. Verbal orders; and
   g. Clarification orders.
3. An occupational therapist is permitted to supervise the following:
   a. Occupational therapy assistant;
   b. Aide;
   c. Temporary occupational therapy licensee;
   d. Temporary occupational therapy assistant licensee; and
   e. Occupational therapy student or occupational therapy assistant student.

State	Citation	Legislative/Regulatory information

Maryland
(cont.)

4. Unless otherwise stated, a supervisor need not be physically present on the premises at all times, but may be available by telephone or by other electronic communication means.

B. Occupational Therapy Assistant

1. Subject to the requirements of this section, an occupational therapy assistant may practice limited occupational therapy only under the periodic supervision of an occupational therapist.

2. In accordance with Regulation .05 of this chapter, an occupational therapy assistant shall document client information as follows:
   a. Progress reports;
   b. Reevaluations;
   c. Discharge summaries; and
   d. Verbal orders.

3. In addition to the other requirements specified by this section, supervision requires that before the initiation of the treatment program and before a planned discharge, the supervising occupational therapist shall provide, by verbal conversation, initial direction to the occupational therapy assistant.

4. In addition to the provisions of §B(2) of this regulation, the supervising occupational therapist working with the occupational therapy assistant shall determine the appropriate amount and type of supervision necessary in response to:
   a. Experience and competence of the occupational therapy assistant;
   b. Change in a client's status; and
   c. Complexity of the treatment program.

5. An occupational therapy assistant, under the direction of the occupational therapist, is permitted to be the primary supervisor for the following:
   a. Aide;
   b. Temporary occupational therapy assistant licensee;
   c. Fieldwork Level I occupational therapy student; and
   d. Fieldwork Level I and Level II occupational therapy assistant student.

6. The occupational therapy assistant may be utilized to facilitate occupational therapy student and occupational therapy assistant student learning experiences in both Level I and Level II fieldwork under the direction of the occupational therapist.

7. The supervising occupational therapist and the occupational therapy assistant shall be jointly responsible for maintaining documentation as set forth in Regulation .05 of this chapter.

Massachu-setts

Statute:
MGL 112 §23A

"Occupational therapy assistant," a person duly licensed in accordance with section twenty-three B and who assists in the practice of occupational therapy who works under the supervision of a duly licensed occupational therapist.

Regulation:
259 CMR 2.01

Direct Supervision

A process by which a supervisor is on the premises and available to provide supervision in the form of aid, direction, and instruction when procedures or activities are performed.

Supervision

A process by which two or more people participate in joint effort to establish, maintain and elevate a level of performance. Supervision requires the physical presence of all parties at regularly scheduled supervision sessions. Supervision is structured according to the supervisee's qualifications, position, level of preparation, depth of experience and the environment within which the supervisee functions.

259 CMR 3.02

Use of Supportive Personnel

1. Responsibility for Supportive Personnel. Primary responsibility for occupational therapy care rendered by supportive personnel rests with the supervising occupational therapist.

2. Supervision of Occupational Therapy Assistants and Occupational Therapy Aides. Adequate supervision of occupational therapy assistants and occupational therapy aides requires, at a minimum, that a supervising occupational therapist perform the following:
   a. Provide initial evaluation;
   b. Interpret available information concerning the individual under care;
   c. Develop plan of care, including long- and short-term goals;
   d. Identify and document precautions, special problems, contraindications, anticipated progress, and plans for re-evaluation;
   e. Select and delegate appropriate tasks in the plan of care;
   f. Designate or establish channels of written and oral communication;
   g. Assess competence of supportive personnel to perform assigned tasks;
   h. Direct and supervise supportive personnel in delegated tasks; and
   i. Re-evaluate, adjust plan of care when necessary, perform final evaluation and establish follow-up plan.

3. Supervision by Occupational Therapists.
   a. Occupational therapists must exercise their professional judgement when determining the number of supportive personnel they can safely and effectively supervise to ensure that quality care is provided at all times.
   b. Licensed occupational therapy personnel must provide adequate staff to patient ratio at all times to ensure the provision of safe, quality care.
   c. An occupational therapist must provide supervision to the following persons rendering occupational therapy services:
      1. occupational therapy assistants; and
      2. temporary license holders.
   d. An occupational therapist must provide direct supervision to the following persons rendering occupational therapy services:
      1. occupational therapist students;
      2. occupational therapy assistant students; and

(Continued)

State	Citation	Legislative/Regulatory information

Massachu-setts
(cont.)

3. occupational therapy aides, rehabilitation aides, or persons known by other similar titles.
4. Performance of Services by Occupational Therapy Assistants.
   a. Occupational therapy assistants may not initiate or alter a treatment program without prior evaluation by and approval of the supervising occupational therapist.
   b. Occupational therapy assistants may, with prior approval of the supervising occupational therapist, adjust a specific treatment procedure in accordance with changes in patient status.
   c. Occupational therapy assistants may not interpret data beyond the scope of their occupational therapy assistant education.
   d. Occupational therapy assistants may respond to inquiries regarding patient status to appropriate parties within the protocol established by the supervising occupational therapist.
   e. Occupational therapy assistants shall refer inquiries regarding patient prognosis to a supervising occupational therapist.
5. Supervision by Occupational Therapy Assistants.
   a. Occupational therapy assistants must exercise their professional judgement when determining the number of supportive personnel they can safely and effectively supervise to ensure that quality care is provided at all times.
   b. An occupational therapy assistant must provide supervision to occupational therapy assistants with temporary licenses.
   c. An occupational therapy assistant must provide direct supervision to the following persons providing occupational therapy services:
      1. occupational therapy assistant students; and
      2. occupational therapy aides, rehabilitation aides or persons known by other similar titles.

259 CMR 3.03

Co-signing of Documentation
1. a. The supervising occupational therapist must co-sign the documentation of occupational therapy students and those holding temporary licenses as occupational therapists.
   b. The supervising occupational therapist or occupational therapy assistant must co-sign the documentation of occupational therapy assistant students, those holding temporary licenses as occupational therapy assistants, and occupational therapy aides, rehabilitation aides, and persons known by other similar titles.
2. Occupational therapy assistants are not required to have their documentation co-signed.
3. Occupational therapy aides, rehabilitation aides, or persons known by other similar titles may not make entries in a patient's record regarding the patient's status. Information describing impairments (such as ROM, strength, cognition, balance, etc.) and function, as well as subjective information (such as patient responses to treatment, report of symptoms and psychological status), is considered to be patient status information which may not be entered in a patient record by aides or persons known by similar titles. Objective information, such as the number of repetitions performed, may be entered on log and flow sheet type documents by aides and such other persons. Entries of objective information by aides and such other persons must be co-signed by the supervising occupational therapist or occupational therapy assistant, in accordance with the requirements of 259 CMR.

Michigan | **Statute:** 333.18301

Definitions; Principles of Construction
a. "Certified occupational therapy assistant" means an individual registered as a certified occupational therapy assistant in accordance with this article.

Regulation:

No relevant regulations.

Minnesota | **Statute:** §148.6402-10

Direct Supervision
"Direct supervision" of an occupational therapy assistant using physical agent modalities means that the occupational therapist has evaluated the patient and determined a need for use of a particular physical agent modality in the occupational therapy treatment plan, has determined the appropriate physical agent modality application procedure, and is available for in-person intervention while treatment is provided.

§148.6402-16

Occupational Therapy Assistant
Except as provided in section 148.6410, subdivision 3, "occupational therapy assistant" means an individual who meets the qualifications for an occupational therapy assistant in sections 148.6401 to 148.6450 and is licensed by the commissioner. For purposes of section 148.6410, subdivision 3, occupational therapy assistant means the employment title of a natural person before June 17, 1996.

§148.6432

Supervision Of Occupational Therapy Assistants
1. Applicability.
   If the professional standards identified in section 148.6430 permit an occupational therapist to delegate an evaluation, reevaluation, or treatment procedure, the occupational therapist must provide supervision consistent with this section. Supervision of occupational therapy assistants using physical agent modalities is governed by section 148.6440, subdivision 6.
2. Evaluations.
   The occupational therapist shall determine the frequency of evaluations and reevaluations for each client. The occupational therapy assistant shall inform the occupational therapist of the need for more frequent reevaluation if indicated by the client's condition or response to treatment. Before delegating a portion of a client's evaluation pursuant to section 148.6430, the occupational therapist shall ensure the service competency of the occupational therapy assistant in performing the evaluation procedure and shall provide supervision consistent with the condition of the patient or client and the complexity of the evaluation procedure.
3. Treatment.
   a. The occupational therapist shall determine the frequency and manner of supervision of an occupational therapy assistant performing treatment procedures delegated pursuant to section 148.6430, based on the condition of the patient or client, the complexity of the treatment procedure, and the proficiencies of the occupational therapy assistant.
   b. Face-to-face collaboration between the occupational therapist and the occupational therapy assistant shall occur, at a minimum, every two weeks, during which time the occupational therapist is responsible for:

State	Citation	Legislative/Regulatory

Minnesota
(*cont.*)

1. planning and documenting an initial treatment plan and discharge from treatment;
2. reviewing treatment goals, therapy programs, and client progress;
3. supervising changes in the treatment plan;
4. conducting or observing treatment procedures for selected clients and documenting appropriateness of treatment procedures. Clients shall be selected based on the occupational therapy services provided to the client and the role of the occupational therapist and the occupational therapy assistant in those services; and
5. ensuring the service competency of the occupational therapy assistant in performing delegated treatment procedures.

    c. Face-to-face collaboration must occur more frequently than every two weeks if necessary to meet the requirements of paragraph (a) or (b).

    d. The occupational therapist shall document compliance with this subdivision in the client's file or chart.

4. Exception.
The supervision requirements of this section do not apply to an occupational therapy assistant who:
1. works in an activities program; and
2. does not perform occupational therapy services. The occupational therapy assistant must meet all other applicable requirements of sections 148.6401 to 148.6450.

Mississippi

Statute:
73-24-3

e. "Occupational therapy assistant" shall mean a person licensed to assist in the practice of occupational therapy under the supervision of or with the consultation of the licensed occupational therapist, and whose license is in good standing.

Regulation:
1.3

"Occupational Therapy Assistant" means a person licensed to assist in the practice of occupational therapy under the supervision of or with the consultation of a licensed occupational therapist, and whose license is in good standing.

"Direct supervision" means the daily, direct, on-site contact at all times of a licensed occupational therapist or occupational therapy assistant when an occupational therapy aide assists in the delivery of patient care.

10.1

An occupational therapy assistant (OTA), shall be defined as an individual who meets the qualifications and requirements as set forth in Section IV of these regulations, and has been issued a license by the Department. The roles and responsibilities of an OTA are

A. To practice only under the supervision of, or in consultation with, an occupational therapist licensed to practice in Mississippi.
B. To assist with but not perform total patient evaluations.
C. To perform treatment procedures as delegated by the occupational therapist.
D. To supervise other supportive personnel as charged by the occupational therapist.
E. To notify the occupational therapist of changes in the patient's status, including all untoward patient responses.
F. To discontinue immediately any treatment procedures which in their judgment appear to be harmful to the patient.
G. To refuse to carry out treatment procedures that they believe to be not in the best interest of the patient.

10.2

Supervision or Consultation
A. An occupational therapy assistant issued a limited permit (see section 4.5).
B. An occupational therapy assistant issued a regular license.
1. Supervision or consultation which means face to face meetings of supervisor and supervisee (OT and OTA) to review and evaluate treatment and progress at the work site, and regular interim communication between the supervisor and supervisee. A face-to-face meeting is held at least once every seventh treatment day or 21 calendar days, whichever comes first.
2. The supervising occupational therapist must be accessible by telecommunications to the occupational therapy assistant on a daily basis while the occupational therapy assistant is treating patients.
3. Regardless of the practice setting, the following requirements must be observed when the occupational therapist is supervising or consulting with the occupational therapy assistant:
    a. The initial visit for evaluation of the patient and establishment of a plan of care must be made by the supervising or consulting occupational therapist.
    b. A joint supervisory visit must be made by the supervising occupational therapist and the occupational therapy assistant with the patient present at the patient's residence or treatment setting once every 7 treatment days or every 21 days, whichever comes first.
    c. A supervisory visit should include
        1. A review of activities with appropriate revision or termination of the plan of care
        2. An assessment of utilization of outside resources (whenever applicable)
        3. Documentary evidence of such visit
        4. Discharge planning as indicated
    d. An occupational therapist may not supervise/consult with more than two (2) occupational therapy assistants except in school settings, or settings where maintenance or tertiary type services are provided, such as the regional treatment centers under the direction of the Department of Mental Health.

Missouri

Statute:
§324.050-8

"Occupational therapy assistant," a person who is licensed as an occupational therapy assistant by the division, in collaboration with the board. The function of an occupational therapy assistant is to assist an occupational therapist in the delivery of occupational therapy services in compliance with federal regulations and rules promulgated by the division, in collaboration with the Missouri board of occupational therapy.

§324.056.2

2. A licensed occupational therapy assistant shall be directly supervised by a licensed occupational therapist. The licensed occupational therapist shall have the responsibility of supervising the occupational therapy treatment program. No licensed occupational therapist shall have under his or her direct supervision more than four occupational therapy assistants.

(Continued)

State	Citation	Legislative/Regulatory information
Missouri (*cont.*)	**Regulation:** 4 CSR 205-4.010	

Supervision of Occupational Therapy Assistants and Occupational Therapy Assistant Limited Permit Holders

1. An occupational therapy assistant and/or occupational therapy assistant limited permit holder shall assist an occupational therapist in the delivery of occupational therapy services in compliance with all state and federal statutes, regulations, and rules.

2. The occupational therapy assistant or occupational therapy assistant limited permit holder may only perform services under the direct supervision of an occupational therapist.

    A. The manner of supervision shall depend on the treatment setting, patient/client caseload, and the competency of the occupational therapy assistant and/or occupational therapy assistant limited permit holder as determined by the supervising occupational therapist. At a minimum, supervision shall include consultation of the occupational therapy assistant and/or occupational therapy assistant limited permit holder with the supervising occupational therapist prior to the initiation of any patient's/client's treatment plan and modification of treatment plan.

    B. More frequent face-to-face supervision may be necessary as determined by the occupational therapist or occupational therapy assistant and/or occupational therapy assistant limited permit holder dependent on the level of expertise displayed by the occupational therapy assistant and/or occupational therapy assistant limited permit holder, the practice setting, and/or the complexity of the patient/client caseload.

    C. Supervision shall be an interactive process between the occupational therapist and occupational therapy assistant and/or occupational therapy assistant limited permit holder. It shall be more than peer review or co-signature. The interactive process shall include but is not limited to the patient/client assessment, reassessment, treatment plan, intervention, discontinuation of intervention, and/or treatment plan.

    D. The supervising occupational therapist or the supervisor's designee must be available for immediate consultation with the occupational therapy assistant and/or occupational therapy assistant limited permit holder. The supervisor need not be physically present or on the premises at all times.

3. The supervising occupational therapist has the overall responsibility for providing the necessary supervision to protect the health and welfare of the patient/client receiving treatment from an occupational therapy assistant and/or occupational therapy assistant limited permit holder. The supervising occupational therapist shall

    A. Be licensed by the board as an occupational therapist, this shall not include a limited permit holder;

    B. Have a minimum of one (1) year experience as a licensed occupational therapist;

    C. Not be under restriction or discipline from any licensing board or jurisdiction;

    D. Not have more than four (4) full-time equivalent (FTE) occupational therapy assistants under his/her supervision at one time;

    E. Be responsible for all referrals of the patient/client;

    F. Be responsible for completing the patient's evaluation/assessment. The occupational therapy assistant and/or occupational therapy assistant limited permit holder may contribute to the screening and/or evaluation process by gathering data, administering standardized tests and reporting observations. The occupational therapy assistant and/or occupational therapy assistant limited permit holder may not evaluate independently or initiate treatment before the supervising occupational therapist's evaluation/assessment;

    G. Be responsible for developing and modifying the patient's treatment plan. The treatment plan must include goals, interventions, frequency, and duration of treatment. The supervising occupational therapist shall be responsible for the outcome of the treatment plan and assigning of appropriate intervention plans to the occupational therapy assistant and/or occupational therapy assistant limited permit holder within the competency level of the occupational therapy assistant and/or occupational therapy assistant limited permit holder;

    H. Be responsible for preparing, implementing, and documenting the discharge plan. The occupational therapy assistant and/or occupational therapy assistant limited permit holder may contribute to the process; and

    I. Ensure that all patient/client documentation becomes a part of the permanent record.

4. The supervising occupational therapist has the overall responsibility for providing the necessary supervision to protect the health and welfare of the patient/client receiving treatment from an occupational therapy assistant and/or occupational therapy assistant limited permit holder. However, this does not absolve the occupational therapy assistant and/or occupational therapy assistant limited permit holder from his/her professional responsibilities. The occupational therapy assistant and/or occupational therapy assistant limited permit holder shall exercise sound judgement and provide adequate care in the performance of duties. The occupational therapy assistant and/or occupational therapy assistant limited permit holder shall

    A. Not initiate any patient/client treatment program or modification of said program until the supervising occupational therapist has evaluated, established a treatment plan and consulted with the occupational therapy assistant and/or occupational therapy assistant limited permit holder;

    B. Not perform an evaluation/assessment, but may contribute to the screening and/or evaluation process by gathering data, administering standardized tests and reporting observations;

    C. Not analyze or interpret evaluation data;

    D. Track the need for reassessment and report changes in status that might warrant reassessment or referral;

    E. Immediately suspend any treatment intervention that appears harmful to the patient/client and immediately notify the supervising occupational therapist; and

    F. Ensure that all patient/client documentation prepared by the occupational therapy assistant and/or occupational therapy assistant limited permit holder becomes a part of the permanent record.

5. The supervisor shall ensure that the occupational therapy assistant and/or occupational therapy assistant limited permit holder provides occupational therapy as defined in section 324.050, RSMo appropriate to and consistent with his/her education, training, and experience.

The Occupational Therapy Assistant: Resources for Practice and Education

Montana	**Statute:** 37-24-103-2	"Certified occupational therapy assistant" means a person licensed to assist in the practice of occupational therapy under this chapter, who works under the general supervision of an occupational therapist in accordance with the provisions of the Essentials for an Approved Educational Program for the Occupational Therapy Assistant, published by the American occupational therapy association and adopted by the board.
	Regulation: 8.35.415	*Supervision—General Statement* 1. The supervisor shall determine the degree of supervision to administer to the supervisee based on the supervisor's estimation of the supervisee's clinical experience, responsibilities, and competence at a minimum. 2. A fully-licensed occupational therapist shall not require supervision. 3. A certified occupational therapist assistant, in accordance with 37-24-103(2), MCA, shall work under the general supervision of a licensed occupational therapist. 4. Temporary practice permit holders under 37-1-305(2), MCA, shall work under the routine supervision of a certified occupational therapist assistant or a licensed occupational therapist. 5. Entry-level practitioners shall be defined as practitioners having less than six months' experience in the specific practice setting and may, on a case-by-case basis, require supervision as determined by the board. 6. Occupational therapy aides under 37-24-103(6), MCA, shall work under the direct supervision of a licensed occupational therapist or a certified occupational therapist assistant. Occupational therapy aides shall have no supervisory capacity.
	8.35.416	*Supervision—Methods* 1. Direct supervision shall require the supervisor to be physically present in the direct treatment area of the client-related activity being performed by the supervisee. Direct supervision requires face-to-face communication, direction, observation and evaluation on a daily basis. 2. Routine supervision requires direct contact at least daily at the site of work, with interim supervision occurring by other methods, such as telephonic, electronic or written communication. 3. General supervision requires face-to-face communication, direction, observation and evaluation by the supervisor of the supervisee's delivery of client services at least monthly at the site of client-related activity, with interim supervision occurring by other methods, such as telephonic, electronic or written communication.
Nebraska	**Statute:** 71-6103-11	Occupational therapy assistant means a person holding an active license as an occupational therapy assistant.
	Regulation: 114-002	Certified occupational therapy assistant means a person who is certified in accordance with guidelines established by the American Occupational Therapy Certification Board.
		Occupational therapy assistant means a person holding an active license as an occupational therapy assistant.
		Supervision means the process by which the quantity and quality of work of an Occupational Therapy Assistant is monitored. Supervision means the directing of the authorized activities of an Occupational Therapy Assistant by a licensed Occupational Therapist and must not be construed to require the physical presence of the supervisor when carrying out assigned duties.
	114-012	*Role Delineation for Occupational Therapy Assistant* A licensed Occupational Therapy Assistant may perform the following duties while under the supervision of a licensed Occupational Therapist or while consulting with a licensed Occupational Therapist:
	114-012.01	Explain overall Occupational Therapy services to client, family, or others who have legitimate interest in the case;
	114-012.02	Solicit referrals from appropriate sources or acknowledge referrals received before or after initial screening for the purpose of initiating Occupational Therapy services by: 1. Responding to a request for service by relaying information or formal referral to the licensed Occupational Therapist; and 2. Entering cases as appropriate to standards of facility, department and profession when authorized by supervising Occupational Therapist.

	114-012.03	Assess need for, nature of, and estimated time of treatment, determining the needed coordination with other persons involved and documenting the activities by:
		1. Screening client to determine client's need for Occupational Therapy services. This may occur before or after referral by:
		  a. Obtaining and reviewing written information about the client from medical records, school records, therapist records, etc.;
		  b. Interviewing client, family, or others with legitimate interest in the case using a structured guide to obtain general history and information about:
		    1. Family history, self-care abilities, academic history, vocational history, play history, and leisure interest and experiences; and
		  c. Organizing, summarizing, and recording data collected by OTA and reporting such data to licensed Occupational Therapist.
		2. Observing client while engaged in individual and/or group activity to collect general data and report on independent living/daily living skills, selected sensorimotor skills, cognitive skills, and psychosocial skills;
		3. Administering standardized and criterion referenced tests as directed by licensed Occupational Therapist to collect data on independent living/daily living skills and performance, sensorimotor developmental status, and cognitive skills and performance in the area of orientation;
		4. Summarizing, recording, and reporting own evaluation data to licensed Occupational Therapist;
		5. Assisting with the evaluation of the data collected; and
		6. Reporting evaluation data as determined by the licensed Occupational Therapist to other appropriate persons.

(Continued)

State	Citation	Legislative/Regulatory information

Nebraska
(*cont.*)
	114-012.04	Assist with the identification and documentation of achievable treatment goals to
		1. Develop, improve, and/or restore the performance of necessary functions; compensate for dysfunction, and/or minimize debilitation in the areas of:
		   a. Independent living/daily living skills and performance;
		   b. Sensorimotor skills and performance in gross and fine coordination, strength and endurance, range of motion, and tactile awareness;
		   c. Cognitive skills and performance; and
		   d. Psychosocial skills and performance.

	114-012.05	Assist in the identification and documentation of treatment methods by
		1. Selecting Occupational Therapy techniques, and media, and determining sequence of activities to attain goals in areas designated under 172 NAC 114-012.04 item 1 by:
		   a. Analyzing activities in reference to client's interests and abilities, major motor processes, complexity, steps involved, and extent to which it can be modified or adapted;
		   b. Adapting techniques/media to meet client need; and
		   c. Discussing Occupational Therapy treatment plan with client, family, others with legitimate interests and staff.

	114-012.06	Assist with implementation or modification of a treatment plan by the use of specific activities or methods which improve or restore performance of necessary functions; compensate for dysfunction; and/or minimize debilitation. The Occupational Therapy Assistant, under the direction of a licensed Occupational Therapist, shall
		1. Engage client in purposeful activity, in conjunction with therapeutic methods, to achieve goals identified in the treatment plan in the following areas:
		   a. Independent living/daily living skills which include physical, psychological, emotional, work, and play;
		   b. Sensorimotor components which include neuromuscular, tactile awareness, and postural balance;
		   c. Cognitive components which include orientation and conceptualization;
		   d. Therapeutic adaptation which includes orthotics, and assistive/adaptive equipment; and
		   e. Prevention which includes energy conservation, joint protection/body mechanics, positioning and coordination of daily living skills.
		2. Orient family and others about the activities being utilized in the treatment plan;
		3. Provide instruction to client, family, and others with a legitimate interest in how to implement the home program developed by the licensed Occupational Therapist; and
		4. Observe medical and safety precautions.

	114-012.07	Assist in determining the need to terminate Occupational Therapy services when the client has achieved the treatment plan goals and/or has achieved maximum benefit from the services. The following steps should be taken 1. Discuss need for treatment plan discontinuation with licensed Occupational Therapist; 2. Assist in preparing occupational therapy discharge plan by recommending adaptations to client's everyday environment; 3. Assist in identifying community resources; and 4. Assist in summarizing and documenting outcome of the Occupational Therapy treatment plan.
	114-012.08	Participate in planning, organizing, and delivery of Occupational Therapy services by 1. Planning daily schedule according to assigned workload; 2. Preparing and maintaining work setting, equipment, and supplies; 3. Ordering supplies and equipment according to established procedures; 4. Maintaining records according to Department procedure; 5. Ensuring safety and maintenance of program areas and equipment; and 6. Assisting with compiling and analyzing data of total Occupational Therapy service.
	114-013	*Requirements for Consulting With or Supervising an Occupational Therapy Assistant* An Occupational Therapy Assistant may assist in the practice of Occupational Therapy under the supervision of or in consultation with an Occupational Therapist.
	114-003.01	If an Occupational Therapist is supervising or consulting with an Occupational Therapy Assistant, s/he must meet the following standards: 1. Evaluate each patient prior to treatment by the Occupational Therapy Assistant; 2. Develop a treatment plan outlining which elements have been delegated to the Occupational Therapy Assistant; 3. Monitor patient's progress; 4. Approve any change in the Occupational Therapy treatment plan; 5. Ensure that the Occupational Therapy Assistant is assigned only to duties and responsibilities for which s/he has been specifically trained and is qualified to perform; 6. Review all documentation written by the Occupational Therapy Assistant; 7. Interpret the results of tests which are administered by the Occupational Therapy Assistant; and 8. Evaluate the treatment plan and determine termination of treatment.
	114-013.02	An Occupational Therapist supervising an Occupational Therapy Assistant must, in addition to the standards outlined in 172 NAC 114-003.01, provide the following: 1. A minimum of four hours per month of on-site supervision if an Occupational Therapy Assistant has more than one year satisfactory work experience as an Occupational Therapy Assistant; or 2. A minimum of eight hours per month of on-site supervision if an Occupational Therapy Assistant has less than one year satisfactory work experience as an Occupational Therapy Assistant.

The Occupational Therapy Assistant: Resources for Practice and Education

State	Citation	Legislative/Regulatory information
Nevada	**Statute:** NRS 640A.060	"Occupational therapy assistant" means a person who is licensed pursuant to this chapter to practice occupational therapy under the general supervision of an occupational therapist.

Regulation:
NAC 640A.250

Practice by Occupational Therapy Assistant

1. An occupational therapy assistant shall not practice occupational therapy without the general supervision of an occupational therapist. Immediate physical presence or constant presence on the premises where the occupational therapy assistant is practicing is not required of the supervising occupational therapist. To provide satisfactory general supervision, the occupational therapist shall:
    a. Give written approval for any initial plan of treatment or program of intervention if the direct care of the patient is being provided principally by the occupational therapy assistant.
    b. Give written approval for any subsequent changes to a plan of treatment or program of intervention if the direct care of the patient is being provided principally by the occupational therapy assistant.
    c. Provide a minimum of 4 hours per month of direct:
        1. Clinical observation and supervision; and
        2. Communication between the occupational therapy assistant and the supervising occupational therapist. The mode and frequency of that communication must be dependent upon the setting for the occupational therapy assistant's practice, the caseload of the occupational therapy assistant and the competency of the occupational therapy assistant as determined by the supervising occupational therapist.
    d. Maintain written records of the direct supervision required by paragraph (c).
2. The supervising occupational therapist and the occupational therapy assistant shall jointly ensure that each record regarding a patient treated by the occupational therapy assistant is signed, dated and reviewed by both the occupational therapy assistant and the supervising occupational therapist. In reviewing the record, the occupational therapist and the occupational therapy assistant shall verify, without limitation:
    a. The accuracy of the record; and
    b. That there is continuity in the services received by the patient pursuant to the plan of treatment or program of intervention.
3. A supervising occupational therapist shall not delegate responsibilities to an occupational therapy assistant which are beyond the scope of his training.
4. The provisions of this section do not prohibit an occupational therapy assistant from responding to acute changes in a patient's condition that warrant immediate assistance or treatment.

640A.260

Supervision and Employment of Occupational Therapy Assistant:
Verification; notice of termination

1. An occupational therapy assistant shall submit verification of his employment and supervision by a licensed occupational therapist to the board within 30 days after a change in his employment or supervision. The verification must be submitted on a form approved by the board.
2. An occupational therapist who is licensed by the board shall notify the board within 30 days after the termination of his supervision of an occupational therapy assistant.

640A.265

Delegation of Duties to Occupational Therapy Assistants and Unlicensed Persons; Limitations

1. An occupational therapist shall supervise any program of treatment which is delegated to an occupational therapy assistant.
2. Only an occupational therapist may:
    a. Interpret the record of a patient who is referred to the occupational therapist by a provider of health care;
    b. Interpret the evaluation of a patient and identify any problem of the patient;
    c. Develop a plan of care for a patient based upon the initial evaluation of the patient, which includes the goal of the treatment of the patient;
    d. Determine the appropriate portion of the program of treatment and evaluation to be delegated to an occupational therapy assistant;
    e. Delegate the treatment to be administered by the occupational therapy assistant;
    f. Instruct the occupational therapy assistant regarding:
        1. The specific program of treatment of a patient;
        2. Any precaution to be taken to protect a patient;
        3. Any special problem of a patient;
        4. Any procedure which should not be administered to a patient; and
        5. Any other information required to treat a patient;
    g. Review the program of treatment of a patient in a timely manner;
    h. Record the goal of treatment of a patient;
    i. Revise the plan of care when indicated;
    j. Supervise the dissemination of any written or oral reports; and
    k. Supervise the final evaluation and discharge summary and determine when treatment should be terminated unless treatment is terminated by a patient or a referring provider of health care.
3. A licensee shall not knowingly delegate to a person who is less qualified than the licensee any program of treatment which requires the skill, common knowledge and judgment of the licensee.
4. An occupational therapist shall not delegate the following duties to an occupational therapy assistant or to a person who is not licensed by the board:
    a. The interpretation of a test or measurement made on a patient; or
    b. The planning of an initial program of treatment and any subsequent program of treatment based on the results of a test performed on a patient.

(Continued)

State	Citation	Legislative/Regulatory information
New Hampshire	**Statute:** RSA §326-C:1	"Occupational therapy assistant" means a person currently licensed to assist in the practice of occupational therapy, under the supervision of an occupational therapist, in the state of New Hampshire.
	Regulation: Med 701.05	"Occupational therapy assistant" (COTA) means a person licensed to assist in the practice of occupational therapy as defined in RSA 326-C:1 IV.
	Med 703.01	*Supervision of COTA* a. Upon accepting responsibility for supervising a COTA, the OTR shall provide formal and informal supervision of the activities of the COTA. b. The supervising OTR shall approve the initial occupational therapy program and any subsequent changes in the program. c. The supervising OTR shall not be required to be physically present while the COTA is performing services within the program, but shall be available to review and approve follow-up treatment and treatment changes. d. The supervising OTR shall provide formal supervision to the COTA for a minimum of 10% of the COTAs work time. Formal supervision shall include, but not be limited to, direct observation of the COTAs performance on a regular basis.
	Med 703.03	*Acceptance of Supervisory Responsibility* a. Any COTA or temporary licensee who practices occupational therapy shall report the name and address of his or her supervisor to the board prior to beginning to practice. b. Any change in supervisor shall be reported to the board within 30 days of such change. c. The OTR who is accepting responsibility for supervision shall notify the board in writing of their willingness to accept that responsibility.
New Jersey	**Statute:** Title 45 45:9-37.53	"Occupational therapy assistant" means a person licensed pursuant to the provisions of this act to assist in the practice of occupational therapy under the supervision of or in collaboration with an occupational therapist on a regularly scheduled basis for the purpose of the planning, review or evaluation of occupational therapy services. "Supervision" means the responsible and direct involvement of a licensed occupational therapist with an occupational therapy assistant for the development of an occupational therapy treatment plan and the periodic review of the implementation of that plan. The form and extent of the supervision shall be determined by the council.
	Regulation:	No relevant regulations.
New Mexico	**Statute:** NM 2000, Chapter 61-12A-1	C. "Certified occupational therapy assistant" means a person having no less than an associate degree in occupational therapy who is certified by the American occupational therapy certification board and licensed in New Mexico to assist a registered occupational therapist in occupational therapy under the supervision of the registered occupational therapist;
	61-12A-5	*Supervision; Required; Defined* No occupational therapy shall be performed by any certified occupational therapy assistant, occupational therapy aide or technician, or by any person practicing on a provisional permit, unless such therapy is supervised by a registered occupational therapist. The board shall adopt regulations defining supervision, which definitions may include various categories such as "close supervision," "routine supervision," and "general supervision."
	Regulations: NMAC 16.15.3.7	*Definitions* A. "Supervision" means the typical oversight required for individuals at the various levels of role performance. Supervision is a shared responsibility. The supervising occupational therapist (OT) has a responsibility to provide supervision to occupational therapy assistants (OTAs), persons practicing on a provisional permit, and occupational therapy aides/technicians. The supervisee has a responsibility to obtain supervision. B. An "entry-level Occupational Therapy Assistant" (OTA) means a new graduate that has not passed the National Board for Certification Occupational Therapy Exam. C. "Entry-level Occupational Therapy Assistant" (OTA) means a new graduate with less than 960 hours of experience who has passed the National Board for Certification in Occupational Therapy (NBCOT) examination, or is new to an area of practice or new to a facility. 960 hours begins on the date of employment with full (non-provisional) licensure. An occupational therapy assistant (OTA) shall also be considered entry-level when moving to a new area of practice. In this case, the occupational therapy assistant (OTA) shall move to intermediate-level status after completing the facility's probationary period. An entry-level occupational therapy assistant (OTA) must demonstrate competency by meeting work performance evaluation criteria in a satisfactory manner. D. "Intermediate-level Occupational Therapy Assistant (OTA)" means an occupational therapy assistant (OTA) that has advanced to this level with up to three (3) years of experience, or a more experienced occupational therapy assistant (OTA) who has recently passed the probationary period in a new area of practice. An intermediate-level occupational therapy assistant (OTA) must demonstrate competency by meeting work performance evaluation criteria in a satisfactory manner. E. "Advanced-level Occupational Therapy Assistant (OTA)" means an occupational therapy assistant (OTA) with a minimum of three years experience in a particular area of practice. An advanced-level occupational therapy assistant (OTA) must demonstrate competency by meeting work performance evaluation criteria in a satisfactory manner. F. "Twenty percent (20%) face-to-face clinical observation" means a minimum of every fifth (5th) contact or 1 out of every 5 shall be direct observation of treatment. G. "Supervision contact" means any form of supervision that is of sufficient length of time to ethically provide guidance.
	16.15.3.8	*Supervision* A. Occupational therapy assistants (OTA) and persons practicing on a provisional permit shall file with the Board a signed current statement of supervision by the occupational therapist or occupational therapists (OT or OTs) who will be responsible for the supervision of the occupational therapy assistant or person practicing on a limited permit. The statement of supervision must be filed

State	Citation	Legislative/Regulatory information

New Mexico
(*cont.*)

with the Board within ten (10) work days of employment and a new statement of supervision must be filed with the Board within ten (10) work days of any change in employment or supervisor.

B. Supervision of persons pending certification as an occupational therapy assistant (OTA) shall consist of specific documentation as detailed in the "Supervision Log." The original of the "Supervision Log" should be kept by the supervisee with a copy kept by the employer and supervisor. A copy of the "Supervision Log" must be submitted to the Board prior to issuance of full licensure.

C. Supervision is an interactive process, more than a paper review or a co-signature, and requires direct in-person contact.

D. Supervision by the occupational therapist (OT) is related to the ability of the occupational therapy assistant (OTA) to safely and effectively provide those interventions delegated by an occupational therapist (OT).

E. An intermediate-level or advanced-level occupational therapy assistant (OTA) may supervise an entry-level occupational therapy assistant (OTA) when his/her job competencies have been assured by the supervising occupational therapist (OT).

F. The occupational therapist (OT) has ultimate overall responsibility for service performance by the occupational therapy assistant (OTA), and for the health and safety of each client in the provision of occupational therapy services.

G. Supervision of the occupational therapy assistant (OTA) shall consist of specific documentation as detailed in the "Supervision Log," Subsection D of 16.15.3.10 NMAC. The original of the "Supervision Log" should be kept by the supervisee with a copy kept by the employer and supervisor. A copy of the "Supervision Log" must be submitted to the Board with each renewal application. For periods of unemployment, a written statement of the time period of unemployment should be attached to the "Supervision Log" and submitted with the renewal form.

H. The Board or its designee has the authority to request a copy of the "Supervision Log" at any time, without prior notice to the supervising therapist or supervisee.

I. The occupational therapist (OT) and the occupational therapy assistant (OTA) shall provide direct supervision to all occupational therapy aides/technicians.

J. Persons practicing on a provisional permit pending certification as an occupational therapy assistant (OTA) or an occupational therapist (OT) are not eligible to supervise.
[06-14-97; 02-14-98; 16.15.3.8 NMAC -Rn & A, 16 NMAC 15.3.8, 06-29-00; A, 04-03-03]

16.15.3.9   *Four Levels of Supervision for OTAs Are Identified*

A. "Direct Supervision" means a minimum of daily direct contact at the site of work with the licensed supervisor physically present within the facility when the supervisee renders care and requires the supervisor to co-sign all documentation that is completed by the supervisee. In a work setting involving multiple sites of work and/or offices, supervision shall occur at one or more of the sites or offices, but not necessarily all sites or offices The occupational therapist (OT) or an intermediate-level or advanced-level occupational therapy assistant (OTA) shall provide direct supervision for persons practicing on a provisional permit pending certification as an occupational therapy assistant. The occupational therapist (OT) and the occupational therapy assistant (OTA) shall provide direct supervision to all occupational therapy aides/technicians.

B. "Close Supervision" means a minimum of daily communication by means of direct contact, telephone, fax, or e-mail. In a single work setting or when involving multiple sites, supervision shall occur at one or more of the sites or offices, but not necessarily at all sites or offices. At a minimum, twenty percent (20%) of close supervision contacts shall be face-to-face clinical observation. Required for entry-level occupational therapy assistants (OTA).

C. "Routine Supervision" means a minimum of direct contact at least every two (2) weeks at the site of work, with interim supervision occurring by other methods such as telephone, fax or e-mail. At a minimum, twenty percent (20%) of routine contacts shall be face-to-face clinical observation. Required for intermediate-level occupational therapy assistants (OTA).

D. "General Supervision" means a minimum of monthly direct contact, with supervision available as needed by other methods such as telephone, fax or e-mail. At a minimum, twenty percent (20%) of general contacts shall be face-to-face clinical observation. Required for advanced-level occupational therapy assistants (OTA).

16.15.3.11   *Task Delegation*

A. As pertains to the occupational therapy assistant (OTA): the occupational therapist (OT) shall evaluate each patient/client before direct care tasks are assigned to the occupational therapy assistant (OTA). The occupational therapist (OT) shall determine and assign only those tasks that can be safely and effectively done by an occupational therapy assistant (OTA). Direct care tasks may include, but are not limited to:
1. Completing data collection procedures such as record review, interviews, general observations, and behavioral checklists;
2. Administering standardized and criterion-referenced tests after service competency has been established;
3. Reporting changes in status that might warrant reassessment or referral;
4. Contributing to treatment plan as developed by the occupational therapist (OT);
5. Providing direct intervention by engaging patient/client in activities related to occupational performance areas;
6. Adjusting and modifying treatment plans subject to final approval by an occupational therapist (OT); and
7. Reporting the factors that warrant discontinuation of intervention orally and in writing.

B. The occupational therapist (OT) must sign the evaluation, the original treatment plan, any change of the treatment plan, and discharge of services.

C. Duties and functions which the occupational therapy assistant (OTA) shall not perform include, but are not limited to:
1. Interpreting referrals or prescriptions for occupational therapy service;
2. Interpreting and analyzing evaluation data;
3. Developing or planning treatment plans independently; and
4. Acting independently without supervision of an occupational therapist (OT);

D. In extenuating circumstances, when the occupational therapy assistant (OTA) is without supervision, the occupational therapy assistant (OTA) may continue carrying out established programs for no longer than thirty (30) calendar days under agency supervision

(Continued)

State	Citation	Legislative/Regulatory information

New Mexico
(*cont.*)

while appropriate occupational therapy supervision is sought. It is the responsibility of the Board to interpret what establishes "extenuating circumstances."

1. The agency and the supervisee must notify the Board office, in writing, of the name of the agency supervisor within twenty-four (24) hours of approval for extenuating circumstances. This notification may be by means of fax or e-mail.
2. The agency supervisor must sign the Supervision Log for each day of supervision.

E. As pertains to the occupational therapy aide/technician: the occupational therapist (OT) shall evaluate each patient/client before direct care tasks are assigned to the occupational therapy aide/technician. Only the occupational therapist (OT) shall determine, assign and modify those tasks that can be safely and effectively performed by the occupational therapy aide/technician.

1. The occupational therapist (OT) or occupational therapy assistant (OTA) shall not document services rendered by an aide or technician as occupational therapy services provided by a licensed practitioner.
2. The occupational therapist (OT) or occupational therapy assistant (OTA) shall supervise those delegated, established routine activities which are performed by the occupational therapy aide/technician.
3. The occupational therapist (OT) and the occupational therapy assistant (OTA) shall not assign or permit occupational therapy aides/technicians to:
   a. interpret referrals or prescriptions for occupational therapy services;
   b. interpret or analyze evaluation data;
   c. develop, plan, adjust, or modify treatment plans;
   d. act on behalf of the occupational therapist (OT) or the occupational therapy assistant (OTA) in any matter related to direct patient/client care which requires judgment or decision making;
   e. act independently without the supervision of an occupational therapist (OT) or an occupational therapy assistant (OTA);
   f. document services provided by an aide or technician as occupational therapy provided by a licensed practitioner; and
   g. represent themselves as an occupational therapist (OT) or occupational therapy assistant (OTA).

New York

Statute:

No relevant statutes .

Regulation:
Part 76, 76.6

Supervision of Occupational Therapy Assistant
The direct supervision required by section 7906(6) of the education law shall include meeting with and observing the occupational therapy assistant on a regular basis to review the implementation of treatment plans and to foster professional development.

North Carolina

Statute:
90-270.67

3. "Occupational therapist assistant" means an individual licensed in good standing to assist in the practice of occupational therapy under this Article, who performs activities commensurate with his education and training under the supervision of a licensed occupational therapist.

Regulation:
"Guide for Supervision of Occupational Therapy Personnel"

The North Carolina Board of Occupational Therapy has adopted as policy the "Guide for Supervision of Occupational Therapy Personnel," as approved by the AOTA Representative, July 1994.

Requirements Of The Licensed Supervising Occupational Therapist
An OT responsible for the supervision of an OTA must notify the Board office in writing within 10 days of any permanent change in that supervisory status. Should you cease supervising an OTA, you will be held responsible for that supervision until official notice is received at the Board office. Failure to notify the Board can subject the OT to disciplinary action. Notice must be in writing with the OT's signature. Telephone notices will not be accepted.

Requirements Of Licensed Occupational Therapist Assistants
OTAs are required to notify the Board office within 10 days of any permanent change in supervision. Should the OT cease supervision and another OT become your supervisor, the OTA and the supervising OT must both notify the Board office in writing of the changes. Failure to notify the Board can subject both the OT and OTA to disciplinary action. Notice must be in writing with signature. Telephone notices will not be accepted.

Supervision is an interactive process. The OTR/L and the OTA/L share responsibility for the supervision of the OTA/L who is providing occupational therapy services. The supervising OTR/L has a legal and ethical responsibility to provide supervision; the OTA/L has a legal and ethical responsibility to obtain supervision. OTA/Ls at all levels require supervision by an OTR/L. This supervision will vary based on the OTA/L's ability to safely and effectively provide intervention delegated by an OTR/L, the employment settings, characteristics of the population being served, the demands of service (i.e., facility standards, state laws and regulations, diagnoses served, techniques used), and primarily the service competency of the OTA/L.

Service competency is the ability to use the identified intervention in a safe and effective manner. It implies that two people can perform the same or equivalent procedures and obtain the same results. This assurance is necessary whenever an OTR/L delegates tasks to an OTA/L (AOTA, 1987). As an example of the employment settings and population characteristics, an OTA/L working with a person whose condition is rapidly changing will require more supervision because of the need for frequent evaluation, reevaluation, and treatment modifications.

Types of supervision occur along a continuum that are close, routine and general. Typically, entry-level OTA/Ls and OTA/Ls new to a particular practice setting will require close supervision; intermediate-level OTA/Ls routine supervision; and advanced-level OTA/Ls general supervision. These typical levels of supervision suggested must be modified based on the critical level of the patient.
- Close supervision requires daily, direct contact at the site of work.
- Routine supervision requires direct contact at least every 2 weeks at the site of work, with interim supervision occurring by other methods, such as telephone or written communication.
- General supervision requires at least monthly direct contact, with supervision available as needed by other methods (AOTA, 1993, p. 1088).

The Occupational Therapy Assistant: Resources for Practice and Education

State	Citation	Legislative/Regulatory information

North Carolina *(cont.)*

In situations where general supervision is indicated, records shall be maintained by both the OTR/L and OTA/L. These records must identify the frequency and type of supervision provided. Documentation may include minutes of staff meetings, performance appraisals, case reviews, and logs indicating the OTR/L's site review of the OTA/L's performance. The effectiveness of the supervision shall be regularly evaluated by both the OTA/L and OTR/L.

Supervision should reflect a review of all aspects of the OTA/L's practice. In any situation, the OTR/L is ultimately responsible for all delegated services. Co-signature on occupational therapy service documentation, often mandated by law or regulation, does not accurately satisfy supervision guidelines. However, many facilities and programs do require a co-signature for reimbursement purposes. Guidelines of external review and accrediting agencies are to be followed.

The supervision of an OTA/L by an OTR/L is an ongoing process that enhances the professional growth of both participants. Each is responsible for knowing and adhering to applicable policies, laws, and guidelines pertaining to OTA/L practice, and each contributes specific skills, resources, perspectives, and knowledge to ensure and enrich the provision of appropriate occupational therapy services.

Administrative supervision can be done by someone other than an OTR/L. Clinical supervision must be done by an OTR/L. If adequate clinical supervision is not available by the OTR/L, the OTA/L may not provide occupational therapy services. The guidelines are not intended to address the supervision needs of OTA/Ls practicing in nontraditional roles such as activity director or educator or in other positions in which they are not providing occupational therapy service.

North Dakota

Statute:
43-40-01

Definitions
3. "Occupational therapy assistant" means a person licensed to assist in the practice of occupational therapy, under this chapter, who works under the supervision of an occupational therapist.

Regulation:
§55.5-02-03-01

Supervision
The occupational therapist shall exercise appropriate supervision over persons who are authorized to practice only under the supervision of the licensed therapist. No occupational therapist may supervise more than three occupational therapy assistants at the same time providing that at least one of the occupational therapy assistants has five or more years of experience in occupational therapy.

1. Supervision is a collaborative process that requires both the licensed occupational therapist and the licensed occupational therapy assistant to share responsibility. Supervision is providing direction in the performance of specific, delineated tasks and responsibilities that are delivered by a licensed occupational therapy assistant and includes the responsibility of reviewing the results of any occupational therapy procedure conducted by the supervisee. Appropriate supervision will include consideration given to factors such as level of skill, the establishment of service competency, experience and work-setting demands, as well as the complexity and stability of the client population to be treated. Supervisors who take a leave of absence or vacation must make arrangements to have their supervisory responsibilities filled by another qualified supervisor.
2. The entry-level occupational therapy assistant who has practiced occupational therapy less than one thousand six hundred fifty hours shall receive onsite supervision from a licensed occupational therapist. Onsite supervision means daily, direct, face-to-face collaboration at least twenty-five percent of the workday and for the remaining seventy-five percent of the workday, the supervisor must be on the premises and readily available by methods such as telephone or electronic communication for face-to-face consultation.
3. The occupational therapy assistant, with greater than one thousand six hundred fifty hours but less than five years of work experience in occupational therapy, shall receive monthly, direct, face-to-face collaboration at the worksite by a licensed occupational therapist at least five percent of the total occupational therapy work as a practicing occupational therapy assistant with interim supervision occurring by other methods such as telephone or electronic communication.
4. The occupational therapy assistant with greater than five years of work experience in occupational therapy shall receive monthly, direct, face-to-face collaboration at the worksite by a licensed occupational therapist a minimum of two and one-half percent of the total supervision occurring by other methods such as telephone or electronic communication.
5. Licensed occupational therapy assistants, regardless of their years of experience, may require closer supervision by the licensed occupational therapist for interventions that are more complex or evaluative in nature and for areas in which service competencies have not been established.
6. Minimal supervision of the occupational therapist and occupational therapy assistant limited permitholder shall include initial and periodic inspection of written evaluation, written intervention plans, patient note, and periodic evaluation of client interaction. Such reviews and evaluations must be conducted in person by a licensed occupational therapist. A minimum of six hours of supervision per week is required. An occupational therapy assistant limited permitholder must have onsite supervision by a licensed occupational therapist.
7. Any documentation written by a limited permitholder for inclusion in the client's official record shall also be signed by the supervising licensed occupational therapist.
8. The supervising occupational therapist shall determine that limited permitholder and occupational therapy assistants hold current permits or licenses to practice or assist in the practice of occupational therapy prior to allowing the limited permitholder and occupational therapy assistants to engage in or assist in the practice of occupational therapy.

Ohio

Statute:
4755.01

Definitions
C. "Occupational therapy assistant" means a person licensed to apply the more standard occupational therapy techniques under the general supervision of an occupational therapist.

Regulation:
4755-7-01

Supervision
Supervision must ensure consumer protection.
A. The following provisions apply to supervision of limited permit holders and occupational therapy assistants:

(Continued)

State	Citation	Legislative / Regulatory information

Ohio
(cont.)

    1. A supervising occupational therapist shall adhere to the following criteria:
        a. Be licensed, and in good standing, by the occupational therapy section of the Ohio occupational therapy, physical therapy and athletic trainers board; and
        b. When maintaining a separate caseload, a 1.0 full-time equivalent (FTE) occupational therapist will supervise no more than four (4) FTE limited permit holders and/or occupational therapy assistants; and
        c. When performing client evaluations and supervision only, with no client treatment responsibilities, a 1.0 FTE occupational therapist will supervise no more than six (6) FTE limited permit holders and/or occupational therapy assistants; and
        d. A supervising occupational therapist with the status of less than 1.0 FTE shall supervise a proportionate number of occupational therapy assistants and limited permit holders.
    2. The supervising occupational therapist shall confirm that the limited permit holder and/or occupational therapy assistant hold current permits or licenses to practice occupational therapy, as provided in section 4755.07 of the Revised Code, prior to allowing the limited permit holder and/or occupational therapy assistant to engage in the practice of occupational therapy.
    3. Any documentation written by an occupational therapy assistant or a limited permit holder for inclusion in the client's official record shall be co-signed by the supervising occupational therapist.

B. Supervision of the limited permit holder, as defined in section 4755.07 of the Revised Code, does not require the supervising occupational therapist to be on-site, but the supervisor must be available for consultation with the limited permit holder at all times. The supervisor and limited permit holder must meet in person a minimum of once per week.
    1. The occupational therapist limited permit holder and the occupational therapy assistant limited permit holder must be supervised by an occupational therapist.
    2. Supervision requires an interactive process between the supervising occupational therapist and the limited permit holder. The interactive process must include, but is not limited to, review of the following: client assessment, reassessment, treatment plan, intervention and the discontinuation of intervention, and/or treatment plan. Co-signing client documentation alone does not meet the minimum level of supervision.
    3. The supervising occupational therapist shall consult with the limited permit holder before the limited permit holder's initiation of any client's treatment plan and/or modification of the treatment plan.
    4. It is the responsibility of the occupational therapy practitioner to establish evidence that the supervision as set forth in rule 4755-7-01 of the Administrative Code has occurred according to the established guidelines. This evidence may be included in the client records or exist as a separate document, such as a supervision log.

C. Supervision of the occupational therapy assistant, as defined in section 4755.01 (C) of the Revised Code, requires initial direction and periodic inspection of the service delivery and relevant in-service training. The supervising occupational therapist need not be on-site, but must be available for consultation with the occupational therapy assistant at all times.
    1. The supervising occupational therapist must provide supervision, a minimum of once per week, to all occupational therapy assistants who are in their first year of practice.

4755-7-03   2. The supervising occupational therapist must provide supervision, a minimum of once per month, to all occupational therapy assistants beyond their first year of practice.
    3. Supervision requires an interactive process between the supervising occupational therapist and the occupational therapy assistant. The interactive process must include, but is not limited to, review of the following: client assessment, reassessment, treatment plan, intervention and the discontinuation of intervention, and/or treatment plan. Co-signing client documentation alone does not meet the minimum level of supervision.
    4. It is the responsibility of the occupational therapy practitioner to establish evidence that the supervision as set forth in rule 4755-7-01 of the Administrative Code has occurred according to the established guidelines. This evidence may be included in the client records or exist as a separate document, such as a supervision log.

Treatments Performed by Occupational Therapy Assistants
The supervising occupational therapist shall determine the occupational therapy treatments that the occupational therapy assistant may perform. In making this determination, the supervising occupational therapist shall consider the following: the clinical complexity of the patient/client, competency of the occupational therapy assistant, the occupational assistant's level of training in the treatment technique, and whether continual reassessment of the patient/client's status is needed during treatment. This rule shall not preclude the occupational therapy assistant from responding to acute changes in the patient/client's condition that warrant immediate action. The occupational therapist shall assume professional responsibility for the following activities, which shall not be wholly delegated, regardless of the setting in which the services are provided:
A. Interpretation of referrals or prescriptions for occupational therapy services.
B. Interpretation and analysis for evaluation purposes.
    1. The occupational therapy assistant may contribute to the evaluation process by gathering data, administering standardized tests and reporting observations. The occupational therapy assistant may not evaluate independently or initiate treatment before the supervising occupational therapist has performed an evaluation/assessment.
C. Development, interpretation, implementation and modifications of the treatment plan and the discharge plan.
    1. The supervising occupational therapist shall be responsible for the development, interpretation, implementation and modification of the treatment plan and delegating the appropriate interventions to the occupational therapy assistant.
    2. The occupational therapy assistant may contribute to the preparation, implementation and documentation of the treatment and discharge summary.

State	Citation	Legislative / Regulatory information
Oklahoma	**Statute:** Title 59 O.S. §888.3	3. "Occupational therapy assistant" means a person licensed to provide occupational therapy treatment under the general supervision of a licensed occupational therapist;
	Regulation: 435.30-1-2	"Direct supervision" means personal supervision and specific delineation of tasks and responsibilities by an Oklahoma licensed occupational therapist and shall include the responsibility for personally reviewing and interpreting the results of any habilitative or rehabilitative procedures conducted by the supervisee. It is the responsibility of the Oklahoma licensed occupational therapist to be onsite during treatment to ensure that the supervisee does not perform duties for which he is not trained.
		"General supervision" means responsible supervision and control, with the Oklahoma licensed occupational therapist providing both initial direction in developing a plan of treatment and periodic inspection of the actual implementation of the plan. Such plan of treatment shall not be altered by the supervised individual without prior consultation with and approval of the supervising occupational therapist. The supervising occupational therapist need not always be physically present or on the premises when the assistant is performing services; however, except in cases of emergency, supervision shall require the availability of the supervising occupational therapist for consultation with and direction of the supervised individual.

	435.30-1-15	*Supervision of Students, New Graduates, Techs, and Aides*
		The Occupational Therapist is responsible and accountable for the overall use and actions of unlicensed personnel under his/her supervision and control.
		1. Students. Supervision of the student must occur by one of the following methods:
		  A. Direct, on-site supervision will be provided by the Oklahoma licensed Occupational Therapist for the Occupational Therapy student in models of healthcare or educational systems. Supervision of the Occupational Therapy Assistant student may be provided by an Oklahoma licensed Occupational Therapy Assistant working under supervision of an Oklahoma licensed Occupational Therapist.
		  B. In emerging occupational therapy models, areas of innovative community-based and social systems-based occupational therapy practice where there is no occupational therapy practitioner on-site, the occupational therapy practitioner must provide a minimum of six hours of weekly supervision. Supervision must include role modeling for the student, direct observation of client interaction, meeting with the student, review of student paperwork, and availability for communication and consultation. The supervisor must be readily available at all other times. It is understood that supervision begins with more direct supervision and gradually decreases to a minimum of six hours weekly as the student demonstrates competence. The supervisor must be cognizant of the individual student's needs and must use judgment in determining when an individual student may need more of the supervisor's time.
		2. New graduates. Direct on-site supervision will be provided by the Occupational Therapist for new Occupational Therapist and Occupational Therapist Assistant graduates practicing under a letter authorizing practice temporarily.
		3. Techs and aides. Direct on-site supervision will be provided by the Occupational Therapist or Occupational Therapy Assistant for aides/technicians providing patient care. Occupational Therapists and Occupational Therapy Assistants will delegate only those tasks that are of a routine nature and do not require interpretation or professional judgment. The occupational therapy practitioner must ensure the aide/technician has demonstrated competency in the delegated tasks.

	435:30-1-16	*Responsible Supervision* a. An occupational therapist will not sign the Form #5, Verification of Supervision, to be the direct clinical supervisor for more than a total of four occupational therapy assistants or applicants for licensure regardless of the type of professional licensure or level of training. b. It shall be the responsibility of the occupational therapist to monitor the number of persons under his/her direct clinical supervision. It shall be the responsibility of the occupational therapy assistant to inquire of the occupational therapist in regards to the number of persons being directly supervised. c. In unique cases, an occupational therapist may petition the Committee to receive permission to supervise additional occupational therapy assistants or applicants. d. If responsible supervision is not practiced, both the occupational therapist and occupational therapy assistant are in violation of this rule.
	435:30-1-17	*Role of Occupational Therapy Assistants in Evaluations* An Occupational therapy assistant's participation in evaluations is not independent. The occupational therapy assistant works in collaboration with and under the supervision of an occupational therapist. It is the occupational therapists responsibility to give appropriate supervision and the occupational therapy assistant's responsibility to seek appropriate supervision. The occupational therapy assistant may have a role in the evaluation process and in the administration of assessment tools and instruments under the supervision of an occupational therapist after competency has been established. It is the occupational therapist who initiates the evaluation process and delegates the appropriate assessment to be carried out by the occupational therapy assistant. The occupational therapy assistant may administer and score these assessments. The occupational therapist interprets the results with input from the occupational therapy assistant to establish a treatment or plan.

(Continued)

State	Citation	Legislative / Regulatory information

Oregon

Statute:
675.210

3. "Occupational therapy assistant" means a person licensed to assist in the practice of occupational therapy under the supervision of an occupational therapist.

Regulation:
339-010-0005

Definitions

1. "Supervision" is a process in which two or more people participate in a joint effort to promote, establish, maintain and/or evaluate a level of performance. The occupational therapist is responsible for the program outcomes and documentation to accomplish the goals and objectives. Levels of supervision:
   a. "Close supervision" requires daily, direct contact in person at the work site;
   b. "Routine supervision" requires the supervisor to have direct contact in person at least every two weeks at the work site with interim supervision occurring by other methods, such as telephone or written communication;
   c. "General supervision" requires the supervisor to have least monthly direct contact in person with the supervisee at the work site with supervision available as needed by other methods.

3. "Licensed occupational therapy practitioner," for purposes of these rules, means an individual who holds a current occupational therapist or occupational therapy assistant license.

339-010-0035

Statement of Supervision for Occupational Therapy Assistant

1. Any person who is licensed as an occupational therapy assistant may assist in the practice of occupational therapy only under the supervision of or with the consultation of a licensed occupational therapist.
2. Before an occupational therapy assistant assists in the practice of occupational therapy, he/she must file with the Board a signed, current statement of supervision of the licensed occupational therapist who will either supervise or consult with the occupational therapy assistant. The signature of the supervising occupational therapist must be notarized.
3. An occupational therapy assistant always requires at least general supervision.
4. The supervising occupational therapist shall provide closer supervision where professionally appropriate.
5. The supervisor, in collaboration with the supervisee, is responsible for setting and evaluating the standard of work performed.

Pennsylvania

Statute:
Act 140, §3

"Occupational therapy assistant." A person licensed to assist in the practice of occupational therapy, under the supervision of an occupational therapist.

Regulation:
Chapter 42, §42.22

Supervision of Occupational Therapy Assistants

a. Section 3 of the act (63 P. S. §1503) provides that licensed occupational therapy assistants may assist in the practice of occupational therapy only under the supervision of an occupational therapist. "Under the supervision of an occupational therapist" means that an occupational therapist currently licensed by the Board:
   1. Evaluates the patient/client.
   2. Prepares a written program plan.
   3. Assigns treatment duties based on that program plan to an occupational therapy assistant currently licensed by the Board who has been specifically trained to carry out those duties.
   4. Monitors the occupational therapy assistant's performance.
   5. Accepts professional responsibility for the occupational therapy assistant's performance.
b. Supervision includes the following:
   1. Communicating to the occupational therapy assistant the results of patient/client evaluation and discussing the goals and program plan for the patient/client.
   2. Periodically reevaluating the patient/client and, if necessary, modifying the program plan.
   3. Case management.
   4. Determining program termination.
   5. Providing information, instruction and assistance as needed.
   6. Observing the occupational therapy assistant periodically.
   7. Preparing on a regular basis, but at least annually, a written appraisal of the occupational therapy assistant's performance and discussing that appraisal with the assistant.
c. Notwithstanding subsections (a)(1) and (b)(2), the supervisor may assign to a competent occupational therapy assistant the administration of standardized tests, the performance of activities of daily living evaluations and other elements of patient/client evaluation and reevaluation that do not require the professional judgment and skill of an occupational therapist.
d. The supervisor shall have supervisory contact with the occupational therapy assistant at least 10% of the time worked by the assistant in direct patient care. "Supervisory contact" means face-to-face individual contact, telephone communication, contact through written reports or group conferences among a supervisor and two or more supervisees. Face-to-face individual contact shall occur onsite at least once a month and shall include observation of the assistant performing occupational therapy. The specific mode, frequency and duration of other types of supervisory contact depend on the treatment setting, the occupational therapy assistant's caseload, the condition of patients/clients being treated by the assistant and the experience and competence of the assistant as determined by the supervisor. The supervisor shall ensure, however, that supervisory contact within each calendar month includes a combination of face-to-face, telephone and written communication.
e. The supervisor shall maintain a supervisory plan and shall document the supervision of each occupational therapy assistant. Documentation shall include evidence of regular supervision and contact between the supervisor and the assistant.
f. A supervisor who is temporarily unable to provide supervision shall arrange for substitute supervision by an occupational therapist currently licensed by the Board. The substitute shall provide supervision that is as rigorous and thorough as that provided by the permanent supervisor.
g. Failure to comply with this section constitutes unprofessional conduct under section 16(a)(2) of the act (63 P. S. § 1516(a)(2)).

State	Citation	Legislative / Regulatory information
Puerto Rico	**Statute:** Chapter 51, §1031.3	"Certified assistant in occupational therapy" is the person who under supervision of an occupational therapist performs proper selected tasks or activities of occupational therapy"
	Regulation: L. Núm 137, §1.3 (translation)	The occupational therapy assistant is the person who assists or helps the occupational therapist in selected tasks or activities that require neither the ability, judgement nor extensive knowledge required of occupational therapists. The occupational therapy assistant's work is made under the immediate direction of the occupational therapist.
	L.Núm 89, Article 1 (translation)	*Definitions* Occupational therapy assistant is the person who under the supervision of an occupational therapist carrys out selected tasks or activities.
Rhode Island	**Statute:** Chapter 5-40.1, §5-40.1-3	10. "Occupational therapy assistant" means a person licensed to practice occupational therapy under the provisions of the Act and the rules and regulations herein. 12. "Supervision" means that a licensed occupational therapist or occupational therapy assistant shall at all times be responsible for supportive personnel and students.

	§5-40.1-21	*Supervision*
		a. A licensed occupational therapist exercises sound judgment and provides adequate care in the performance of duties. A licensed occupational therapist is permitted to supervise the following: occupational therapists, occupational therapy assistants, occupational therapy aides, care extenders, occupational therapy students, and volunteers.
		b. A licensed occupational therapy assistant exercises sound judgment and provides adequate care in the performance of duties. A licensed occupational therapy assistant is permitted to supervise the following: occupational therapy aides, care extenders, students, and volunteers.
		c. Subject to the requirements of this section, a licensed occupational therapy assistant may practice limited occupational therapy only under the supervision of a licensed occupational therapist. Supervision requires at a minimum that the supervising licensed occupational therapist meet in person with the licensed occupational therapy assistant to provide initial direction and periodic on-site supervision. The supervising licensed occupational therapist working with the licensed occupational therapy assistant determines the amount and type of supervision necessary in response to the experience and competence of the licensed occupational therapy assistant and the complexity of the treatment program. The supervisor and the licensed occupational therapy assistant are jointly responsible for maintaining records, including patient records, to document compliance with this regulation.
		d. A licensed occupational therapy assistant:
		  1. May not initiate a treatment program until the patient has been evaluated and the treatment planned by the licensed occupational therapist;
		  2. May not perform an evaluation, but may assist in the data gathering process and administer specific assessments where clinical competency has been demonstrated, under the direction of the licensed occupational therapist;
		  3. May not analyze or interpret evaluation data;
		  4. May participate in the screening process by collecting data and communicate the information gathered to the licensed occupational therapist;
		  5. Monitors the need for reassessment and report changes in status that might warrant reassessment or referral under the supervision of the licensed occupational therapist; and
		  6. Immediately discontinues any treatment procedure which appears harmful to the patient and immediately notifies the supervising occupational therapist.
		1. An occupational therapy aide is a worker trained on the job. A licensed occupational therapist or licensed occupational therapy assistant using occupational therapy aide personnel to assist with the provision of occupational therapy services must provide close supervision in order to protect the health and welfare of the consumer.
		2. The primary function of an occupational therapy aide functioning in an occupational therapy setting is to perform designated routine tasks related to the operation of an occupational therapy service. These tasks may include, but are not limited to, routine department maintenance, transporting patients/clients, preparing or setting up treatment equipment and work area, assisting patients/clients with their personal needs during treatment, assisting in the construction of adaptive equipment, and carrying out a predetermined segment or task in the patient's care.
		f. The licensed occupational therapist or occupational therapy assistant shall not delegate to an occupational therapy aide:
		  1. Performance of occupational therapy evaluation procedures;
		  2. Initiation, planning, adjustment, modification, or performance of occupational therapy procedures requiring the skills or judgment of a licensed occupational therapist or licensed occupational therapy assistant;
		  3. Making occupational therapy entries directly in patients' or clients' official records; and
		  4. Acting on behalf of the occupational therapist in any matter related to occupational therapy which requires decision making or professional judgment.

	Regulation: R5-40.1-OCC, §1.8	"Occupational therapy assistant" means a person licensed to practice occupational therapy under the provisions of the Act and the rules and regulations herein.
	§1.10	"Supervision" means that a licensed occupational therapist or occupational therapy assistant shall at all times be responsible for supportive personnel and students.
	§5.5.2	A licensed occupational therapy assistant shall exercise sound judgment and provide adequate care in the performance of duties.

(Continued)

State	Citation	Legislative / Regulatory information
Rhode Island (*cont.*)		a. A licensed occupational therapy assistant is permitted to supervise the following: – Occupational therapy aides; – Care extenders; – Students; and – Volunteers.
	§5.5.3	Subject to the requirements of this section, a licensed occupational therapy assistant may practice limited occupational therapy only under the supervision of a licensed occupational therapist.
	§5.5.4	Supervision requires, at a minimum, that the supervising licensed occupational therapist meet in person with the licensed occupational therapy assistant to provide initial direction and periodic on-site supervision.
	§5.5.5	The supervising licensed occupational therapist working with the licensed occupational therapy assistant shall determine the amount and type of supervision necessary in response to experience and competence of the licensed occupational therapy assistant and complexity of the treatment program.
	§5.5.6	The supervisor and the licensed occupational therapy assistant are jointly responsible for maintaining records, including patient records, to document compliance with these regulations.
	§5.5.7	A licensed occupational therapy assistant: a. may not initiate a treatment program until the patient has been evaluated and the treatment planned by the licensed occupational therapist; b. may not perform an evaluation, but may assist in the data-gathering process and administer specific assessments where clinical competence has been demonstrated, under the direction of the licensed occupational therapist; c. may not analyze or interpret evaluation data; d. may participate in the screening process by collecting data and shall communicate the information gathered to the licensed occupational therapist; e. shall monitor the need for reassessment and report changes in status that might warrant reassessment or referral under the supervision of the licensed occupational therapist; and f. shall immediately discontinue any treatment procedure which appears harmful to the patient and immediately notify the supervising occupational therapist.
South Carolina	**Statute:** Chapter 36, §40-36-20	4. "Direct supervision" means personal, daily supervision, and specific delineation of tasks and responsibilities by an occupational therapist and includes the responsibility for personally reviewing and interpreting the results of a supervisee on a daily basis. 9. "Occupational therapy assistant" means a person licensed to assist in the practice of occupational therapy under the supervision of an occupational therapist. 10. "On-site" means the same premises while direct client treatment is being performed. 12. "Supervision" means personal and direct involvement of an occupational therapist in a supervisee's professional experience which includes evaluation of the supervisee's performance with respect to each client treated by the supervisee.
	§40-36-300	*Responsibilities and Duties of Occupational Therapy Assistants and Aides; Restrictions* A. An occupational therapy assistant only shall assist in the practice of occupational therapy under the supervision of a licensed occupational therapist and shall: 1. only accept those duties and responsibilities for which the assistant has been specifically trained and is qualified to perform; 2. consult with the supervising occupational therapist every seven treatments or thirty days, whichever is first, for each client; 3. inform the occupational therapist of any changes in a client that may require reevaluation or change in treatment; 4. contribute to a client evaluation by gathering data, administering structured tests, and reporting observations but may not evaluate a client independently or initiate treatment before a licensed occupational therapist's evaluation. B. An occupational therapy aide may perform duties associated with nontreatment aspects of occupational therapy including, but not limited to, transporting clients, preparing treatment areas, attending to the personal needs of clients during treatment sessions, and clerical or housekeeping activities under the direct on-site supervision of a licensed occupational therapist or licensed occupational therapy assistant. When performing these duties, the occupational therapy aide must be clearly identified by using "O.T./Aide" or another designation approved by the board; C. An occupational therapy aide may not: 1. perform an activity or task which requires licensure under this chapter; 2. perform an activity or task which requires the exercise of the professional judgment of an occupational therapist; or 3. develop or model client treatment plans or discharge plans. D. An occupational therapy student may perform duties or functions commensurate with the student's training and experience under the direct on-site supervision of a licensed occupational therapist.
	Regulation:	No relevant regulations.
South Dakota	**Statute:** Title 36, 36-31-1	6. "Occupational therapy assistant," any person licensed to assist in the practice of occupational therapy, under the supervision of or with the consultation of a licensed occupational therapist and whose license is in good standing;
	Regulation: 20:64:01:01	2. "Direct supervision," the physical presence of an occupational therapist or occupational therapy assistant in the immediate room when redemptive tasks are being performed by an occupational therapy aide; 3. "Supervision," the physical presence of an occupational therapist on the premises where a patient is being cared for by an occupational therapy assistant.

The Occupational Therapy Assistant: Resources for Practice and Education

State	Citation	Legislative / Regulatory information

South Dakota *(cont.)* 20:64:03:02

Supervision of Occupational Therapy Assistant

An occupational therapy assistant with less than one year of experience in the assistant's present area of practice must receive a minimum of 10 hours of supervision from an occupational therapist for each 40 work hours or 25 percent of the total scheduled work hours. An occupational therapy assistant with more than one year of experience in the assistant's present area of practice must receive a minimum of 4 hours of supervision from an occupational therapist for each 40 work hours or 10 percent of the total scheduled work hours. The supervising occupational therapist shall evaluate each patient with input from the occupational therapy assistant as appropriate, prepare a written treatment plan outlining the tasks and responsibilities that may be performed by the occupational therapy assistant, monitor patient progress and reevaluate the treatment plan, and determine the termination of treatment. The frequency and manner of supervision is determined by the supervising licensed occupational therapist based on the condition of the patient or client, the proficiencies of the occupational therapy assistant, and the complexity of the therapy method. If the supervision agreement is terminated, the occupational therapy assistant must notify the board in writing within 15 days of such termination. In addition, the supervising occupational therapist must also notify the board in writing within 15 days if the supervision agreement is terminated.

Tennessee

Statute:
§63-13-103

4. "Certified occupational therapy assistant" (COTA) means an individual who has passed the entry level licensure examination of NBCOT for an occupational therapy assistant or who was licensed as an occupational therapy assistant prior to June 1977, and who is licensed to practice occupational therapy pursuant to this chapter under the supervision of an occupational therapist

10. "Occupational therapy assistant" means a person licensed to assist in the practice of occupational therapy under the supervision of an occupational therapist

12. "On-site supervision" means the supervising physical therapist or physical therapist assistant must:
   a. Be continuously on-site and present in the department or facility where assertive personnel are performing services;
   b. Be immediately available to assist the person being supervised in the services being performed; and
   c. Maintain continued involvement in appropriate aspects of each treatment session in which a component of treatment is delegated to assertive personnel.

§63-13-206

Supervision of a COTA and Temporary Licensees

a. Supervision of a "COTA" means initial directions and periodic inspection of the service delivery and provisions of relevant in-service training. The supervising licensed occupational therapist shall determine the frequency and nature of the supervision to be provided based on the client's or patient's required level of care and the COTA's caseload, experience and competency.

Regulation:
1150-2-.01

8. Certified Occupational Therapy Assistant (OTA)—Any person who has met the qualifications for certified occupational therapy assistant and holds a current, unsuspended or unnerved, certificate which has been lawfully issued by the committee. Such person assists and works under the supervision of a certified occupational therapist.

27. Supervision is defined as the following:
   a. Close: Daily direct contact at the site of treatment.
   b. Routine: Direct contact at least every two (2) weeks at the site of treatment, with interim supervision occurring by other methods such as telephone or written communication.
   c. General: At least monthly direct contact with supervision available as needed by other methods.
   d. Minimal: Provided only on a need basis, and may be less than monthly.
   e. Continuous: Within sight of the individual being supervised.

1150-2-.10

Supervision

The committee adopts, as if fully set out herein, and as it may from time to time be amended, the current "Guide for Supervision of Occupational Therapy Personnel in the Delivery of Occupational Therapy Services" issued by the American Occupational Therapy Association. Information to acquire a copy may be obtained by contacting either of the following:

American Occupational Therapy Association
4720 Montgomery Lane
Bethesda, MD 20824-1220
Telephone: (301) 652-2682
T.D.D.: (800) 377-8555
Fax: (301) 652-7711
Fax On Request: (800) 701-7735 (for a specific document)
Internet: www.aota.org

Tennessee Board of Occupational and Physical Therapy Examiners
Committee of Occupational Therapy
First Floor, Cordell Hull Building
425 Fifth Avenue North
Nashville, TN 37247-1010
Telephone: (615) 532-3202 ext. 25135
Telephone: (888) 310-4650 ext. 25135
Fax: (615) 532-5164
Internet: www.state.tn.us/health

1. Supervision of an Occupational Therapist on a limited permit shall include initial and periodic inspection of written evaluations, written treatment plans, patient notes and periodic evaluation of performance. The supervison must be conducted in person by a licensed occupational therapist and shall be as follows:

(Continued)

State	Citation	Legislative / Regulatory information

Tennessee
(*cont.*)

a. Routine supervision with direct contact every 2 weeks at the site of treatment, with interim supervision occurring by other methods such as the telephone, conferences, written communication, and e-mail.

b. Supervision must include observation of the individual treatment under a limited permit in order to assure service competency in carrying out evaluation, treatment planning and treatment implementation.

c. The frequency of the face-to-face collaboration between the person treating under a limited permit and the supervising therapist should exceed direct contact every 2 weeks if the condition of the patient/client, complexity of treatment, evaluation procedures, and proficiencies of the person practicing under the limited permit warrants it.

d. Appropriate records must be maintained to document compliance.

e. A co-signature by supervising Occupational Therapist is required on evaluations, treatment plans, and discharge summaries.

2. Supervision of an Occupational Therapy Assistant on a limited permit means initial directions and periodic inspection of the service delivery and provisions of relevant in-service training. The supervising licensed occupational therapist shall determine the frequency and nature of the supervision to be provided based on the client's or patient's required level of care and the OTA's caseload, experience and competency. Supervision of an Occupational Therapy Assistant on a limited permit shall include initial and periodic inspection of patient notes and periodic evaluation of performance. The supervision must be conducted in person by a licensed occupational therapist and shall be as follows:

a. The Occupational Therapist shall be responsible for the evaluation of the patient and development of the patient/client treatment plan. The Occupational Therapy Assistant on a limited permit may contribute information from observations and standardized test procedures to the evaluation and the treatment plans.

b. The Occupational Therapy Assistant can implement and coordinate intervention plan under supervision of a licensed Occupational Therapist.

c. The Occupational Therapy Assistant can provide direct services that follow a documented routine and accepted procedure under the supervision of the licensed Occupational Therapist.

d. The Occupational Therapy Assistant can adapt activities, media, environment according to needs of patient/client under supervision of the licensed Occupational Therapist.

e. Documentation provided by the Occupational Therapy Assistant while on a limited permit must be co-signed by a licensed Occupational Therapist.

4. Supervision of an Occupational Therapy Assistant with permanent licensure means initial directions and periodic inspection of the service delivery and provisions of relevant in-service training. The supervising licensed occupational therapist shall determine the frequency and nature of the supervision to be provided based on the client's or patient's required level of care and the OTA's caseload, experience and competency. Supervision of an Occupational Therapy Assistant with permanent licensure shall be as follows:

a. The frequency of the face-to-face collaboration between the Occupational Therapy Assistant and the supervising Occupational Therapist should exceed direct contact of once a month if the condition of the patient/client, complexity of treatment, evaluation procedures, and proficiencies of the person practicing warrants it.

b. The Occupational Therapist shall be responsible for the evaluation of the patient and the development of the patient/client treatment plan. The Occupational Therapy Assistant may contribute information from observations and standardized test procedures to the evaluation and the treatment plans.

c. The Occupational Therapy Assistant can implement and coordinate intervention plan under the supervision of the licensed Occupational Therapist.

d. The Occupational Therapy Assistant can provide direct services that follow a documented routine and accepted procedure under the supervision of the Occupational Therapist.

e. The Occupational Therapy Assistant can adapt activities, media, environment according to the needs to the patient/client, under the supervision of the licensed Occupational Therapist.

f. Appropriate records must be maintained to document compliance.

4. Supervision of an Occupational Therapy Aide/Tech shall be as follows:

a. There shall be close supervision with daily, direct contact at site of treatment, which demands physical presence of a licensed Occupational Therapist or Occupational Therapy Assistant, whenever the Aide/Tech assists in the practice of Occupational Therapy.

b. There shall be personal instruction, observation and evaluation by the licensed Occupational Therapist or licensed Occupational Therapy Assistant.

c. There shall be specific delineation of tasks and responsibilities by the licensed Occupational Therapist or licensed Occupational Therapy Assistant who is responsible for reviewing and interpreting the results of care. The licensed Occupational Therapist or licensed Occupational Therapy Assistant must ensure that the Aide/Tech does not perform duties for which he is not trained.

1. A licensed occupational therapy practitioner may delegate to unlicensed personnel, including but not limited to Aides/Techs, specific routine tasks associated with nontreatment aspects of occupational therapy services which are neither evaluative, assessive, task selective, or recommending in nature, nor which require decision-making or making occupational therapy entries in official patent records, if the following conditions are met:

i. The occupational therapy practitioner accepts professional responsibility for the performance of that duty by the personnel to whom it is delegated. In the case of duties delegated by a OTA, both the OTA and the OT who supervises the technician will be responsible; and

ii. The unlicensed personnel do not perform any duties which require licensure under this act; and

iii. The occupational therapy practitioner ensures that the unlicensed personnel have been appropriately trained for the performance of the tasks.

2. Tasks which may be delegated may include

i. Transporting of patients;

The Occupational Therapy Assistant: Resources for Practice and Education

State	Citation	Legislative / Regulatory information

Tennessee *(cont.)*

    ii. Preparing or setting up a work area or equipment;

    iii. Routine department maintenance or housekeeping activities;

    iv. Taking care of patients' personal needs during treatments; and

    v. Clerical, secretarial or administrative duties.

    d. Appropriate records must be maintained to document compliance. The licensed Occupational Therapist or licensed Occupational Therapy Assistant must countersign all Aide/Tech documentation.

    e. Intensity of supervision is determined by nature of task to be performed, the needs of the consumer, and the capability of the Aide/Tech.

5. Supervision parameters

    a. Supervision is a collaborative process that requires both the licensed occupational therapist and the licensed occupational therapy assistant to share responsibility. Appropriate supervision will include consideration given to factors such as level of skill, the establishment of service competency (the ability to use the identified intervention in a safe and effective manner), experience and work setting demands, as well as the complexity and stability of the client population to be treated.

    b. Supervision is an interactive process that requires both the licensed occupational therapist and the licensed occupational therapy assistant or other supervisee to share responsibility for communication between the supervisor and the supervisee. The licensed occupational therapist should provide the supervision and the supervisee should seek it. An outcome of appropriate supervision is to enhance and promote quality services and the professional development of the individuals involved.

    c. Supervision of occupational therapy services provided by a licensed occupational therapy assistant is recommended as follows:

        1. Entry level occupational therapy assistants are persons working on initial skill development (less than 1 year of work experience) or who are entering new practice environments or developing new skills (one or more years. of experience) and should require close supervision.

        2. Intermediate level occupational therapy assistants are persons working on increased skill development, mastery of basic role functions (minimum one–three years of experience or dependent on practice environment or previous experience) and should require routine supervision.

        3. Advanced level occupational therapy assistants are persons refining specialized skills (more than 3 years work experience, or the ability to understand complex issues affecting role functions) and should require general supervision.

        4. Licensed occupational therapy assistants, regardless of their years of experience, may require closer supervision by the licensed occupational therapist for interventions that are more complex or evaluative in nature and for areas in which service competencies have not been established.

        5. Certain occupational therapy assistants may only require minimal supervision when performing non-clinical administrative responsibilities.

Texas

Statute: 454.002

6. "Occupational therapy assistant" means a person licensed by the board as an occupational therapy assistant who assists in the practice of occupational therapy under the general supervision of an occupational therapist.

Regulation: §362.1

6. Certified Occupational Therapy Assistant (COTA)—An alternate term for a Licensed Occupational Therapy Assistant. An individual who uses this term must hold a regular or provisional license to practice or represent self as an occupational therapy assistant in Texas and must practice under the general supervision of an OTR or LOT. An individual who uses this term is responsible for ensuring that he or she is otherwise qualified to use it.

27. Licensed Occupational Therapy Assistant (LOTA)—A person who holds a valid regular or provisional license to practice or represent self as an occupational therapy assistant in Texas and who is required to practice under the general supervision of an OTR or LOT.

36. Occupational Therapy Assistant (OTA)—A person who holds a Temporary License to practice as an occupational therapy assistant in the state of Texas, who is waiting to receive results of taking the first available Examination, and who is required to be under continuing supervision of an OTR or LOT.

§373.2

Supervision of a Temporary Licensee

    a. Supervision of an occupational therapist with a temporary license includes:

        1. frequent communication between the supervising occupational therapist and the temporary licensee by telephone, written report or conference, including the review of progress of patients/clients assigned, plus

        2. encounters twice a month where the OTR or LOT directly observes the temporary licensee providing services to one or more patients/clients with face-to-face, real time interaction.

    b. Supervision of an occupational therapy assistant with a temporary license includes;

        1. sixteen hours of supervision a month of which at least twelve hours are through telephone, written report or conference, including the review of progress of patients/clients assigned; plus

        2. four or more hours of supervision a month which are face-to-face, real time supervision with the temporary licensee providing services to one or more patients/clients.

    c. Temporary licensees may not supervise anyone.

    d. All documentation completed by an individual holding a temporary license which becomes part of the patient's/client's permanent file, must be approved and co-signed by the supervising occupational therapist.

    e. A temporary licensee works under the supervision of an regular licensed occupational therapist, whose name and license number are on file on the board's "Supervision of a Temporary Licensee" form.

    f. A temporary licensee does not become a regular licensee with those privileges until the regular license is in hand.

(Continued)

State	Citation	Legislative / Regulatory information

Texas (*cont.*)	§373.3	*Supervision of a Licensed Occupational Therapy Assistant*
		a. Supervision per month of eight hours includes:
		  1. A minimum of six hours a month of frequent communication between the supervising OTR(s) or LOT(s) and the COTA or LOTA by telephone, written report, email, conference etc., including review of progress of patient's/client's assigned.
		  2. A minimum of two hours of supervision a month of face-to-face, real time interaction with the OTR(s) or LOT(s) observing the COTA or LOTA providing services with patients/clients.
		b. Part-time licensees may pro-rate these hours, but shall document no less than four hours of supervision per month, one hour of which includes face-to-face, real time interaction by the OTR(s) and LOT(s) observing the COTA or LOTA providing services with patients/clients.
		c. COTAs or LOTAs with more than one employer must have a supervisor at each job whose name is on file with the board.

Utah	**Statute:** 58-42a-102	3. "Certified occupational therapy assistant" or "COTA" means a person certified as a certified occupational therapy assistant by the American Occupational Therapy Certification board. 8. "Occupational therapy assistant" or "OTA" means a person licensed in the state to practice occupational therapy under the supervision of an occupational therapist as set forth in Section 58-42a-306.
	58-42a-305	Limitation upon occupational therapy services provided by an occupational therapist assistant. 1. An occupational therapist assistant shall perform occupational therapy services under the supervision of an occupational therapist as set forth in Section 58-42a-306. 2. a. An occupational therapist assistant may not write an individual treatment plan or approve or cosign modifications to a treatment plan. b. An occupational therapist assistant may contribute to and maintain a treatment plan.
	58-42a-306	*Supervision Requirements* The supervising occupational therapist shall perform the following functions: 1. Write or contribute to an individual treatment plan; 2. Approve and cosign on all modifications to the treatment plan; 3. Perform an assessment of the patient before referring the patient to a supervised occupational therapist assistant for treatment; 4. Meet face-to-face with the supervised occupational therapist assistant as often as necessary but at least once every two weeks, to adequately provide consultation, advice, training, and direction; 5. Meet with each patient who has been referred to a supervised occupational therapist assistant at least once each month, unless otherwise approved by the division in collaboration with the board, to further assess the patient, evaluate the treatment, and modify the individual's treatment plan; 6. Limit supervision to not more than two occupational therapist assistants unless otherwise approved by the division in collaboration with the board; and 7. Remain responsible for patient treatment provided by the occupational therapist assistant.

	Regulation:
	R156-42a-102
		1. "General supervision" as used in Section 58-42a-304 and Subsection R156-42a-302b(2) means the supervising occupational therapist is:
		  a. present in the area where the person supervised is performing services; and
		  b. immediately available to assist the person being supervised in the services being performed.

Vermont	**Statute:** Title 26, §3351	2. "Occupational therapy assistant" means a person who is licensed to assist in the practice of occupational therapy under the supervision of an occupational therapist.

	Regulation:
	§3.7
		Supervision Standards
		a. As used in this rule:
		Supervision means the responsible periodic review and inspection of all aspects of occupational therapy services by the appropriate licensed occupational therapist.
		Close supervision means daily, direct, face-to-face contact at the site of work and applies only to occupational therapists with initial skill development proficiencies or occupational therapy assistants, as appropriate for the delivery of occupational therapy services.
		Routine supervision means direct face-to-face contact at least every two weeks at the site of the work, with interim supervision occurring by other methods, such as telephonic, electronic, or written communication and applies only to occupational therapy assistants General supervision means at least monthly direct face-to-face contact, with interim supervision available as needed by other methods, and applies only to occupational therapists with increased skill development and mastery of basic role functions or occupational therapy assistants, as appropriate, for the delivery of occupational therapy services.
		b. Supervision is a collaborative process that requires both the licensed occupational therapist and the licensed occupational therapy assistant to share responsibility. Appropriate supervision will include consideration given to such factors as level of skill, the establishment of service competency (the ability to use the identified intervention in a safe and effective manner), experience and work setting demands, as well as the complexity and stability of the client population to be treated.
		c. The supervision of the occupational therapy assistant is a process that is aimed at ensuring the safe and effective delivery of occupational therapy services and fosters professional competence and development.
		d. For effective supervision to occur that will ensure safety and effectiveness of service delivery and that will support the occupational therapy assistant's professional growth, a variety of types and methods of supervision should be used by the occupational therapist. Examples of methods or types of supervision include observation, co-treatment, dialogue/discussion, and teaching/instruction.
		e. The occupational therapist develops a plan for supervision that includes input from the OTA in regard to the following:
		  1. the frequency of supervisory contact
		  2. the method(s) or type(s) of supervision

The Occupational Therapy Assistant: Resources for Practice and Education

Vermont
(*cont.*)

   3. the content areas addressed

  f. The supervisory plan is documented and a log of supervisory contacts is kept by both parties. The log includes the frequency and methods of supervision used.

  g. Supervision of occupational therapy services provided by a licensed occupational therapy assistant shall be implemented as follows:

    1. Entry level occupational therapy assistants are persons working on initial skill development (less than 1 year of work experience) or who are entering new practice environments or developing new skills (one or more years of experience) and shall require close supervision.

    2. Intermediate level occupational therapy assistants are persons working on increased skill development, mastery of basic role functions (minimum one–three years of experience or dependent on practice environment or previous experience) and shall require routine supervision.

    3. Advanced level occupational therapy assistants are persons refining specialized skills (more than 3 years work experience, or the ability to understand complex issues affecting role functions) and shall require general supervision.

    4. Licensed occupational therapy assistants, regardless of their years of experience, may require closer supervision by the licensed occupational therapist for interventions that are more complex or evaluative in nature and for areas in which service competencies have not been established.

  h. General statements regarding roles and responsibilities during the delivery of occupational therapy services:

    1. The occupational therapist is responsible for the overall delivery of occupational therapy services and is accountable for the safety and effectiveness of the occupational therapy service delivery process.

    2. The occupational therapy assistant delivers occupational therapy services under the supervision of the occupational therapist.

    3. It is the responsibility of the occupational therapist to be directly involved in the delivery of services during the initial evaluation and regularly throughout the course of intervention.

    4. Services delivered by the occupational therapy assistant are specifically selected and delegated by the occupational therapist. When delegating to the occupational therapy assistant, the occupational therapist considers the following factors:

      A. the complexity of the client's condition and needs

      B. the knowledge, skill, and competence of the occupational therapy assistant.

      C. the nature and complexity of the intervention.

    5. Prior to delegation of any aspect of the service delivery process to the occupational therapy assistant, service competency must be demonstrated and documented between the occupational therapist and occupational therapy assistant. Service competency is demonstrated and documented for clinical reasoning and judgment required during the service delivery process as well as for the performance of specific techniques, assessments, and intervention methods used. Service competency must be monitored and reassessed regularly.

    6. The role delineation and responsibilities of the occupational therapist and the occupational therapy assistant remain unchanged regardless of the setting in which occupational therapy services are delivered (i.e., traditional, non-traditional, or newly emerging practice settings).

  i. An occupational therapist or occupational therapy assistant practicing under a temporary license must have daily, direct, on-site supervision by a licensed occupational therapist for the duration of the temporary license. The supervisor is available for advice and intervention, and will sign all notes entered into the patient's medical record.

Virginia

Statute:

No relevant statutes.

Regulation:
18VAC
85-80-10

"Occupational therapy personnel" means appropriately trained individuals who provide occupational therapy services under the supervision of a licensed occupational therapist

18VAC
85-80-110

Supervisory Responsibilities

A. Delegation to unlicensed occupational therapy personnel.

    1. An occupational therapist shall be responsible for supervision of occupational therapy personnel who work under his direction.

    2. An occupational therapist shall not delegate the discretionary aspects of the initial assessment, evaluation or development of a treatment plan for a patient to unlicensed occupational therapy personnel nor shall he delegate any task requiring a clinical decision or the knowledge, skills, and judgment of a licensed occupational therapist.

    3. Delegation shall only be made if, in the judgment of the occupational therapist, the task or procedures does not require the exercise of professional judgment, can be properly and safely performed by appropriately trained unlicensed occupational therapy personnel, and the delegation does not jeopardize the health or safety of the patient.

    4. Delegated tasks or procedures shall be communicated on a patient-specific basis with clear, specific instructions for performance of activities, potential complications, and expected results.

B. The occupational therapist providing clinical supervision shall meet with the occupational therapy personnel to review and evaluate treatment and progress of the individual patients at least once every fifth treatment session or 21 calendar days, whichever occurs first.

(Continued)

State	Citation	Legislative / Regulatory information
Washington	**Statute:** RCW 18.59.020	4. "Occupational therapy assistant" means a person licensed to assist in the practice of occupational therapy under the supervision or with the regular consultation of an occupational therapist
		6. "Occupational therapy practitioner" means a person who is credentialed as an occupational therapist or occupational therapy assistant.
	Regulation: WAC 246-847-010	2. "Supervision" and "regular consultation" of an occupational therapy assistant by an occupational therapist in RCW 18.59.020(4) and "direct supervision" of a person holding a limited permit by an occupational therapist in RCW 18.59.040(7) shall mean face-to-face meetings between the occupational therapist and occupational therapy assistant and between the occupational therapist and holder of a limited permit occurring at intervals as determined necessary by the occupational therapist to establish, review, or revise the client's treatment objectives. The meetings shall be documented and the documentation shall be maintained in each client's treatment record. The failure to meet to establish, review, or revise the client's treatment objectives at sufficient intervals to meet the client's needs shall be grounds for disciplinary action against the occupational therapist's license and/or the occupational therapy assistant's license to practice in the state of Washington and/or the limited permit pursuant to WAC 246-847-160 (4) and (14), 246-847-170 (2) and (3) and RCW 18.59.100 for conduct occurring prior to June 11, 1986 and pursuant to RCW 18.130.180 for conduct occurring on or after June 11, 1986.
West Virginia	**Statute:** §30-28-3	f. "Occupational therapy assistant" means a person licensed to assist in the practice of occupational therapy under the general supervision of the licensed occupational therapist, and whose license is in good standing. As contained in this section, the term "general supervision" means initial direction and periodic inspection of the actual activities; however, the supervising licensed occupational therapist need not always be physically present or on the premises when the licensed assistant is performing services.
	Regulation: Title 13, §13-1-2	1.7. "Direct Supervision" means the actual physical presence of a licensed supervisor and the specific delineation of tasks and responsibilities for personally reviewing and interpreting the results of any habilitative or rehabilitative procedures conducted by the limited permit holder, occupational therapy student, or aide. It is the responsibility of the licensed supervisor to ensure that the limited permit holder, occupational therapy student, or aide does not perform duties for which he or she is not trained. The supervising licensed occupational therapist or licensed occupational therapy assistant shall be physically present when the limited permit holder, occupational therapy student, or aide is performing the patient or consumer service. An occupational therapist practicing under a limited permit shall be supervised by a licensed occupational therapist.
		2.10. "General Supervision" means initial direction, periodic inspection of service delivery, periodic meetings to review the outcome of service delivery, and the personal and direct involvement of the supervisor in the certified occupational therapy assistant's professional experience which includes evaluation of his or her performance. The supervisor need not be present or on the premises at all times where the licensed certified occupational therapy assistant is performing the professional services.
		2.19. "Occupational Therapy Assistant" means a person licensed to assist in the practice of occupational therapy under the general supervision of the licensed occupational therapist and whose license is in good standing.
Wisconsin	**Statute:** Chapter 448, §448.96	6. "Occupational therapy assistant" means an individual who is licensed by the affiliated credentialing board to assist in the practice of occupational therapy under the supervision of an occupational therapist.
	Regulation: Med 19.02	17. "Supervision" of an occupational therapy assistant means a process in which an occupational therapy assistant performs duties delegated by an occupational therapist in a joint effort to promote, establish, maintain, and evaluate the occupational therapy assistant's level of performance and service.
	Med 19.09	*Practice by Occupational Therapy Assistants* An occupational therapy assistant may not practice without the supervision of an occupational therapist unless the occupational therapy assistant is providing screening, habilitation, prevention, patient consultation or patient education outside of rehabilitation.
	Med 19.10	1. Supervision of an occupational therapy assistant by an occupational therapist shall be either close or general. The supervising occupational therapist shall have responsibility for the outcome of the performed service. 1. a. When close supervision is required, the supervising occupational therapist shall have daily, direct contact on the premises with the occupational therapy assistant. The occupational therapist shall provide initial direction in developing the plan of treatment and shall periodically inspect the actual implementation of the plan. The occupational therapist shall counter sign all patient related documents prepared by the occupational therapy assistant. 1. b. When general supervision is allowed, the supervising occupational therapist shall have direct contact on the premises with the occupational therapy assistant at least once each month. In the interim between direct contacts, the occupational therapist shall maintain contact with the occupational therapy assistant by telephone, written reports and group conferences. The occupational therapist shall record in writing a specific description of the supervisory activities undertaken for each occupational therapy assistant. 1. c. Close supervision is required for all rehabilitative services provided by an entry level occupational therapy assistant. All other occupational therapy services provided by an occupational therapy assistant may be performed under general supervision, if the supervising occupational therapist determines, under the facts of the individual situation, that general supervision is appropriate using established professional guidelines. 2. In extenuating circumstances, when the supervising occupational therapist is absent from the job, the occupational therapy assistant may carry out established programs for 30 calendar days. The occupational therapist must provide up-to-date documentation prior to absence.

State	Citation	Legislative / Regulatory information
Wyoming	**Statute:** Chapter 40, §33-40-102	*Definitions* a. ii. "Certified occupational therapy assistant" means a person licensed to assist in the practice of occupational therapy, under this act, and who works under the supervision of a registered occupational therapist.
	Regulation: Chapter 1, §1	e. "Close supervision" mean daily, direct contact at the site of work and applies only to OT/OTRs with initial skill development proficiencies or OTA/COTAs, as appropriate, for the delivery of occupational therapy services.
		h. "General supervision" means at least monthly direct contact with interim supervision available as needed by other methods, an applies only to OT/OTRs with increased skill, development and mastery of basic role functions or OTA/COTAs as appropriate, for the delivery of occupational therapy services.
		m. "Occupational therapy assistant" means an occupational therapy assistant who has met all educational requirements for an occupational therapy assistant, and was initially certified as a Certified Occupational Therapy Assistant (COTA) by NBCOT, and did not renew the certification but remains in good standing.
		p. "Routine supervision" means direct contact at least every two weeks at the site of work, with interim supervision occurring by other methods, such as telephonic, electronic or written communication and applies only to OTA/COTAs.

	Chapter 3, §1	*Delineation of Roles*
		 a. An occupational therapist currently licensed by the Board:
		   i. Evaluates the patient/client.
		   ii. Prepares a written program plan and provides treatment as appropriate.
		   iii. Assigns treatment duties based on that program plan to an occupational therapy assistant currently licensed by the Board who has been specifically trained to carry out those duties.
		   iv. Monitors the occupational therapy assistant's performance.
		   v. Accepts professional responsibility for the occupational therapy assistant's performance.
		 b. An occupational therapy assistant currently licensed by the board assists in the practice of occupational therapy and performs treatment and delegated assessment commensurate with their education and training.

	§2	*Supervision of Certified Occupational Therapy Assistants/Occupational Therapy Assistants*
		 a. A licensed COTA/OTA may assist in the practice of occupational therapy only under the supervision of an OTR/OT.
		 b. The supervisor shall have supervisory contact with the COTA/OTA at least 5% of the time worked by the assistant in direct patient care. Additional supervisory guidelines are as follows:
		   i. Entry-level COTA/OTA (working on initial skill development or entering new practice). Close supervision by OTR/OT is recommended. "Close Supervision" means daily, direct contact at the site of work.
		   ii. Intermediate-level COTA/OTA (working on increased skill development and mastery of basic role functions and demonstrates ability to respond to situations based on previous experience). Routine supervision by an OTR/OT is recommended. "Routine supervision" means direct contact at least every two weeks at the site of work, with interim supervision occurring by other methods, such as telephonic, electronic or written communication.
		   iii. Advanced-level COTA/OTA (refining specialized skills with the ability to understand complex issues affecting role functions). General supervision is recommended. "General Supervision" means at least monthly direct contact, with interim supervision available as needed by other methods.
		 c. The supervisor shall maintain a supervisory plan and shall document the supervision of each COTA/OTA. Documentation shall include evidence of regular supervision and contact between the supervisor and the assistant and may be subject to Board review upon request. Supervision includes the following:
		   i. Communicating to the COTA/OTA the results of patient/client evaluation and discussing the goals and program plan for the patient/client.
		   ii. Providing information, instruction and assistance as needed.
		   iii. Preparing on a regular basis, but at least annually, a written appraisal of the COTA/OTA's performance and discussing appraisal.
		   iv. The supervisor may assign to a competent COTA/OTA the administration of standardized tests, the performance of activities of daily living evaluations and other elements of patient/client evaluation and reevaluation that do not require the professional judgment and skill of an occupational therapist.
		   v. More frequent supervision may be necessary as determined by the OTR/OT or the COTA/OTA, dependent on the level of expertise displayed by the COTA/OTA, the setting and the population characteristics.
		 d. A supervisor who is temporarily unable to provide supervision shall arrange for substitute supervision by an OTR/OT currently licensed by the Board. The substitute shall provide supervision that is as rigorous and thorough as that provided by the permanent supervisor.
		 e. Failure to comply with this section constitutes unprofessional conduct.

Chapter 8

A Guide for Managers and Supervisors to Develop a System for Assessment of Competencies

Administration & Management Special Interest Section (2000–2003):

Brent Braveman, PhD, OTR/L, FAOTA

Patricia Gentile, MS, OTR/L, BCN

Janet Stafford, OT/L

Michael Berthelette, MSM, OTR/L

Linda Learnard, OTR/L

Introduction

The Administration & Management Special Interest Section (AMSIS) Standing Committee has developed this guide as a resource for occupational therapy managers and supervisors to assist in the process of establishing and evaluating specific competencies for occupational therapy personnel. Any person who is responsible for evaluating the performance of others to ensure that the care received by occupational therapy consumers is delivered in a safe and standardized manner may benefit from the use of this guide. The process of developing and implementing a system for assessment of competencies may be particularly helpful in settings accredited by an agency such as the Joint Commission on Accreditation of Healthcare Organizations (JCAHO) or the Commission on Accreditation of Rehabilitation Facilities (CARF).

Focus

The focus of this guide is on the *process* of developing and implementing a system for the assessment of competencies. Although exemplars are provided to illustrate steps in this process, specific competencies are always driven by the actual job tasks and responsibilities assigned to a specific staff member and documented within the individual's job description. Using this guide requires that the user apply the process to his or her own setting and organization. As noted earlier, the guide is developed primarily for settings that include assessment of competencies in response to accreditation processes but may be adapted and used for any setting.

Terminology

Users of this guide should be aware that multiple organizations related to health care delivery are concerned with developing and maintaining *competency* of staff. The American Occupational Therapy Association (AOTA), the National Board for Certification in Occupational Therapy (NBCOT), JCAHO, CARF, and many state professional regulatory boards, among other organizations, have programs, policies, or efforts under way related to competency issues. Therefore, users of this guide must always be aware of the context in which terminology is used. For example, AOTA's Professional Development Tool (PDT) distinguishes between the terms *competence* (an individual's capacity to perform job responsibilities) and *continuing competency* (the development of capacity and competency characteristics needed for the future as a component of ongoing professional development or lifelong learning). Managers and supervisors who are interested in learning more about developing their own continued competency and helping staff that they supervise with that process should consult the PDT. This tool can be found in the "Professional Development" section of the AOTA Web site at www.aota.org.

This guide focuses on the process of establishing and measuring *specific competencies* (explicit statements that define specific areas of expertise and are related to effective performance within a specific job) as part of the role of managers or supervisors in hiring and evaluating competent occupational therapy personnel. Readers are encouraged to review the glossary of terms found in Table 1 before proceeding with use of the guide and to use terms accurately in their day-to-day practice.

Relationship of Assessment of Competencies to Other Management Functions

The process of establishing and assessing specific competencies is related to a number of other critical management

TABLE 1. Glossary of Terms

Term	Definition
Competent (adjective)	Successfully performing a behavior or task as measured according to a specific criterion (Hinojosa, Bowen, Case-Smith, Epstein, Moyers, & Schwope, 2000). For example: "Using the rules of English composition, I am competent to write this sentence."
Competency (noun)	"Competency focuses on an individual's actual performance in a particular situation" (McConnell, 2001, p. 14). Competency implies a determination that one is competent. For example: "My evaluator indicates I have adequately demonstrated the sentence-writing competency needed to perform my job duties."
Competencies (plural of competency)	Competencies are explicit statements that define specific areas of expertise and are related to effective or superior performance in a job (Spencer & Spencer, 1993). For example: "I have demonstrated several competencies needed for adequate performance of my job duties. One of these competencies is sentence writing."
Competency characteristics	The capabilities that the person brings to the job task that include motives, traits, self-concept, knowledge, and skills (Spencer & Spencer, 1993). For example: "I show an enthusiasm for and a knowledge of sentence writing."
Competence (noun)	"Competence refers to an individual's capacity to perform job responsibilities" (McConnell, 2001). For example: "My job performance evaluation indicates that I demonstrate competence in sentence writing."
Continuing competence	Continuing competence involves the development of capacity and competency characteristics needed for the future and is a component of ongoing professional development or lifelong learning. For example: "If I hope to write more effectively, I need to maintain a continuing competence in sentence writing."
Professional development	May include a program of continuing competence but also includes a focus on one's career development in terms of achieving excellence or achieving independent practitioner and expert role status, and in terms of assuming new, more complex roles and responsibilities. For example: "Because I hope to write for publication, a formal writing course is part of my professional development plan."

functions. Maintaining a broader view of assessment of competencies is useful to recognize the connections between these management functions and to create synergies and efficiencies in completing management work tasks. This section of the guide overviews the various management or supervisory functions and the role that assessment of competencies plays in each related work task.

Creation of Job Descriptions

Job descriptions should be specific to the essential functions performed by each category of personnel (e.g., occupational therapy aide, occupational therapy assistant, occupational therapist). Elements of these essential functions should be reflected in specific competencies developed for an employee, and in turn, consideration of competencies may help managers to write or update job descriptions to be more accurate. For example, including "evaluation, recommendation, and fabrication of adaptive equipment, splints, or orthotics" in a job description might indicate the need for development of competencies related to splint fabrication. In turn, knowing that a staff member frequently fabricates splints might indicate the need to add this task as an essential function within the individual's job description.

Recruitment of New Employees

Having a well-developed job description and a system for the assessment of competencies can be useful in the process of recruiting and hiring new employees. For example, assessment of specific competencies may help managers and supervisors determine the skills, training, and education required for persons being hired to fill a specific vacancy and can therefore guide them in writing recruitment materials and screening and interviewing applicants.

Assessment of Initial Competency

Accreditation bodies such as JCAHO require documentation of a comprehensive orientation of new employees. An important part of new employee orientation for occupational therapists includes initial assessment of competencies for all essential job functions. This is true in settings subject to accreditation, as well as in settings such as community-based agencies or private businesses not subject to an accreditation process but in which the manager or supervisor wishes to ensure provision of quality care and to safeguard to whatever extent possible against malpractice litigation. Assessment of initial competency in essential job functions or for high-risk job tasks (e.g., transferring patients, working with a patient with cardiac precautions) or job functions requiring advanced competency (e.g., physical agent modalities) should occur before the employee independently completes these job tasks. Finding out during the orientation process that an employee cannot demonstrate competence in an essential job function allows the manager or supervisor to safeguard consumers by taking steps to assist the staff member to develop competence in essential job function before the end of the orientation period.

Annual Assessment of Competence

An annual assessment of competencies related to accreditation requirements (e.g., blood-borne pathogen training or fire and safety training as required by the Occupational Safety and Health Administration [OSHA]) or to essential job functions should be included as part of the annual appraisal of staff performance. Competency statements included in an annual assessment of competence might include those required of all staff (e.g., OSHA compliance) or competencies related to a specific employee's job tasks or skills (e.g., competencies related to advanced practice skills, such as the use of physical agent modalities). Competencies included in annual assessments may build on established knowledge, skills, and capacities reflecting the ever-changing nature of some jobs in light of an organization's mission and goals. These competencies reflect new, changing, high-risk, and problem-prone aspects of the job as it evolves over time:

- Developing ongoing competencies based on new initiatives, procedures, technologies, policies, or practices
- Changes in procedures, technologies, policies, or practices
- High-risk job functions
- Problematic job functions identified by continuous quality improvement efforts, consumer or staff surveys, incident reports, or any other formal or informal evaluation processes.

Continuing Education and Professional Development

Developing, assessing, and documenting demonstration of competencies related to essential job functions and planning and promoting the professional development of staff are related but separate processes. This guide for managers focuses on competencies, but as a result of implementing a comprehensive system for assessment of competencies, a manager may become aware of acute or more long-term needs of staff related to continuing education or professional development. A system for assessment of competencies may help a manager identify needed inservice training or other continuing education opportunities that would benefit staff. In conjunction with a performance appraisal system, managers and staff can also identify goals for individual professional development. As mentioned earlier, AOTA's PDT may be helpful to both managers and staff in this process.

Staffing Plans, Including Per Diem or Registry Staff

In situations in which an organization may purchase services from an outside agency or vendor or maintain their own registry of per diem staff, the organization must obtain information from that outside agency or vendor to verify that the contracted staff have the proper credentials (e.g., licensure as required by a state practice act). A human resources professional may complete this function, but consultation by the occupational therapy manager may ensure that accurate checks are completed. The hiring organization is responsible for verifying that the contract or per diem staff can demonstrate competencies related to essential job functions. Although the process of orienting and assessing

competencies for contract or per diem staff adds considerable expense for the hiring organization, contract and per diem staff must undergo the same assessment of competencies as permanent staff to ensure the safety of consumers and the quality of care being delivered within the organization. To minimize expense, documentation of some competencies prior to beginning work (e.g., CPR certification, bloodborne pathogen training) might be written into contracts with agencies or may be made to be the responsibility of per diem staff to be completed during nonpaid time.

A system for the assessment of competencies may also assist with the overall staffing plan for a department, and in fact, some accrediting agencies may require that a system be in place. For example, identifying that only two staff members have documented competencies related to children under the age of 7 might help a manager determine that additional training must be provided to other staff to ensure that adequate numbers of competent staff are available if these two staff members are on vacation, or for weekends if there is decreased coverage on these days. Accrediting bodies may require that the same level of care be provided regardless of the day of the week that patients are admitted to the facility.

Agency Accreditation and Licensure

Managers working in accredited and licensed facilities and programs must ensure that their programs for assessment of competencies meet all accrediting and licensing standards. Complying with these outside standards may be a challenge because, over the last several years, accrediting and licensing bodies have become increasingly focused on competency issues.

Managers should be aware that, although there are some commonalities, standards related to competency may vary from one accrediting body to another and may change over time. Managers should carefully review competency standards from each accrediting body when developing competency programs for their staff. The most common accrediting bodies occupational therapy managers may be involved with are JCAHO and CARF. Standards related to the assessment of competencies for both JCAHO Leadership and CARF Business Practices are primarily found in the Human Resource Section of their manuals. Managers should carefully review these standards when developing competency programs for their staff.

Quality Control and Continuous Quality Improvement Efforts

A synergy may be created between a system for assessment of competencies and quality control and quality improvement processes. Quality control measures such as the intermittent use of a check sheet to evaluate custom-made splints fabricated by staff may highlight problem areas and signal the need for establishment of a specific assessment of competencies related to splinting or for further training or education to ensure that staff are able to meet pre-established competencies. Similarly, continuous quality improvement efforts that include a focus on process improvement may indicate the need to establish new competencies or revisit established measures of competencies by providing targeted training for staff.

Outcomes Evaluation and Management

It must be recognized that many factors influence the outcomes of occupational therapy intervention. A system for assessing competencies related to essential job functions will, in itself, not ensure adequate outcomes. Other factors related to the patients or clients, such as their support, their medical condition, and the length and type of intervention provided, may all affect the outcome of occupational therapy intervention. Occupational therapy managers are most likely aware that the process of evaluating a *single* outcome with an individual patient or client calls for very different procedures than evaluating *program* outcomes or outcomes of occupational therapy intervention at the population level. However, ensuring that staff members can demonstrate specific competencies in regard to discrete essential job functions can help to prevent unusual cases or "outliers" from influencing the overall variability found in outcome measures.

Competencies and Domains of Knowledge

In developing a comprehensive system for assessing competencies, managers will need to consider a wide range of objectives that reflect the cognitive domain (knowing), affective domain (appreciating and valuing), and the psychomotor domain (physical performance). For a helpful reference on writing objectives for various domains, see Gronlund and Linn (1990). Table 2 includes examples of competency statements related to the cognitive, affective, and psychomotor domains.

An alternative approach is to utilize the *Standards for Continuing Competence* developed by AOTA's Commission on Continuing Competence and Professional Development (CCCPD). These standards overlap with the domains of knowledge just discussed but also include standards related to ethical and critical reasoning. The *Standards for Continuing Competence* are intended to

assist occupational therapy practitioners to assess, maintain, and document competence in all the roles they assume. The core of occupational therapy includes an understanding of occupation, its influence on performance, and the importance of purposeful activity; unique skills such as activity analysis and adaptation and critical and ethical reasoning; and core values and attitudes related to holistic intervention and the right of the individual to be self-determining. The core is developed as a result of a socialization process wherein the knowledge, skills, and attitudes fundamental to the profession are integrated and internalized as part of one's professional self-image. Regardless of the roles one assumes this core is present and guides beliefs and actions. (AOTA, 1994)

The standards include those specific to occupational therapy and are related to each of five areas: (1) knowledge, (2) critical reasoning, (3) interpersonal attitudes, (4) performance skills, and (5) ethical reasoning. The standards may be accessed on the AOTA Web site as part of the PDT.

Examples of Types of Competencies

Age-Related Competencies

This category of competencies documents that employees have the knowledge and skills to work with patients of a specific age group. For example, employees who work in a neonatal intensive care unit require one set of knowledge and skills specific to that age group, whereas employees who work with older adults in a skilled nursing facility require a

TABLE 2. Examples of Competency Statements From the Cognitive, Affective, and Psychomotor Domains for a Pediatric Therapist

Cognitive domain (knowing)	The therapist will be able to state key developmental milestones in children ages 0–3.
	The therapist will be able to state resources available to assist families in accessing needed services in their community.
Affective domain (appreciating and valuing)	The therapist's documentation reflects an appreciation for cultural influences on approaches to parenting.
	The therapist demonstrates valuing the involvement of parents in the process of planning occupational therapy intervention by asking their opinions and using information-seeking behaviors.
Psychomotor domain (physical performance)	The therapist will be able to safely remove an infant from the incubator when performing an assessment.
	The therapist will create a positioning plan for chronically ill children in the pediatric intensive care unit.

different set of knowledge and skills specific to older adults. Remember that, in situations in which staff are rotated to different units or programs and are asked to provide intervention to a different age group, they should be assessed on competencies for this new group before they intervene independently.

Equipment-Related Competencies

This category relates to the skills involved with using specific equipment in performance of job duties. These competencies may be part of initial competency assessment in some settings (e.g., use of mobile arm supports on a spinal cord injury unit), or they may be used in assessment of advanced competencies in other settings (e.g., the use of a computerized work simulation unit).

Advanced Practice or Specialized Practice Competencies

The use of advanced practice skills, such as advanced application of neurorehabilitation techniques, or specialized practice skills, such as physical agent modalities, requires specific education and training. Employees who use advanced practice skills or specialized practice skills should be evaluated specifically for competencies in these skills. Documentation of assessment of these competencies should become a formal part of employee records. Because techniques and equipment change frequently, advanced or specialized practice competencies should be reevaluated for appropriateness and updated frequently. For more information regarding physical agent modalities, refer to the AOTA official document "Physical Agent Modalities Position Paper" (AOTA, 2003).

Competencies Related to Specific Skills or Procedures

Depending on the setting and the types of clients seen by occupational therapists, there may be specific skills or procedures related to the process of assessing and intervening with clients for which specific assessment of competencies is appropriate. Examples might include competencies related to the administration of specific standardized assessments, competencies in procedures routinely performed (e.g., the fabrication of certain types of splints), or competencies in an intervention (e.g., serial casting), or in procedures related to a setting (e.g., safety precautions on a mental health unit).

Documenting Assessment of Competencies

Managers and supervisors must realize that as far as an accreditation reviewer or legal entity is concerned, assessment of competencies that are not documented in a permanent written format may as well not have occurred at all. Assessments of competencies should be documented in a formal and standardized way, and it is recommended that documentation become a permanent part of each employee's personnel file. Documentation of assessments of competencies may be completed in concert with, or as part of, other elements of managerial documentation, including
- New employee orientation forms,
- Annual performance appraisal forms, and
- Quality control and improvement forms such as check sheets and audits.

Elements of Effective Documentation

Documentation of assessment of competencies should include the following elements:
- Written specific statements reflecting essential job functions that identify specific and measurable tasks or behaviors
- The method(s) to assess each competency
- The person(s) who assessed each competency
- The date(s) on which a competency was assessed
- An action plan for competencies for which the employee is deemed less than fully competent
- The date for the next assessment of the competency.

Specific Methods for Assessing Competencies

Specific competencies may be assessed in a variety of manners, and an assessment approach that matches the domain of knowledge reflected in the competency statement should be chosen. The following should be considered when choosing specific methods to assess competencies:
- Different assessment methods are required to assess different competencies based upon the primary domains of knowledge reflected in the competency statements
- A single method of assessment seldom captures all of the domains (cognitive, affective, and psychomotor)
- Some competencies (e.g., CPR or responding to ethical dilemmas) may not easily be assessed in real-life situations and may need to be assessed through case studies or role-playing that simulate situations that might be encountered. These competencies should still be included, however, to document that training was provided
- Avoid using only checklists and posttests. Although these approaches are cost effective, these methods do not assess critical thinking or interpersonal skills
- Base your program for assessment of competencies on sound adult learning principles, including
  - Informing the employee why he or she needs to know specific information or be able to demonstrate specific skills;
  - Recognizing that adults bring prior learning and experience to all learning situations and building on the employee's prior experience;

- Allowing sufficient time for learning;
- Allowing for presentation of new material in multiple formats (e.g., oral, written, and/or observation);
- Using a task-oriented, problem-solving approach to learning; and
- Using self-directed learning as a learning option when possible, especially with assessment of competencies related to advanced skills such as equipment or physical agent modality competencies.

Methods for Assessment of Competencies

The following are suggested methods for assessing competencies and factors to consider when using each method of assessment. Again, managers are reminded that methods for assessing competencies should be matched with the domain of knowledge related to each competency and to use multiple methods whenever possible.

- Posttests, including written tests or quizzes, oral exams, surveys, worksheets, calculation tests, crossword puzzles, and some forms of games
  - Posttests work well to measure cognitive skills (an individual's comprehension of basic knowledge).
  - Posttests are not effective in measuring behavioral performance (psychomotor skills).
- Return demonstration (demonstrating a set of skills to another skilled observer)
  - Appropriate for measuring behavioral performance (psychomotor domain)
  - May occur in an artificial environment (skills lab) or in a real-world setting and may be done immediately following instruction or at a later time
  - Must go beyond description—describing an action may reflect the cognitive domain (knowing), but performance is required to assess competencies in the psychomotor domain
  - Most effective if a standard set of guidelines or criteria for evaluation (competency checklist) is used
  - The observer must be familiar with the criteria for evaluation and have demonstrated the indicated competency to another trained observer (within the facility or via a training or continuing education venue) prior to the observation.
- Observation of daily work
  - Appropriate for measuring skills in the behavioral (psychomotor) and affective (appreciating and valuing) domains
  - Both supervisors and peers can be used for these types of observation.
- Case studies (provide individuals with a situation and ask them to explain their responses or choices in that situation)
  - Appropriate for assessing critical thinking skills

- Manager or supervisor must create a check sheet or other evaluation tool to document specific competencies that are based on predetermined criteria related to the case content
- Can be prepared in many different ways
- Create a story of a clinical situation and ask questions that capture the nature of the competency you are measuring
- Can be used with individuals or discussion groups to facilitate teambuilding and group problem solving.
- Exemplars (a story you tell or write yourself describing a situation you have experienced or describing a rationale you thought about and choices you made in a situation)
  - Appropriate to measure critical thinking skills and interpersonal skills
  - Can capture actions that are NOT taken when not taking action is the competency choice in a given situation
  - Appropriate for use with a variety of personnel and are great for both staff and leadership positions
  - Very useful for personnel who must establish trust with a client, provide customer service, or deal with sensitive issues.
- Peer reviews
  - Appropriate for assessment of interpersonal skills and critical thinking skills
  - Staff should be prepared via a thorough orientation to the process, including suggestions for giving constructive feedback so that receiving feedback from peers is viewed as a positive rather than a negative experience
  - May be provided in a written format using check sheets or a written summary or in a verbal "face-to-face" format.
- Self-assessment
  - Appropriate for assessment of critical thinking skills
  - Appropriate for assessment of values, beliefs, opinions, and attitudes because it engages individuals in a reflective exercise that allows employees to put into words their conscious and unconscious thoughts
  - Has limited utility for assessment of psychomotor skills, and an additional method should always be used for high-risk procedures or skills that could result in harm to patients or clients.
- Discussion groups
  - Appropriate for assessment of all three skill domains, especially critical thinking skills, if paired with demonstrations, etc.
  - Include preparation activities on giving and receiving feedback in a constructive and respectful way
  - Promotes group cohesiveness and support
  - Allows a group of individuals to share their thoughts and strategies on an issue and discuss the merits and consequences of various plans of action
  - Promotes problem solving

- Competency assessment criteria should be prepared ahead of time
- There should be a facilitator who explains the expectations of the competency and how it is used as an assessment method
- Select a case study that has meaning to all members of the group or bring a situation that they have recently encountered, such as dealing with a difficult customer.

Putting It All Together—Examples of Synthesis of Assessment and Documentation Components for Competencies

Table 3 includes examples to illustrate how a sample of categories of competencies, specific competency statements, and methods of assessing competencies and documenting assessment are combined. Sample forms for the documentation of the assessment of competencies are included at the end of this guide.

Summary

This guide is intended as a introduction to the development of a system for the assessment and documentation of competencies as a benefit for members of AOTA. Members using this guide are encouraged to supplement it by referring to other resources mentioned within the guide and to seek additional assistance by liaising with other occupational therapy managers experienced in the assessment of competencies.

TABLE 3. Examples of Synthesis of Assessment and Documentation of Competencies

Category of Competency	Example of Competency Standard	Example of Evaluation Method	Documentation Methodology
Initial evaluation of competence	Safely completes transfer from wheelchair to bed, etc.	Observation by supervisor	Checklist of initial competencies showing "competent" or need for intervention and action taken
Annual evaluation of competence	Identifies electrical safety hazards and steps to be taken to rectify the situation	Watch a videotape combined with a posttest	Copy of posttest placed in personnel record signed by qualified reviewer
Age-related competence	Differentiates between chronological and developmental age	Peer review of cases, including observation of treatment and chart review	Peer evaluation form signed by employee, observer, and supervisor, including any intervention plan
Equipment-related competence	Completes safety check of a computerized work simulator before use	Self-review using checklist	Checklist turned into supervisor and placed in personnel record
Physical agent modality competence	Identifies all contraindications for use of ultrasound	Posttest after training module	Copy of posttest placed in personnel record signed by qualified reviewer

References

American Occupational Therapy Association. (1999). Standards for continuing competence. *American Journal of Occupational Therapy, 53,* 599–600.

American Occupational Therapy Association. (2003). *Physical agent modalities: A position paper.* Bethesda, MD: Author.

Gronlund, N. E., & Linn, R. L. (1990). *Measurement and evaluation in teaching* (6th ed.) New York: Macmillan.

Hinojosa, J., Bowen, R., Case-Smith, J., Epstein, C. F., Moyers, P., & Schwope, C. (2000). Standards for continuing competence for occupational therapy practitioners. *OT Practice, 5*(20), CE-1–CE-8.

McConnell, E. A. (2001). Managers fast track, competence v. competency. *Nursing Management, 32*(5), 14.

Spencer, L. M., & Spencer, S. M. (1993). *Competence at work.* New York: Wiley.

JAMAICA HOSPITAL MEDICAL CENTER
JAMAICA, NEW YORK
DEPARTMENT OF PHYSICAL MEDICINE AND REHABILITATION
OCCUPATIONAL THERAPY DIVISION

Annual Observation
Technical Application Superficial Thermal Physical Agent Modality
PARAFFIN

Name _____   Date _____

Reviewer_____   Patient Observed: (initials)_____

A.	*SELECTION*	*YES*	*NO*	*N/A*	*COMMENTS*
1.	Verbalizes clinical rationale for use of paraffin				
B.	*APPLICATION*	*YES*	*NO*	*N/A*	*COMMENTS*
1.	Instructed patient to wash hand prior to application				
2.	Checked skin prior to application				
3.	Oriented patient to modality, including effects and precautions				
4.	Chose appropriate application techniques for body part being treated				
5.	Used appropriate wrapping				
6.	Positioned patient comfortably after paraffin applied				
7.	Checked time of initial application or used timer				
8.	Removed paraffin when intervention was complete				
9.	Checked skin upon removal				
10.	Asked patient about effect of paraffin post application (e.g., pain relief, pliability)				
C.	*DOCUMENTATION*	*YES*	*NO*	*N/A*	*COMMENTS*
1.	Type of modality				
2.	Location/method of application				
3.	Skin inspection (before, during, after)				
4.	Response				

COMPETENCY MET   ☐ *yes*   ☐ *no*

If no:

Action Plan: _____

Following Action Plan: COMPETENCY MET ☐ *yes* ☐ *no*

Reviewer's Signature: _____

Staff Signature: _____

JAMAICA HOSPITAL MEDICAL CENTER
JAMAICA, NEW YORK
DEPARTMENT OF PHYSICAL MEDICINE AND REHABILITATION
OCCUPATIONAL THERAPY DIVISION

Annual Observation
Technical Application Superficial Thermal Physical Agent Modality
HOT PACKS
Name _____   Date _____
Reviewer_____   Patient Observed: (initials)_____

A.	SELECTION	YES	NO	N/A	COMMENTS
1.	Verbalizes clinical rationale for use of hot pack				
B.	APPLICATION	YES	NO	N/A	COMMENTS
1.	Checked skin prior to application				
2.	Oriented patient to modality, including effects and precautions				
3.	Chose appropriate size for body part being treated				
4.	Used appropriate layers of towels (6–8) to wrap hot pack				
5.	Positioned patient comfortably for hot pack application				
6.	Draped hot pack correctly onto body part				
7.	Checked time of initial application or used timer				
8.	Checked patient's skin within 5–10 minutes of application				
9.	Based on skin check, when warranted adjusted layers/draping accordingly				
10.	Removed hot pack when time was up				
11.	Checked skin upon removal				
12.	Asked patient about effect of hot pack post-application (e.g., pain relief, pliability)				
C.	DOCUMENTATION	YES	NO	N/A	COMMENTS
1.	Type of modality				
2.	Location/method of application				
3.	Skin inspection (before, during, after)				
4.	Response				

COMPETENCY MET   ☐ *yes*   ☐ *no*
If no:
Action Plan: _____
Following Action Plan: COMPETENCY MET ☐ *yes* ☐ *no*
Reviewer's Signature: _____
Staff Signature: _____

JCAHO COMPETENCY STANDARDS CHECKLIST

The following checklist may be helpful in determining whether your program is meeting current JCAHO competency standards:

____   Staff competency in the following areas has been assessed as part of the initial orientation process:

     ____   Age-related competencies

     ____   Equipment/safety-related competencies

     ____   High-volume, high-risk skills sets

____   When a change in assignment/job category occurs, staff competency is reassessed in the following areas:

     ____   Age-related competencies

     ____   Equipment/safety-related competencies

     ____   High-volume, high-risk skills sets

____   Competency assessment is ongoing and includes, at a minimum, an annual performance appraisal with competency assessment in the following areas:

     ____   Age-related competencies

     ____   Equipment/safety-related competencies

     ____   High-volume, high-risk skills sets

____   In cases where competence has not been met, a specific, objective action plan with target dates has been developed for the employee.

     ____   Staff learning needs are assessed annually

     ____   Trends related to overall staff competency are monitored and addressed

University of Illinois at Chicago Medical Center

Job Classification _____

Methodology for Validation _____   *Times Per Year* _____

Competency	High Risk	High Volume	Problem Prone	High Risk Low Volume	Link to Quality Plan	Professional Standard	Methodology for Validation	Times Per Year
Mandatory All Employees								
Patient Confidentiality	X							
Fire Safety	X							
Electrical Safety	X							
Hazard Communication	X							
Infection Control	X							
Emergency Management	X							
Mandatory Patient Contact								
Age-Appropriate Care								
TB & PPE								
Signs of Abuse								
Restraints								
Blood-Borne Pathogens								
Mandatory as Needed								
Radiation Safety								
CPR								
Defibrillator								

Methodology for Validation	Times Per Year
1. Return Demonstration	1. 1 × annually
2. Cognitive Test	2. 1 × every 2 years
3. Observation	3. Semiannually
4. Peer Review	4. Other
5. Chart Review–Audit	
6. Other	

The Occupational Therapy Assistant: Resources for Practice and Education

Chapter 9

AOTA Standards for Continuing Competence

These standards will assist occupational therapy practitioners to assess, maintain, and document competence in all the roles that they assume. The core of occupational therapy includes an understanding of occupation, its influence on performance, and the importance of purposeful activity; unique skills such as activity analysis and adaptation, and critical and ethical reasoning; and core values and attitudes related to holistic intervention and the right of an individual to be self-determining. The core is developed as a result of a socialization process wherein the knowledge, skills, and attitudes that are fundamental to the profession are integrated and internalized as a part of one's professional self-image. Regardless of the roles one assumes, this core is present and guides beliefs and actions.

Standard 1. Knowledge

Occupational therapy practitioners shall demonstrate understanding and comprehension of the information required for the multiple roles they assume. The individual must

- Integrate mastery of the core of occupational therapy into the multiple roles assumed,
- Maintain up-to-date knowledge of appropriate professional Association documents and demonstrate application of this information to practice,
- Demonstrate a commitment to lifelong learning,
- Document subject matter expertise associated with primary roles,
- Demonstrate an understanding of current literature related to primary roles and to the consumer population(s) served, and
- Demonstrate knowledge of legislative, legal, and regulatory issues related to practice and the roles assumed.

Standard 2. Critical Reasoning

Occupational therapy practitioners shall employ reasoning processes to make sound judgments and decisions within the context of their roles. The individual must

- Apply deductive and inductive reasoning in making decisions specific to roles and functions;
- Demonstrate problem-solving skills required in assumed roles;
- Assess, and when necessary and feasible, modify contextual factors that influence performance;
- Integrate information from a variety of sources to formulate actions and to make decisions; and
- Reflect on one's own practice to develop revised strategies for action, to make future decisions, and to guide professional development needs.

Standard 3. Interpersonal Abilities

Occupational therapy practitioners shall develop and maintain their professional relationships with others within the context of their roles. The individual must

- Demonstrate effective communication skills;
- Use methods of communication that match the abilities, learning styles, and therapeutic needs of consumers[1] and others;
- Demonstrate professional behavior;
- Use feedback from consumers, families, supervisors, and colleagues to modify one's professional behavior; and
- Collaborate with consumers, families, and professionals to attain consumer outcomes.

Standard 4. Performance Skills

Occupational therapy practitioners shall demonstrate the expertise, aptitudes, proficiencies, and abilities to competently fulfill their roles. The individual must

- Demonstrate practice grounded in the core of occupational therapy,

---

[1]*Consumer* is used in this document to refer to individuals who receive occupational therapy services and includes, but is not limited to, children, students, clients, patients, customers, and agencies.

- Demonstrate the skilled performances required to succeed in roles,
- Use resources needed to perform roles,
- Evaluate and incorporate technology as appropriate, and
- Update performance based on current research and literature.

Standard 5. Ethical Reasoning

Occupational therapy practitioners shall identify, analyze, and clarify ethical issues or dilemmas in order to make responsible decisions within the changing context of their roles. The individual must

- Understand and adhere to the profession's *Code of Ethics* (AOTA, 1994) as well as other applicable codes of ethics;
- Accept responsibility for self-directed learning by defining learning objectives, planning a professional development program, and evaluating progress;
- Identify ethical principles and core values and attitudes that are applicable to changing situations and use these principles to resolve ethical dilemmas;
- Identify and examine ethical dilemmas using ethical reasoning to guide decisions and actions; and
- Reflect on the results of ethical decision making.

Reference

American Occupational Therapy Association. (1994). Occupational therapy code of ethics. *American Journal of Occupational Therapy, 48,* 1037–1038.

PREPARED BY THE CONTINUING COMPETENCE TASK FORCE
Jim Hinojosa, OT, PhD, FAOTA, Chairperson
Robin Bowen, EdD, OTR, FAOTA
Jane Case-Smith, EdD, OT/L, FAOTA
Cynthia Epstein, MA, OTR, FAOTA
Carole Schwope, MA, COTA/L
Penny Moyers, EdD, OTR, FAOTA, Executive Board Liaison
Brena Manoly, PhD, OT, National Office Liaison
George W. Rowley, MA, OTR/L, National Office Liaison

for

THE AOTA EXECUTIVE BOARD
Karen Jacobs, EdD, OTR/L, CPE, FAOTA, President

Adopted by the Representative Assembly (1999M33)

Previously published and copyrighted in 1999 by the American Occupational Therapy Association in the *American Journal of Occupational Therapy, 53,* 599–600.

Chapter 10

Model Continuing Competence Guidelines for Occupational Therapists and Occupational Therapy Assistants: A Resource for State Regulatory Boards

Purpose

The purpose of these model guidelines for continuing competence of occupational therapists and occupational therapy assistants is to provide a template for use by occupational therapy regulatory boards and state agencies when drafting or amending regulations addressing participation in continuing competence activities. The model is intended to help safeguard the public health, safety, and welfare by establishing minimum guidelines that are consistent with the American Occupational Therapy Association's (AOTA's) *Standards for Continuing Competence* and accepted practice in the profession of occupational therapy.

Continuing education (CE) has been widely accepted as a method of maintaining and enhancing professional competence. AOTA recognizes, however, that there are multiple methods by which an individual may demonstrate pursuit of continuing competence. The following model guidelines for regulation encourage use of a variety of continuing competence activities including continuing education, academic coursework, independent study, mentorship, participation in research, and other activities. Optional provisions are provided to encourage licensees to conduct a self-assessment and implement a professional development plan for continuing competence.

Chapter 01. General Regulations

01. Definitions

A. In this chapter, the following terms have the meanings indicated.

1. *AOTA Approved Provider Program* refers to a voluntary process of review and approval of continuing education (CE) providers by the American Occupational Therapy Association (AOTA) based on established criteria and guidelines that assess a provider's ability to develop and implement CE activities that are relevant to the practice of occupational therapy. Providers who are approved by AOTA will be authorized to offer AOTA CEUs for continuing education activities.

2. *AOTA CEU* means a standard unit of measure for participation in an organized continuing education activity that meets the AOTA Approved Provider criteria for relevance to the foundation and/or practice of occupational therapy. One AOTA CEU is equivalent to 10 contact hours of participation in an organized CE activity, excluding meals and breaks.

3. *Board* means the [state or jurisdiction] Occupational Therapy Regulatory Board.

4. *Contact Hour* means a unit of measure for a continuing education activity. One contact hour equals 60 minutes in a learning activity, excluding meals and breaks.

5. *Continuing Competence* means a dynamic, multidimensional process in which an occupational therapist or an occupational therapy assistant develops and maintains the knowledge, performance skills, interpersonal abilities, critical reasoning skills, and ethical reasoning skills necessary to perform his or her professional responsibilities.

6. *Continuing Education* means structured educational experiences beyond entry-level academic degree work that are intended to provide advanced or enhanced knowledge in a particular area.

7. *Continuing Education Credit* means credit given for a formalized activity in the form of contact hours or continuing education units.

8. *Continuing Education Unit (CEU)* means a unit of measure for continuing education. One CEU is defined as 10 contact hours of participation in a learning activity excluding meals and breaks.

9. *Peer Reviewed* means any written work that is blind reviewed by more than one person under uniform criteria.

10. *Points* means an assigned unit of measure for each continuing competence activity as defined in Section 05.

02. Continuing Competence Requirements for Licensure

A. Licensees applying for license renewal shall complete a minimum of _____ points of qualified activities for maintaining continuing competence during the preceding biannual renewal period. Licensees who are issued a license for a period less than 24 months shall prorate the number of points to _____ point(s) for each month licensed.

B. Applicants for licensure who are or have previously been licensed in another state that does not have continuing education or continuing competence requirements for license renewal shall show evidence of completing _____ points of qualified activities for maintaining continuing competence within the 1 year of submitting the application for licensure.

C. Applicants for licensure who were previously licensed by the Board and whose license has lapsed for _____ years or less from the time the application is filed shall obtain _____ points of qualified activities for maintaining continuing competence for each year in which the license has been in the lapsed status.

D. Applicants for licensure who were previously licensed by the Board and whose license has lapsed for more than _____ years shall obtain _____ points of qualified activities for maintaining continuing competence and may be required by the Board to fulfill additional requirements that show evidence of competency to practice as an occupational therapist or occupational therapy assistant on a case-by-case basis.

03. Exceptions to Requirements

A. Applicants for initial licensure as an occupational therapist or occupational therapy assistant who apply for licensure within 1 year of successfully completing the entry-level certification exam are exempt from continuing competence activity requirements.

B. Applicants for licensure by endorsement from a state or jurisdiction which has continuing education or continuing competence activity requirements for license renewal are exempt from continuing competence activity requirements.

04. Approval of Activities for Maintaining Continuing Competence

A. Provider Pre-Approval
1. Provided that the activities are consistent with the provisions of these regulations, the Board shall grant pre-approval to

a. Activities sponsored or approved by the [state or jurisdiction] occupational therapy association;
b. Activities sponsored or approved by AOTA; and
c. Activities sponsored by AOTA Approved Providers.

B. Approval of Provider Activities
1. A provider who wishes to obtain Board approval of activities for maintaining continuing competence, consistent with Section 05, shall submit to the Board at least _____ days in advance of the program all required information, including
a. Course description;
b. Learning outcomes;
c. Target audience;
d. Content focus;
e. Detailed agenda for the activity;
f. Amount of credit offered;
g. Qualifications for the presenter(s);
h. Sample documentation for demonstrating satisfactory completion by course participants such as certificate of completion.

2. Upon review of the completed application, the Board shall notify the provider as to whether or not the program has been approved and, if approved, the number of points that will be awarded.

3. A provider of a continuing competence activity shall furnish documentation for demonstrating satisfactory completion to all participants, specifying the following information:
a. Name of the participant;
b. Name of the provider;
c. Dates of the activity and completion;
d. Title and location of the activity;
e. Number of points awarded by the Board; and
f. Signature of the provider or representative.

C. Approval of Other Activities
1. A licensee may obtain Board approval of continuing education credits for activities not already approved. Activities must be consistent with Section 05. In order to obtain Board approval, the licensee shall submit to the Board the following materials:
a. Course description;
b. Learning outcomes;
c. Target audience;
d. Content focus;
e. Detailed agenda for the activity;
f. Qualifications for the presenter(s);
g. Sample documentation for demonstrating satisfactory completion by course participants such as certificate of completion.

2. Upon review of the completed application, the Board shall notify the licensee as to whether or not the activ-

ity has been approved and, if approved, the number of points awarded.

05. Scope of Qualified Activities for Maintaining Continuing Competence

A. To be accepted by the Board, activities must be related to a licensee's current or anticipated roles and responsibilities in occupational therapy and must directly or indirectly serve to protect the public by enhancing the licensee's continuing competence.

B. Subject matter for qualified activities include research; theoretical or practical content related to the practice of occupational therapy; or the development, administration, supervision, and teaching of clinical practice or service delivery programs by occupational therapists or occupational therapy assistants.

06. Qualified Activities for Maintaining Continuing Competence

A. Continuing Education Courses
1. Includes attendance and participation as required at a live presentation such as a workshop, seminar, conference, or in-service educational program. May also include participation in other continuing education activities that require a formal assessment of learning. Examples include electronic or Web-based courses, AOTA Self-Paced Clinical Courses or other formalized self-study courses, AOTA Continuing Education Articles, etc.
2. A licensee may earn _____ point(s) for each contact hour or equivalent unit that is awarded by the provider.
3. Documentation shall include a certificate of completion or similar documentation including name of course, date, author/instructor, sponsoring organization, location, and number of hours attended and amount of continuing education credit earned.

B. Academic Coursework
1. Includes participation in on-site or distance learning academic courses from a university, college, or vocational technical adult education course related to the practice of occupational therapy.
2. A licensee may earn _____ point(s) per credit hour.
3. Documentation shall include an original official transcript indicating successful completion of the course, date, and a description of the course from the school catalogue or course syllabus.

C. Independent Study
1. Includes reading books, journal articles, reviewing videos, etc.
2. A licensee may earn _____ point(s) for _____ hour(s) spent in an independent study activity.

3. Documentation shall include title, author, publisher, time spent, and date of completion. Licensee must include a statement that describes how the activity relates to a licensee's current or anticipated roles and responsibilities.

D. Mentorship
1. Participation as Mentee
a. Participation in a formalized mentorship agreement with a mentor as defined by a signed contract between the mentor and mentee that outlines specific goals and objectives and designates the plan of activities that are to be met by the mentee.
b. A licensee may earn _____ point(s) for _____ hour(s) spent in activities directly related to achievement of goals and objectives. The Board may accept formalized mentorship programs for the amount of credit recommended by the mentor or as deemed appropriate by the Board.
c. Documentation shall include name of mentor and mentee, copy of signed contract, dates, hours spent and focus of mentorship activities, and outcomes of mentorship agreement.
2. Participation as Mentor
a. Participation in a formalized mentorship agreement with a mentee as defined by a signed contract that designates the responsibilities of the mentor and specific goals and objectives that are to be met by the mentee.
b. A licensee may earn _____ point(s) for each _____ hour(s) spent in mentorship activities as a mentor.
c. Documentation shall include name of mentor and mentee, copy of signed contract, dates, hours spent and focus of mentorship activities, and outcomes of mentorship agreement.

E. Fieldwork Supervision
1. Participation as the primary clinical fieldwork educator for Level II OT or OTA fieldwork students.
2. A licensee may earn _____ point(s) for supervision of a fieldwork student. Documentation shall include verification provided by the school to the fieldwork educator with the name of student, school, and dates of fieldwork or the signature page of the completed student evaluation form. Evaluation scores and comments should be deleted or blocked out.

F. Professional Writing
1. Publication of a peer-reviewed or non-peer-reviewed book, chapter, or article.
2. A licensee may earn
a. _____ point(s) as an author of a book,
b. _____ point(s) as author of a chapter,

c. ____ point(s) as author peer-reviewed article,

d. ____ point(s) as author of a non-peer-reviewed article,

e. ____ point(s) as an editor of a book.

3. Documentation shall consist of full reference for publication, including title, author, editor, and date of publication, or copy of acceptance letter if not yet published.

G. Presentation and Instruction

1. First time or significantly revised presentation of an academic course or peer-reviewed or non-peer-reviewed workshop, seminar, in-service, electronic or Web-based course, etc.

2. A licensee may earn ____ point(s) for each hour of credit that is awarded for an activity.

3. Documentation shall include a copy of official program/schedule/syllabus, including presentation title, date, hours of presentation, and type of audience or verification of such signed by the sponsor.

H. Research

1. Development of or participation in a research project.

2. A licensee may earn ____ point(s) for each ____ hour(s) spent working on a research project.

3. Documentation includes verification from the primary investigator indicating the name of research project, dates of participation, major hypotheses or objectives of the project, and licensee's role in the project.

I. Grants

1. Development of a grant proposal.

2. A licensee may earn ____ point(s) for each ____ hour(s) spent working on a grant proposal.

3. Documentation includes name of grant proposal, name of grant source, purpose and objectives of the project, and verification from the grant author regarding licensee's role in the development of the grant if not the author.

J. Professional Meetings and Activities

1. Consistent with Section 05, participation in board or committee work with agencies or organizations in professionally related areas to promote and enhance the practice of occupational therapy.

2. A licensee may earn ____ point(s) for participation on a committee or board for 1 year or a minimum of ____ hours.

3. Documentation includes name of committee or board, name of agency or organization, purpose of service, and description of licensee's role. Participation must be validated by an officer or representative of the organization or committee.

07. Waiver of Requirements

A. Under extenuating circumstances, the Board may waive all or part of the continuing competence activity requirements of these regulations if an occupational therapist or occupational therapy assistant submits written request for a waiver and provides evidence to the satisfaction of the Board of an illness, injury, financial hardship, family hardship, or other similar extenuating circumstance which precluded the individual's completion of the requirements on a case-by-case basis.

08. Documentation/Reporting Procedures

A. Licensees shall maintain the required proof of completion for each continuing competence activity as specified in these regulations. The required documentation shall be retained by the licensee for a minimum of 2 years following the last day of the license renewal period for which the continuing competence activities were earned.

B. Licensees should not send their continuing competence activity documentation to the Board unless audited or otherwise requested by the Board.

09. Audit of Continuing Competence Activities

A. The Board shall perform a random audit or full review of licensees' continuing competence activity requirements at least once during each licensing period.

B. A licensee who is audited shall complete the requirements of the audit by the deadline specified by the board.

C. A licensee who fails to comply with the continuing competence activity requirements of these regulations may be subject to disciplinary action that may include suspension or revocation of license.

10. Other Provisions

A. Licensees may not carry over continuing competence activity points from one licensure period to the next.

B. Licensees may not receive credit for the same continuing competence activity more than once.

Chapter 02. Optional Provisions

01. Definitions

A. In this chapter, the following terms have the meanings indicated.

1. *AOTA Continuing Competence Plan for Professional Development* means AOTA's self-initiated plan to assist occupational therapists and occupational therapy assistants in addressing competence in their various responsibilities and career stages. It encourages occu-

pational therapists and occupational therapy assistants to examine each area of responsibility relative to their practice and perform a self-assessment of professional development strengths and needs in order to develop and implement an effective continuing competence plan for professional development.

2. *AOTA's Professional Development Tool* refers to an AOTA resource that facilitates the process of assessing individual learning needs and interests, creating a professional development plan, and documenting professional development activities.

3. *AOTA Standards for Continuing Competence* means standards adopted for the profession by the AOTA Representative Assembly that establish the principal criteria by which individual occupational therapists and occupational therapy assistants can examine their own competence. The Standards for Continuing Competence address knowledge, critical reasoning, interpersonal abilities, performance skills, and ethical reasoning.

4. *Portfolio* means an organized system for gathering a record of work history, professional accomplishments, and professional and learning activities, as well as documentation of the activities identified to meet individual professional development needs.

5. *Professional Development* means the ongoing process by an occupational therapist or occupational therapy assistant to actively engage in activities that improve skills necessary for meeting the behaviors or tasks inherent in each of his or her professional responsibilities.

6. *Self-assessment* means the process of reflecting on one's professional responsibilities in relationship to the knowledge, skills, behaviors, and attitudes already acquired and those needed in order to demonstrate competence in the individual's areas of responsibility.

02. Continuing Competence Plan for Professional Development

A. It is the responsibility of each licensee to design and implement his or her own strategy for developing and demonstrating continuing competence. Each licensee has current and/or anticipated roles and responsibilities that require specific knowledge, attitude, abilities, and skills. It is incumbent upon each licensee to examine his or her unique responsibilities, assess his or her continuing competence needs related to these responsibilities, and develop and implement a plan to meet those needs.

B. The Board recognizes the American Occupational Therapy Association (AOTA) as the standard setting body for the profession of occupational therapy and endorses the use of AOTA's voluntary Professional Development Tool.

C. A licensee may seek recognition by the Board for an alternative professional development plan for maintaining continuing competence provided that the proposed plan is consistent with the provisions of these regulations and includes

1. The completion of a formal self-assessment process;

2. The establishment of professional development goals and objectives; and

3. A portfolio approach to organize and document continuing competence activities related to the licensee's plan.

D. Licensees who voluntarily implement a plan for continuing competence during the current license period can receive credit toward their continuing competence activity requirements.

1. A licensee may earn _____ point(s) for completion of activities related to the development and implementation of a continuing competence plan for professional development.

2. Documentation shall include a signed document by the licensee attesting to the fact that he or she has used AOTA's Professional Development Tool consistent with the provisions of these regulations.

03. Board Certification and Specialty Certification

A. The Board shall recognize completion of activities that result in board certification or specialty certification by AOTA during the current licensure period.

B. A licensee may seek prior approval by the Board for recognition of an alternative board or specialty certification.

C. A licensee may earn up to _____ point(s) for each board certification or specialty certification credential earned or re-certified during the current licensure period.

D. Documentation includes certificate of completion or other documentation from the recognized certifying body that identifies satisfactory completion of requirements for obtaining board certification or specialty certification.

Approved by the Representative Assembly November 2003

Chapter 11

Competency Checklists

PRACTITIONER COMPETENCY CHECKLIST

Note change in rating scale: Infrequently (less than 50%); Frequently (51–94%); Consistently (95–100%).

Applicable to OTRs	COTAs*	Practitioner Competency Items	Infrequently	Frequently	Consistently	Comments	Need to Increase
X	X	Consider age and developmental level; gender; education; cultural background; and socioeconomic, medical, and functional status when providing OT services.					
X		Select assessments to determine the individual's functional abilities and problems as related to occupational performance areas; occupational performance components; physical, social, and cultural environments; performance safety; and prevention of dysfunction.					
X	X	Administer standardized tests according to defined protocol.					
X	X	Administer criterion-referenced tests according to defined protocol.					
X	X	Use skilled observations, interview, record review, and unstructured tests.					
X	X	Administer specialized evaluations according to defined protocol.					
X	X	Interpret occupational therapy assessment data.					
X	**	Analyze and summarize collected evaluation data to indicate the individual's current functional status.					
X	X	Assess and incorporate effect of the environment/context of performance in patient care.					
X	**	Estimate potential for response to OT intervention.					
X	**	Develop goals and recommendations based on assessment results that are clear, measurable, behavioral, functional, and appropriate to the individual's needs, personal goals, and expected outcomes after intervention.					
X	**	Establish goals in collaboration with individual.					
X	**	Update goals as performance changes.					
X	**	Establish measurement methods for determining achievement of goals.					
X	**	Determine the frequency and duration of occupational therapy services.					
X	**	Refer individuals to other appropriate resources when the therapist determines that the knowledge and expertise of other professionals is indicated.					

*Under supervision of OTR.

**Contributes to the process in collaboration with an OTR.

WORK AND BEHAVIOR COMPETENCY CHECKLIST

All of the items apply to both OTRs and COTAs.

Maintaining and Updating Clinical Competency Items	Infrequently	Frequently	Consistently	Comments	Need to Increase
State functional outcome in documentation that is meaningful and appropriate to individual patient/client.					
Document clearly, timely, and meet facility policies and procedures and applicable regulations.					
Use time efficiently and do job tasks in a reasonable amount of time.					
Handle multiple work demands and variable schedules and caselaods.					
Monitor own performance and identify supervisory needs.					
Actively participate and responsibly respond in the supervisory relationship.					
Accommodate to change and modify own behavior according to the demands of the situation.					
Accommodate personal style to work effectively with a variety of people.					
Accommodate priorities according to the needs of the program, department, and others.					
Actively contribute information in meetings, conferences, and informal interactions.					
Appraise and communicate the value of occupation therapy to a variety of audiences.					
Identify consultation needs and effectively negotiate with appropriate sources to receive needed consultation.					
Function according to the AOTA *Code of Ethics* and *Standards of Practice* of the profession.					
Comply with the institution's protocols, policies, and procedures.					
Demonstrate an understanding of the financial implications of treatment costs and resources on occupational therapy services.					
Synthesize and analyze the information from federal, state, and local laws that has a direct impact on the delivery of occupational therapy services.					
Participate in quality improvement activities.					

The Occupational Therapy Assistant: Resources for Practice and Education

Chapter 12

Sample State Occupational Therapy Supervision Logs

NEW MEXICO BOARD OF EXAMINERS FOR OCCUPATIONAL THERAPY
SUPERVISION LOG

CIRCLE ONE: OT OTA COTA

Print name of **supervisee**: _____ License No. _____

Print name(s) of **supervisor**(s): _____ License No. _____

Employer/Worksite: _____ Phone _____

Address: _____

Please check the <u>Level of Supervision</u> that is provided on each form. NOTE: The supervisor should begin a new supervision log each time the supervisee advances to a new level.

☐ Direct   ☐ Close   ☐ Routine   ☐ General

Complete instructions appear on the reverse side of this form. Fill in the amount of time spent in minutes in each category. The supervisor must initial in the last column. Supervision must include a combination of site and office contacts, and observations. Twenty percent (20%) of **all contacts** shall be face-to-face clinical observation. **This is a two-sided form. Please copy both sides.**

Date	Clinical Observation	Documentation Review	Case Review	Direct Training	Non-Direct Contact*	Description of Activities	Initials

Non-Direct Contact means telephone, fax, or e-mail.

Random audits may be performed at any time.

I certify that the information contained in this supervision log is true and correct. I further understand that my license could be in jeopardy if I have knowingly made any incomplete/false entries in the completion of this log.

Supervisee Signature _____ License # _____ Date _____

Supervisor Signature _____ License # _____ Date _____ Initials _____

INSTRUCTIONS

Copy the Blank Log.

You may make as many copies as you need. Be sure to copy both sides of the log.

Fill in Identified Information

Complete one log for each practitioner (OT, OTA, or COTA)

Definitions: **OT**—Occupational Therapist pending certification from NBCOT and practicing under a provisional license
OTA—Occupational Therapy Assistant pending certification from NBCOT and practicing under a provisional license
COTA—Certified Occupational Therapy Assistant

If the practitioner works for more than one employer, complete a separate log for each employer. Fill in the name of the practitioner being supervised (supervisee) and the name of the supervisor(s). If more than one person provides supervision, or if supervisors change during the year, add each supervisor's name to the log. If multiple supervisors make it difficult to record information, attach additional logs with names, signatures, and initials of other supervisor(s).

Record Supervision

In the blank columns, indicate amount of time (in minutes) spent in each category on the day supervision occurs. Supervisor must initial the last column.

Sign the Log

The supervisee must sign the log when the log is full, or upon leaving employment, whichever comes first.
The supervisor must sign the log when the log is full, or upon leaving employment or at the end of supervision responsibilities, whichever comes first. Include initials, as used on the log, with the signature.

Keep the Log and Copies

A copy of the log must be maintained by the facility where the services are provided. The supervisee must keep the original supervision log. It is recommended that the supervisee retain the log for 3 or more years. ***A copy of the log must be submitted to the Board prior to issuance of full licensure, prior to renewal of any COTA license, and at any time upon request by the Board.***

For complete rules and regulations related to supervision, refer to

Occupational Therapy Rules and Regulations
Title 16, Chapter 15, Part 3

The following information is abbreviated and intended for general reference. Refer to the above-referenced Rules document for complete descriptions.

"Direct Supervision" means a minimum of daily direct contact at the site of work with the licensed supervisor physically present within the facility when the supervisee renders care and requires the supervisor to co-sign all documentation that is completed by the supervisee. In a work setting involving multiple sites of work and/or offices, supervision shall occur at one or more of the sites or offices, but not necessarily all sites or offices. The registered occupational therapist (OTR/L) or an intermediate-level or advanced-level certified occupational therapy assistant shall provide direct supervision for persons practicing on a provisional permit pending certification as a certified occupational therapy assistant (COTA/L). The registered occupational therapist (OTR/L) and the certified occupational therapy assistant (COTA/L) shall provide direct supervision to all occupational therapy aides/technicians.

"Close Supervision" means a minimum of daily communication by means of direct contact, telephone, fax, or e-mail. In a single work setting or when involving multiple sites, supervision shall occur at one or more of the sites or offices, but not necessarily at all sites or offices. Twenty percent (20%) of close supervision contacts shall be face-to-face clinical observation. Required for entry-level certified occupational therapy assistants (COTA/L).

"Routine Supervision" means a minimum of direct contact at least every two (2) weeks at the site of work, with interim supervision occurring by other methods such as telephone, fax, or e-mail. Twenty percent (20%) of routine contacts shall be face-to-face clinical observation. Required for intermediate-level certified occupational therapy assistants (COTA/L).

"General Supervision" means a minimum of monthly direct contact, with supervision available as needed by other methods such as telephone, fax, or e-mail. Twenty percent (20%) of general contacts shall be face-to-face clinical observation. Required for advanced-level certified occupational therapy assistants (COTA/L).

Supervision of OTs practicing on a provisional permit pending certification as an OTR/L.

Supervision shall be provided by an OTR/L and must occur on-site. In work settings involving multiples sites of work, supervision shall occur at one or more of the sites, but not necessarily all sites. Supervision shall occur three (3) or more times per week for persons working five (5) days per week, two (2) or more times per week for persons working four (4) days per week, one(1) or more times per week for persons working three (3) or less days per week.

Texas Board of Occupational Therapy Examiners
Occupational Therapy Supervision Log

Please read reverse side for instructions and information

Make copies of this page as needed for your own documentation

Name of Licensee: _____

License #: _____

Temporary License   or   Regular License

Name of Supervisor(s) & License(s) #: _____

_____

_____

Employer or Facility: _____

1	2–3		4–5		6	7
Year	Direct observation of the provision of OT services to patients/clients		Other supervision		Total hours supervision	Hours worked/ notes
	Hours	Supervisor's initials	Hours	Supervisor's initials		
Jan.						
Feb.						
March						
April						
May						
June						
July						
Aug.						
Sept.						
Oct.						
Nov.						
Dec.						

Supervision Log, Revised July 2001.

The Occupational Therapy Assistant: Resources for Practice and Education

- The Log is a good way to maintain a record of your supervision for your and your employer's records.
- Copy the blank log. Make as many copies as you need.
- Complete your documentation each month.

Licensees maintain and retain their own log. If you work for more than one employer, complete a separate log for each. Fill in your name, the year, and the name(s) of the supervising occupational therapist(s).

If you change supervisors during the year, either fill out a new Supervisor's Form, or write or fax the Board within 30 days. Information about a change of your address or work information must also be given to the Board within 30 days.

INSTRUCTIONS

In Columns 1, record the year reflected in this log.

In Columns 2 and 3, record the hours you are observed working directly with patients.

In Columns 4 and 5, record the number of hours of any other supervision (not the direct supervision), such as documentation and case review, telephone contact, email, etc. The supervising occupational therapist should sign.

In Column 6, record the total hours of supervision for that month—the sum of columns 2 and 4.

In Column 7 you can reflect the average or shorted workweek or notes to remind you of special circumstances.

SUPERVISION RULES
Read Chapter 373-Supervision

Supervision of a OTA With a
Temporary License

Sixteen (16) hours of supervision a month of which at least 12 hours are through telephone, written report, or conference, including the review of progress of patients/clients assigned, plus

Four (4) or more hours of supervision a month which are face-to-face, real-time supervision with the temporary licensee providing services to one or more patients/clients.

Supervision of a Licensed
Occupational Therapy Assistant

A minimum of six (6) hours a month of frequent communication with the supervising occupational therapist(s) and the occupational therapy assistant by telephone, written report, email, conference etc., including review of progress of patients/clients assigned, plus,

A minimum of two (2) hours of supervision a month of face-to-face, real-time interaction observing the occupational therapy assistant providing services with patients/clients.

- Part-time licensees may pro-rate these hours but shall document no less than 4 hours of supervision per month, 1 hour of which includes face-to-face, realtime interaction with patients.
- Check the website for changes in rules and other information at http://www.ecptote.state.tx.us

---

**Do not mail Supervision Log with your renewal,
retain for your records**

Supervision Log, Revised July 2001

A) A certified occupational therapy assistant shall practice only under the supervision of a registered occupational therapist. Supervision is a process in which 2 or more persons participate in a joint effort to establish, maintain, and elevate a level of performance and shall include the following criteria:

1. To maintain high standards of practice based on professional principles, supervision shall connote the physical presence of the supervisors and the assistant at regularly scheduled supervision sessions.

2. Supervision shall be provided in varying patterns as determined by the demands of the areas of patient/client service and the competency of the individual assistant. Such supervision shall be structured according to the assistant's qualifications, position, level of preparation, depth of experience, and the environment within which he/she functions.

3. The supervisors shall be responsible for the standard of work performed by the assistant and shall have knowledge of the patients/clients and the problems being discussed.

4. *A minimum guideline of formal supervision is as follows:*

   a. The occupational therapy assistant who has *less than 1 year of work experience or who is entering new practice environments or developing new skills shall receive a minimum of 5% on-site face-to-face supervision from a registered occupational therapist per month.* On-site supervision consists of direct, face-to-face collaboration in which the supervisor must be on the premises. The remaining work hours must be supervised.

   b. The occupational therapy assistant with *more than 1 year of experience in his/her current practice shall have a minimum of 5% direct supervision from a registered occupational therapist per month. The 5% direct supervision shall consist of 2% direct, face-to-face collaboration.* The remaining supervision shall be a combination of telephone or electronic communication or face-to-face consultation.

B) *Record Keeping.* It is the responsibility of the occupational therapy assistant to maintain on file at the job site signed documentation reflecting supervision activities. This supervision documentation shall contain the following: date of supervision, means of communication, information discussed, and the outcomes of the interaction. Both the supervising occupational therapist and the occupational therapy assistant must sign each entry.

(Source: Amended at 26 Ill. Reg. 18330, effective December 13, 2002)

SAMPLE—Occupational Therapy Assistant Supervision Log*

Name of Licensee:

License #:

Level of Experience:*

☐ Less than 1 year in current practice area   ☐ More than 1 year in current practice area

Name of Supervisor(s) and Licensure #:

Employer or Facility:

Year	Direct observation of the provision of OT services to individuals		Other supervision Ex: combination of telephone or electronic media or face-to-face communication		Total hours of supervision	Hours worked	Type/topic of supervision Example: Treatment discussion, service competency issues, documentation, etc...
200_	Time	Supervisor's initials	Time	Supervisor's initials			
January							
February							
March							
April							
May							
June							

(continued)

Year 200_	Direct observation of the provision of OT services to individuals		Other supervision Ex: combination of telephone or electronic media or face-to-face communication		Total hours of supervision	Hours worked	Type/topic of supervision Example: Treatment discussion, service competency issues, documentation, etc...
	Time	Supervisor's initials	Time	Supervisor's initials			
July							
August							
September							
October							
November							
December							

Comments:

_____

_____

_____

Refer to the IDPR Occupational Therapy Practice Act—Rule Section #1315.163

The Occupational Therapy Assistant: Resources for Practice and Education

Chapter 13

Forging OTA–OT Partnerships That Work

With rapid changes in health care on the horizon, we as occupational therapy practitioners must solidify our positions by performing our jobs as efficiently and effectively as possible. And one key to accomplishing this goal is by establishing strong and effective OTA–OT partnerships.

The profession as a whole must recognize the value of OTAs in such partnerships if we are to provide quality health care services. And it is equally important for occupational therapy practitioners to understand the individual roles of each player in the partnership. According to the "OT Roles Document," such understanding must encompass knowledge of *major functions* (primary purpose of the role), *scope of role* (delineating the range of responsibility and complexity that typically occurs within the role), and *key performance areas* (common activities and expectations associated with role function).

It is important to note that the OTA–OT relationship is one of partnership, not one of power and intimidation. It should be built on mutual respect and trust and based on accountability. In effective OTA–OT partnership, the skills of each practitioner should be enhanced by the other. This type of partnership allows each practitioner to use their capabilities and skills optimally. Members of a partnership have a common goal—to provide the best occupational therapy services possible to each client effectively and safely—and both must contribute toward that goal.

Partnerships, like individuals, are unique; what works for one team may not work for another. Since it is unlikely you will remain in a single relationship throughout your career, the need to establish and reestablish partnerships can be a continuing process. Here are a few key points on how to successfully foster effective and rewarding OTA–OT partnerships:

1. *Trust and respect*—A strong knowledge of your partner's background and a genuine positive regard for differences each practitioner brings to the relationship are an excellent starting point. It also helps to be in touch with your own strengths and weaknesses, your limits and abilities, and your needs and desires—a lifelong process for some of us. In addition, it is vital that each partner clearly understands the role of the other in a given situation and respects the differences in these roles.

While it is a fact that OTAs work under the supervision of an OT, members of each partnership must establish how this relationship will play out in a clinical setting—keeping in mind state regulations, facility policies, and AOTA standards of practice.

2. *Communication*—This is a key element in any successful partnership. In their time of uncertainty and discomfort, our clients look to us for a sense of safety, trust, support, and understanding. We learn to adapt on an individual basis our communication with clients so as to maximize the benefits of our interventions. The same communication skills are necessary in the interaction between an OTA and an OT working as a team.

Only about 30% of communication between individuals is verbal; the majority occurs on the nonverbal level. If members of an OT–OTA partnership can achieve effective communication on the verbal and nonverbal levels, they can avoid second guessing one another or filling in the gaps with assumptions—practices that increase the risk of harming, rather than helping, our clients.

3. *Responsibility and accountability*—There are numerous guidelines to consider in the process of the OTA–OT supervision. It is the responsibility of each individual to keep abreast of the guidelines. It is equally important for each individual to take responsibility for the supervision process. When I refer to supervision, I am referring to a process well beyond co-signing notes and discussion of patient care plans. In the eyes of AOTA, supervision has a much greater role in professional and personal development. According to AOTA's *Guide for Supervision of Occupational Therapy Personnel in the Delivery of Occupational Therapy Services* (AOTA, 1999), *supervision* is defined as a "mutual undertaking between the super-

visor and the supervisee that fosters growth and development; assures appropriate utilization of training and potential; encourages creativity and innovation; and provides guidance, education, support, encouragement, and respect while working toward a goal. In a truly healthy partnership, this type of supervision is a two-way street that benefits both parties personally and professionally.

In a time of uncertainty and changes in health care, practitioners may feel that their jobs or positions are threatened. There is enough pressure from other disciplines challenging our role as OT practitioners. We need to focus on dissolving this threat if we are to better our position in this difficult marketplace.

With a clear understanding of the roles and better utilization of the OTA and OT, we can more effectively and efficiently serve our clients' needs. Both parties in a partnership must strive to achieve this understanding if the collaboration is to succeed. We must confront the changing health care environment provocatively and demonstrate to others that our system is better with the OTA–OT partnership than without.

Reference

American Occupational Therapy Association. (1999). Guide for supervision of occupational therapy personnel in the delivery of occupational therapy services. *American Journal of Occupational Therapy, 53.*

Originally published as Campbell, K. J. (1998). OTA focus: Forging OTA–OT partnerships that work. *OT Week, 12*(21), 10.

Chapter 14

Medicare Supervision Requirements for Reimbursement

When determining the level of supervision required, consider two sources. First, check your state practice act and regulations. Second, check the policy of the patient's payer. You must comply with both policies. If one policy requires a more stringent level of supervision, then you must follow that guidance.

—AOTA Reimbursement and Regulatory Policy Department

Setting/Payer	Assistant	Medicare Coverage of Services Provided by Therapy Students	Type and Level of Supervision of Student Required
Medicare Part A *Hospital and Inpatient Rehabilitation*	General supervision.	HCFA has not issued specific rules.	HCFA has not issued specific rules. See relevant state law for further guidance on supervision for the services to be considered occupational therapy.
Medicare Part A *Skilled-Nursing Facility (SNF)*	General supervision. OT must be accessible while the assistant is providing services to the beneficiary. The OTA cannot supervise a therapy aide.	The minutes of therapy services provided by Occupational Therapy and Occupational Therapy Assistant students may be recorded on the MDS as minutes of therapy received by the beneficiary.	Services of Occupational Therapy and Occupational Therapy Assistant students must be provided in the "line of sight" of the Occupational Therapist. Occupational Therapy Assistants can provide clinical supervision to OTA students; however, if the services are to be recorded for payment purposes, they must be performed in "line of sight" of an Occupational Therapist.
Medicare Part A *Hospice*		HCFA has not issued specific rules.	HCFA has not issued specific rules. See relevant state law for further guidance on supervision for the services to be considered occupational therapy.
Medicare Part B *Partial Hospitalization*		HCFA has not issued specific rules.	HCFA has not issued specific rules. See relevant state law for further guidance on supervision for the services to be considered occupational therapy.
Medicare Part A *Home Health*	General supervision.	Regulations (§484.115) specifically cite definitions for "qualified personnel," which do not include students. However, HCFA has not issued specific restrictions regarding students providing services in conjunction with a qualified Occupational Therapist or Occupational Therapy Assistant.	Services by students can be provided (as allowed by state law) as part of a home health visit, when the student is supervised by an Occupational Therapist or Occupational Therapy Assistant in the home.
Medicare Part B *Private Practice, Hospital Outpatient, SNF, CORF, ORF, Rehabilitation agency, and other Part B providers including home health agencies when providing Part B services*	General supervision.	Medicare does not cover services of students provided to patients receiving occupational therapy under the Part B outpatient benefit. Outpatient therapy services are defined as direct, one-to-one patient services provided by the practitioner.	No level of supervision is adequate to allow for payment of student services under Part B.

Chapter 15

HIPAA Guidelines for Fieldwork

Per HIPAA guidelines, students cannot report this information in fieldwork assignments such as case studies presentations:

- Name
- Location—includes anything smaller than a state, such as street address
- Dates—all, including date of birth, admission, and discharge dates
- Telephone numbers
- Fax numbers
- Electronic e-mail addresses
- Social security numbers
- Medical record numbers
- Health plan beneficiary numbers
- Account numbers
- Certificate and/or license numbers
- Vehicle identification numbers and license plate numbers
- Device identifiers and their serial numbers
- Web universal resource locators (URLs)
- Internet protocol (IP) address numbers
- Biometric identifiers, including finger and voice prints
- Full-face photographic images and any comparable images
- Any other unique identifying number, characteristic, or code.

For written reports, the following information *can* be shared:

- Age (ages 90 and older must be aggregated to prevent the identification of older individuals)
- Race
- Ethnicity
- Marital status
- Codes (a random code may be used to link cases, as long as the code does not contain, or be a derivative of, e.g., the person's social security number, date of birth, phone/fax numbers).

Students, as well as practitioners, often keep "working files" in their desk. This is still allowed under HIPAA guidelines; however, this information must be locked in a file cabinet when not in use and must be shredded when no longer needed.

PART III

Reimbursement

The majority of occupational therapy clients rely on federal or state reimbursement to receive occupational therapy services. After state regulatory laws and rules, practitioners must follow reimbursement rules, because they are written into federal and state statutes. Major reimbursers of occupational therapy services include but are not limited to Medicare Parts A and B, Medicaid; Early Intervention Programs; 3–21 Programs in the schools and community; state developmental disabilities or mental health programs; and CHAMPUS/TRICARE.

Medicare offers specific supervision language for occupational therapy assistants:

> Only a qualified occupational therapist has the knowledge, training, and experience required to evaluate and, as necessary, re-evaluate a patient's level of function; determine whether an OT program could reasonably be expected to improve, restore, or compensate for loss of function; and where appropriate, recommend to the physician a plan of treatment. However, while the skills of a qualified occupational therapist are required to evaluate the patient's level of function and develop a plan of treatment, a qualified occupational therapy assistant functioning under the general supervision of the qualified occupational therapist may also carry out the implementation of a plan. General supervision "requires initial direction and periodic inspection of the actual activity." However, the supervisor need not always be physically present or on the premises when the assistant is performing the services." (Medicare, Intermediary Benefits, Sec. 3101.9(7))

Medicare requires that occupational therapists be involved with a client from start to finish of services. Occupational therapy assistants can implement a plan under general supervision. Even though the occupational therapist is considered the qualified professional completing assessments, the occupational therapy assistant can contribute parts of the assessment as long as the therapist is completing aspects, directing process, interpreting results, and developing the plan. Assistants may work with patients under Medicare if the team and administration establish standardized protocols and competency assessments that could be used by the occupational therapy assistants.

For the Medicare SNF PPS, physical and occupational therapy assistants may provide rehabilitation services under the supervision of a professional therapist who is accessible while the assistant is providing those services to the client. The therapy assistant cannot supervise a therapy aide. The professional therapist is responsible for ensuring that the assistant is capable of performing therapy services without the more stringent "line-of-sight" level of supervision required for therapy aides.

Medicare requirements have changed related to occupational therapy assistants in private practice. The American Occupational Therapy Association (AOTA) was successful in working with the Centers for Medicare and Medicaid in removing the requirement for close, in-sight supervision for occupational therapy assistants, who now can operate under general supervision. This was a victory for occupational therapy assistants and an excellent example of the benefits of belonging to occupational therapy's professional organization.

For Medicaid, each state varies in its supervision language. Occupational therapy assistants are encouraged to contact their state for specifics. Medicaid now is a reimbursement source for qualified children in school, which is a major area of occupational therapy employment.

Occupational therapy assistants also can rely on AOTA's Reimbursement Department for the most up-to-date information, especially changes in reimbursement and regulations and how these may affect occupational therapy (check www.aota.org for updates). AOTA lobbies to ensure that occupational therapy is a covered service and has been successful in delaying implementation of a moratorium on the $1,500 Medicare cap on occupational therapy services.

The following resources can help occupational therapy assistants manage the complexities of reimbursement:

- Chapter 16. Reimbursement for OTA Services
- Chapter 17. Guidelines for Documentation of Occupational Therapy
- Chapter 18. Sample Medicare Forms
- Chapter 19. Sample Occupational Therapy Assistant Supervision Grid
- Chapter 20. Medicare SNF PPS and Consolidated Billing
- Chapter 21. State Medicaid Offices, Health Departments, and Workers' Compensation Departments
- Chapter 22. Regulations for OTAs Using *CPT* Codes.

Chapter 16

Reimbursement for OTA Services

Do All Third-Party Payers Have the Same Rules Pertaining to the Coverage of and Payment for Occupational Therapy Services?

No. In fact there is little consistency from payer to payer in the types of services covered, who they consider qualified to provide services and how they pay. Most public payers, like Medicare, Medicaid, and CHAMPUS, have some written guidelines that can be obtained from public sources. For private payers, each must be contacted individually in order to understand their rules.

Medicare

Medicare, a Federal entitlement program providing health insurance to the elderly and people with disabilities, publishes national coverage rules. However, the Centers for Medicare and Medicaid Services (CMS), the agency that regulates Medicare, invests authority for administration of a large portion of the Medicare program to local insurance companies. For traditional Medicare enrollees, *Fiscal Intermediaries* (FIs) provide medical review services and pay claims for services provided by all "institutional" providers, including hospitals, home health agencies, and nursing homes. Medicare contractors who provide the same function for physicians and occupational therapists in private practice are referred to as *Carriers*. In addition, Medicare beneficiaries may enroll in a variety of *Medicare Advantage Plans* (MCPs), including managed care and other options. Each FI, carrier, and MCP can develop its own local coverage guidelines within the scope of national rules.

Medicaid

Medicaid, a joint Federal–State program for low-income individuals, is largely implemented by State policy. Each State has a Medicaid office from which to get information. Also, many States have contracted with individual *managed care health plans* to deliver care to a portion or all of their Medicaid populations. These plans, thus, have the authority to determine specific rules by which Medicaid members receive care within guidance set by the state.

Other Public Health Programs

There are other state and federal health care programs through which your patients may receive services. For example, the U. S. Department of Defense determines overall policies for CHAMPUS/TRICARE, the health plan for civilian dependents of military personnel. In addition, a large segment of the U.S. population receives health care under the Federal Employees Health Benefit Program (FEHBP) operated by the Office of Personnel Management (OPM), but administered by a wide range of insurance companies. Many states provide specific services under the authority of the health department, and some have started new programs to provide health care access to children under the State Child Health Insurance Program (SCHIP), which is a joint effort with the federal government. Each state also manages its own workers compensation program through a state board or commission.

Private Insurers

The term "private insurer" can refer to any non-governmental entity that provides or administers health care plans, including Blue Cross plans, commercial insurers, and any type of managed care organization. Each private insurer generally offers a wide range of insurance products to employers. Therefore, a Blue Cross plan offered by one employer will not necessarily provide the same coverage as that of another employer who contracts with the same Blue Cross plan. Health care practitioners should always ascertain the exact plan coverage and limitations for each patient before assuming that services will be paid by insurance.

What Do I Need to Know About Supervision Requirements?

First, you need to know the laws in your state regarding practice. No matter what other requirements a payer may have, you must always comply with state regulation. Recent Medicare changes have clarified supervision requirements across settings. In Medicare settings, an occupational therapy assistant must practice under the "general" supervision (i.e., initial direction and periodic inspection) of an occupational therapist. That is, the therapist must be accessible while the assistant is providing services. The American Occupational Therapy Association (AOTA) interprets accessibility to include situations where the therapist is not on-site, but can be easily reached by phone, pager, etc.

Before providing services to patients with other State-based (e.g., workers compensation, Medicaid) or private insurance, you should obtain specific information from the payer regarding credentialing of practitioners and supervision requirements.

What Do I Need to Know About Coding and Billing?

Most medical payers require two types of codes, diagnoses and procedures. The diagnosis coding most used in the United States is the *International Classification of Diseases, 9th Revision, Clinical Modification*, more commonly called *ICD-9-CM*. These codes describe diseases, conditions, symptoms, or other bases for medical services. Generally, occupational therapy practitioners should use *ICD-9-CM* codes that relate to the reason for therapy. Since most diagnosis codes are medically, not functionally oriented, occupational therapy practitioners should assure that their documentation reflects the functional relationship between the diagnosis and treatment provided.

The *Current Procedural Terminology (CPT)* is the most widely used procedure system. Occupational therapy professionals generally use the Physical Medicine and Rehabilitation (PM&R) section of codes to describe treatment. If you are required to provide CPT codes for your services, you should always ask for a list of preferred codes for each payer being billed. The *CPT* is updated every year, but not all payers update their systems to accommodate new and revised codes. Medicare always requires the current version of *CPT*. Your billing department may be able to help you obtain the correct coding information for each payer.

What Questions Should I Ask an Insurer to Find Out What I Need to Know?

When trying to get answers from a government agency or a private company, the most difficult activity is finding the person who has the answers. This often means spending time speaking to many different people. Most private companies have a Provider Relations Department, which is a good place to start. Your billing department may already have information or contact names within each payer organization that they bill.

Your first step should be to ask for whatever packet of information they provide to prospective providers and members. This may answer many of your questions. Also, after you have read this material, you will understand the company better and know what answers were not provided. When you can say, "I read your material before calling," it is then easier to get information over the phone. When speaking to an insurer, always ask for the person's name. Following are some of the facts that you need to help you begin a dialogue with an insurer.

- What is the insurer's definition of occupational therapy?
- What specific credentials do they require for occupational therapy practitioners?
- Do they have a specific list of codes that providers should use to bill for occupational therapy services?
- Do they have any specific requirements for supervision or documentation of occupational therapy?
  If contact is a Medicare intermediary or carrier,
- Have they developed any local medical review policy for occupational therapy or for services that are likely to be provided by occupational therapy practitioners?

What About the Balanced Budget Act of 1997?

The Balanced Budget Act of 1997 (BBA) made many critical and important changes to modernize payment under Medicare. Following is a general summary of the most significant changes of the BBA affecting occupational therapy practitioners. However, policy changes occur frequently and readers are encouraged to monitor the AOTA Web site, OT Practice, and other resources to stay apprised of specific Medicare requirements in their areas of practice.

Skilled Nursing Facility (SNF), Part A Services

For those Medicare patients who qualify for the skilled nursing facility benefit, payment for all care, including rehabilitation services, is now made under a prospective payment system (PPS). Under the PPS, patients are classified into broad Resource Utilization Groups (RUG) based on each person's minimum data set assessment. SNFs are paid a per diem amount which has been computed for each RUG category. The SNF must provide all necessary services to a patient, but receives no more than the designated per diem rate for a set period of time.

Outpatient (Including SNF Part B)

The BBA requires that all Medicare Part B therapy (OT, PT, and SLP) be coded using *CPT* codes and, beginning January 1, 1999 be paid under a fee schedule. HCFA has adopted use of the Medicare Physician Fee Schedule, under which OTs in private practice have been paid since 1992. The fee schedule now applies to all outpatient therapy, including Part B services for patients residing in nursing homes who do not qualify for the SNF Part A benefit.

Additionally, the BBA imposed a $1,500 per patient per year cap on OT services and a $1,500 cap on PT/SLP combined services for treatment received in all settings except hospital outpatient departments. However, the cap has not yet been fully implemented.

Home Health Benefit

Several interim changes were proscribed by the BBA for home health services, including an aggregate per patient cap. Congress required a home health prospective payment system be in place by October 2000. Therapy services provided to patients who do not qualify for the home health benefit (e.g., not homebound or do not need nursing, physical therapy, or speech-language pathology) by a HHA are considered Medicare outpatient services and subject to the outpatient Part B rules.

Other Rehabilitation Settings

Payment changes continue to occur. It is clear that we can expect many major Medicare changes over the next several years, as CMS attempts to assure appropriate utilization and payment.

How Can I Stay Up-to-Date on Reimbursement Issues?

Reimbursement policies change frequently. Each year Congress enacts new or amended laws that affect the amounts that providers are paid for occupational therapy and other health care services. As government agencies, such as the CMS (for Medicare and Federal Medicaid) and U.S. Department of Defense (for CHAMPUS/TRICARE), develop regulations to implement these laws, details become available through daily public notices in the *Federal Register*.

Health care program changes by states (e.g., Workers' Compensation, Medicaid, Child Health Insurance) occur in a similar way. The state legislature passes laws that are implemented by state agencies, such as the health department, insurance commission, or Medicaid. States also have a *State Register* in which notices of proposed regulatory changes are published. If you have trouble finding resources in your state, check your public library for information. Your state legislator or representative's office also should be able to help you locate the correct state or county office.

Additional sources of health care policy and program changes are

CMS, www.cms.gov

CHAMPUS/TRICARE, www.ochampus.mil/

Federal Employers Health Benefit Program, www.opm.gov/insure/98/index.htm

U.S. Government Printing Office (*Federal Register* notices and other public records), www.gpo.gov

State Governments: Most states have a Web site that may include links to government sites, such as the state legislature, insurance commission, or health department.

Individual Blue Cross and Blue Shield plans and commercial insurance companies, such as AETNA and Prudential, may have Web sites that provide information about their plans or names of staff to whom you can address questions.

Chapter 17

Guidelines for Documentation of Occupational Therapy

Documentation is necessary whenever professional services are provided to a client. Occupational therapists and occupational therapy assistants under the supervision of an occupational therapist determine the appropriate type of documentation and document the services provided within their scope of practice. This document, based on the *Occupational Therapy Practice Framework: Domain and Process* (American Occupational Therapy Association [AOTA], 2002), describes the components and the purpose of professional documentation used in occupational therapy. AOTA's *Standards of Practice for Occupational Therapy* (1998) state: "An occupational therapy practitioner documents the occupational therapy services provided within the time frames, format, and standards established by the practice settings, agencies, external accreditation programs, and payers." In this document, *client* may refer to an individual, family/caregivers, group, or population.

The purpose of documentation is to

- Articulate the rationale for provision of occupational therapy services and the relationship of this service to the client's outcomes
- Reflect the therapist's clinical reasoning and professional judgment
- Communicate information about the client from the occupational therapy perspective
- Create a chronological record of client status, occupational therapy services provided to the client, and client outcomes.

Types of Documentation

The following box outlines common types of reports. Depending on the service delivery and setting, reports may be named differently or combined and reorganized to meet the specific needs of the setting. Occupational therapy documentation should always record the professional's activity in the areas of evaluation, intervention, and outcomes (AOTA, 2002).

Process Areas	Type of Report
I. Evaluation	A. Evaluation or Screening Report
	B. Reevaluation Report
II. Intervention	A. Intervention Plan
	B. Occupational Therapy Service Contacts
	C. Progress Report
	D. Transition Plan
III. Outcomes	A. Discharge/Discontinuation Report

Content of Reports

I. Evaluation

  A. Evaluation or Screening Report

    1. Documents the referral source and data gathered through the evaluation process. Includes

      a. Description of the client's occupational profile

      b. Analysis of occupational performance and identification of factors that hinder and support performance in areas of occupation

      c. Delineation of specific areas of occupation that will be targeted for intervention and outcomes expected.

    2. An abbreviated evaluation process (e.g., screening) documents only limited areas of occupation applicable to the client and to the situation.

    3. Suggested content with examples:

      a. *Client information*—name/agency, date of birth, gender, applicable medical/educational/developmental diagnoses, precautions, and contraindications

      b. *Referral information*—date and source of referral, services requested, reason for referral, funding source, and anticipated length of service

      c. *Occupational profile*—client's reason for seeking occupational therapy services, current areas of occupation that are successful and areas that are problematic, contexts that support or hinder occupations, medical/educational/work history, occupational history (e.g., patterns of living, interest, values), client's priorities, and targeted outcomes

  d. *Assessments used and results*—types of assessments used and results (e.g., interviews, record reviews, observations, and standardized or nonstandardized assessments), description of the client factors, contextual aspects or features of the activities that facilitate or inhibit performance, and confidence in test results

  e. *Summary and analysis*—interpretation and summary of data as it is related to occupational profile and referring concern

  f. *Recommendation*—judgment regarding appropriateness of occupational therapy services or other services **Note:** Intervention goals addressing anticipated outcomes, objectives, and frequency of therapy are listed on the Intervention Plan.

B. Reevaluation Report
 1. Documents the results of the reevaluation process. Frequency of reevaluation depends upon the needs of the setting and the progress of the client.
 2. Suggested content with examples:
  a. *Client information*—name/agency, date of birth, gender, applicable medical/educational/developmental diagnoses, precautions, and contraindications
  b. *Occupational profile*—updates on current areas of occupation that are successful and that are problematic, contexts that support or hinder occupations, summary of any new medical/educational/work information, and updates or changes to client's priorities and targeted outcomes
  c. *Reevaluation results*—focus of reevaluation, specific types of assessments used, and client's performance and subjective responses
  d. *Summary and analysis*—interpretation and summary of data as related to referring concern, and comparison of results with previous evaluation results
  e. *Recommendations*—changes to occupational therapy services, revision or continuation of goals and objectives, frequency of occupational therapy services, and recommendation for referral to other professionals or agencies where applicable.

II. Intervention
 A. Intervention Plan
  1. Documents the goals, intervention approaches, and types of interventions to be used to achieve the client's identified targeted outcomes based on results of evaluation or reevaluation processes. Includes recommendations or referrals to other professionals and agencies.
  2. Suggested content with examples:
   a. *Client information*—name/agency, date of birth, gender, precautions, and contraindications
   b. *Intervention goals*—measurable goals and short-term objectives directly related to the client's ability to engage in desired occupations
   c. *Intervention approaches and types of interventions to be used*—intervention approaches that include: create/promote, establish/restore, maintain, modify, and prevent; types of interventions that include: consultation process, education process, therapeutic use of activities to enhance occupation, and therapeutic use of self
   d. *Service delivery mechanisms*—service provider, service location, and frequency and duration of services
   e. *Plan for discharge*—discontinuation criteria, location of discharge, and follow-up care
   f. *Outcome measures*—outcomes that include improved occupational performance, client satisfaction, role competence, improved health and wellness, prevention of further difficulties, and improved quality of life
   g. *Professionals responsible and date of plan*—names and positions of persons overseeing intervention plan, date plan was developed, and date when plan was modified or reviewed.
 B. Occupational Therapy Service Contacts
  1. Documents contacts between the client and the occupational therapist or the occupational therapy assistant. Records the types of interventions used and client's response. Includes telephone contacts, interventions, and meetings with others.
  2. Suggested content with examples:
   a. *Client information*—name/agency, date of birth, gender, diagnosis, precautions, and contraindications
   b. *Therapy log*—date, type of contact, names/positions of persons involved, summary or significant information communicated during contacts, client attendance and participation in

intervention, reason service is missed, types of interventions used, client's response, environmental or task modification, assistive or adaptive devices used or fabricated, statement of any training education or consultation provided, and the persons present.

C. Progress Report
1. Summarizes intervention process and documents client's progress toward goals achievement. Includes new data collected; modifications of treatment plan; and statement of need for continuation, discontinuation, or referral.
2. Suggested content with examples:
   a. *Client information*—name/agency, date of birth, gender, diagnosis, precautions, and contraindications
   b. *Summary of services provided*—brief statement of frequency of services and length of time services have been provided; techniques and strategies used; environmental or task modifications provided; adaptive equipment or orthotics provided; medical, educational, or other pertinent client updates; client's response to occupational therapy services; and programs or training provided to the client or caregivers
   c. *Current client performance*—client's progress toward the goals, and client's performance in areas of occupations
   d. *Plan or recommendations*—recommendations and rationale as well as client's input to changes or continuation of plan.

D. Transition Plan
1. Documents the formal transition plan and is written when client is transitioning from one service setting to another within a service delivery system.
2. Suggested content with examples:
   a. *Client information*—name/agency, date of birth, gender, diagnosis, precautions, and contraindications
   b. *Client's current status*—client's current performance in occupations
   c. *Transition plan*—name of current service setting and name of setting to which client will transition, reason for transition, time frame in which transition will occur, and outline of activities to be carried out during the transition plan
   d. *Recommendations*—recommendations and rationale for occupational therapy services, modifications or accommodations needed, and assistive technology and environmental modifications needed.

III. Outcomes
A. Discharge Report—Summary of Occupational Therapy Services and Outcomes
1. Summarize the changes in client's ability to engage in occupations between the initial evaluation and discontinuation of services and make recommendations as applicable
2. Suggested content with examples:
   a. *Client information*—name/agency, date of birth, gender, diagnosis, precautions, and contraindications
   b. *Summary of intervention process*—date of initial and final service; frequency, number of sessions, summary of interventions used; summary of progress toward goals; and occupational therapy outcomes—initial client status and ending status regarding engagement in occupations, client's assessment of efficacy of occupational therapy services
   c. *Recommendations*—recommendations pertaining to the client's future needs; specific follow-up plans, if applicable; and referrals to other professionals and agencies, if applicable.

APPENDIX A. Fundamental Elements of Documentation

Each occupational therapy client has a client record maintained as a permanent file. The record is maintained in a professional and legal fashion (i.e., organized, legible, concise, clear, accurate, complete, current, grammatically correct, and objective). The following elements are present in all documentation:

1. Client's full name and case number (if applicable) on each page of documentation
2. Date and type of occupational therapy contact
3. Identification of type of documentation, agency, and department name
4. Occupational therapist's or occupational therapy assistant's signature with a minimum of first name or initial, last name, and professional designation
5. When applicable on notes or reports, signature of the recorder directly at the end of the note without space left between the body of the note and the signature
6. Countersignature by an occupational therapist on documentation written by students and occupational therapy assistants when required by law or the facility
7. Acceptable terminology defined within the boundaries of setting
8. Abbreviations usage as acceptable within the boundaries of setting

9. When no facility requirements are listed, errors corrected by drawing a single line through an error and by initialing the correction (liquid correction fluid and erasures are not acceptable)
10. Adherence to professional standards of technology, when used to document occupational therapy services
11. Disposal of records within law or agency requirements
12. Compliance with confidentiality standards
13. Compliance with agency or legal requirements of storage of records.

References

American Occupational Therapy Association. (2002). Occupational therapy practice framework: Domain and process. *American Journal of Occupational Therapy, 56,* 609–639.

American Occupational Therapy Association. (1998). Standards of practice for occupational therapy. *American Journal of Occupational Therapy, 52,* 866–869.

Authors

Gloria Frolek Clark, MS, OTR/L, FAOTA
Mary Jane Youngstrom, MS, OTR/L, FAOTA

for

COMMISSION ON PRACTICE
Sara Jane Brayman, PhD, OTR/L, FAOTA, Chairperson

Adopted by the Representative Assembly 2003M16

This document replaces the 1994 *Elements of Clinical Documentation* (previously published and copyrighted in 1995 by the *American Journal of Occupational Therapy, 49,* 1032–1035).

Chapter 18

Sample Medicare Forms

Occupational therapy assistants can fill out the CMS-700/701 forms if there is sufficient written treatment plan information. Medicare coverage rules state that the occupational therapist is primarily responsible for evaluating the patient and developing the treatment plan. If an occupational therapy assistant completes the form, the countersignature of the occupational therapist is an indicator to Medicare that the occupational therapist carried out the evaluation/reevaluation. Effective July 1, 2003, CMS no longer requires the use of the CMS-700/701 form for reporting purposes, because patient plan of care information must already be included in the patient's medical record. Any written format or variation of this form may be used as long as all the required information is identifiable to the payer for reimbursement purposes.

CPT is a trademark of the American Medical Association. All *CPT* codes, descriptions, numeric modifiers, instructions, and other materials are copyrighted by the American Medical Association.

The following are sample CMS-700/701 forms.

PLAN OF TREATMENT FOR OUTPATIENT REHABILITATION
(COMPLETE FOR INITIAL CLAIMS ONLY)

1. PATIENT'S LAST NAME	FIRST NAME	M.I.	2. PROVIDER NO.	3. HICN
4. PROVIDER NAME	5. MEDICAL RECORD NO. *(Optional)*		6. ONSET DATE	7. SOC. DATE

8. TYPE	9. PRIMARY DIAGNOSIS *(Pertinent Medical D.X.)*	10. TREATMENT DIAGNOSIS	11. VISITS FROM SOC.
☐ PT ☐ OT ☐ SLP ☐ CR ☐ RT ☐ PS ☐ SN ☐ SW			

12. PLAN OF TREATMENT FUNCTIONAL GOALS

GOALS *(Short Term)*

OUTCOME *(Long Term)*

PLAN

13. SIGNATURE *(professional establishing POC including prof. designation)*

14. FREQ/DURATION *(e.g., 3/Wk. x 4 Wk.)*

I CERTIFY THE NEED FOR THESE SERVICES FURNISHED UNDER THIS PLAN OF TREATMENT AND WHILE UNDER MY CARE ☐ N/A

15. PHYSICIAN SIGNATURE

16. DATE

17. CERTIFICATION

FROM   THROUGH   N/A

18. ON FILE *(Print/type physician's name)*
☐

20. INITIAL ASSESSMENT *(History, medical complications, level of function at start of care. Reason for referral.)*

19. PRIOR HOSPITALIZATION

FROM   TO   N/A

21. FUNCTIONAL LEVEL *(End of billing period)* PROGRESS REPORT   ☐ CONTINUE SERVICES **OR**   ☐ DC SERVICES

22. SERVICE DATES
FROM   THROUGH

Form CMS-700-(11-91)

INSTRUCTIONS FOR COMPLETION OF FORM CMS-700

(Enter dates as 6 digits, month, day, year)

1. **Patient's Name** - Enter the patient's last name, first name and middle initial as shown on the health insurance Medicare card.

2. **Provider Number** - Enter the number issued by Medicare to the billing provider *(i.e., 00–7000)*.

3. **HICN** - Enter the patient's health insurance number as shown on the health insurance Medicare card, certification award, utilization notice, temporary eligibility notice, or as reported by SSO.

4. **Provider Name** - Enter the name of the Medicare billing provider.

5. **Medical Record No.** - *(optional)* Enter the patient's medical/clinical record number used by the billing provider.

6. **Onset Date** - Enter the date of onset for the patient's primary medical diagnosis, if it is a new diagnosis, or the date of the most recent exacerbation of a previous diagnosis. If the exact date is not known enter 01 for the day *(i.e., 120191)*. The date matches occurrence code 11 on the UB-92.

7. **SOC** *(start of care)* **Date** - Enter the date services began at the billing provider (the date of the first Medicare billable visit which **remains the same on subsequent claims** until discharge or denial corresponds to occurrence code 35 for PT, 44 for OT, 45 for SLP and 46 for CR on the UB-92).

8. **Type** - Check the type therapy billed; i.e., physical therapy (PT), occupational therapy (OT), speech-language pathology (SLP), cardiac rehabilitation (CR), respiratory therapy (RT), psychological services (PS), skilled nursing services (SN), or social services (SW).

9. **Primary Diagnosis** - Enter the pertinent written medical diagnosis resulting in the therapy disorder and relating to 50% or more of effort in the plan of treatment.

10. **Treatment Diagnosis** - Enter the written treatment diagnosis for which services are rendered. For example, for PT the primary medical diagnosis might be Degeneration of Cervical Intervertebral Disc while the PT treatment DX might be Frozen R Shoulder or, for SLP, while CVA might be the primary medical DX, the treatment DX might be Aphasia. If the same as the primary DX enter SAME.

11. **Visits From Start of Care** - Enter the **cumulative total** visits *(sessions)* completed since services were started at the billing provider for the diagnosis treated, through the last visit on this bill. *(Corresponds to UB-92 value code 50 for PT, 51 for OT, 52 for SLP, or 53 for cardiac rehab.)*

12. **Plan of Treatment/Functional Goals** - Enter brief current plan of treatment goals for the patient for this billing period. Enter the major short-term goals to reach overall long-term outcome. Enter the major plan of treatment to reach stated goals and outcome. Estimate time-frames to reach goals, when possible.

13. **Signature** - Enter the signature *(or name)* and the professional designation of the professional establishing the plan of treatment.

14. **Frequency/Duration** - Enter the current frequency and duration of your treatment; e.g., 3 times per week for 4 weeks is entered 3/Wk x 4Wk.

15. **Physician's Signature** - If the form CMS-700 is used for certification, the physician enters his/her signature. **If certification is required and the form is not being used for certification, check the ON FILE box in item 18.** If the certification is not required for the type service rendered, check the N/A box.

16. **Date** - Enter the date of the physician's signature only if the form is used for certification.

17. **Certification** - Enter the inclusive dates of the certification, **even if the ON FILE box is checked in item 18.** Check the N/A box if certification is not required.

18. **ON FILE** (Means certification signature and date) - Enter the **typed/printed name of the physician** who certified the plan of treatment that is on file at the billing provider. If certification is not required for the type of service checked in item 8, type/print the name of the physician who referred or ordered the service, **but do not check the ON FILE box.**

19. **Prior Hospitalization** - Enter the inclusive dates of recent hospitalization *(1st to DC day)* **pertinent** to the patient's current plan of treatment. Enter N/A if the hospital stay does not relate to the rehabilitation being rendered.

20. **Initial Assessment** - Enter only **current relevant history** from records or patient interview. Enter the major functional limitations stated, if possible, in objective measurable terms. Include only relevant surgical procedures, prior hospitalization and/or therapy for the same condition. Include only pertinent baseline tests and measurements from which to judge future progress or lack of progress.

21. **Functional Level** (end of billing period) - Enter the pertinent progress made and functional levels obtained at the end of the billing period compared to levels shown on initial assessment. Use objective terminology. Date progress when function can be consistently performed. When only a few visits have been made, enter a note indicating the training/treatment rendered and the patient's response if there is no change in function.

22. **Service Dates** - Enter the From and Through dates which represent this billing period *(should be monthly)*. Match the From and Through dates in field 6 on the UB-92. DO NOT use 00 in the date. Example: 01 08 91 for January 8, 1991.

The Occupational Therapy Assistant: Resources for Practice and Education

UPDATED PLAN OF PROGRESS FOR OUTPATIENT REHABILITATION

(Complete for Interim to Discharge Claims. Photocopy of CMS-700 or 701 is required.)

1. PATIENT'S LAST NAME	FIRST NAME	M.I.	2. PROVIDER NO.	3. HICN

4. PROVIDER NAME	5. MEDICAL RECORD NO. *(Optional)*	6. ONSET DATE	7. SOC. DATE

8. TYPE ☐ PT ☐ OT ☐ SLP ☐ CR ☐ RT ☐ PS ☐ SN ☐ SW	9. PRIMARY DIAGNOSIS *(Pertinent Medical D.X.)*	10. TREATMENT DIAGNOSIS	11. VISITS FROM SOC.
	12. FREQ/DURATION *(e.g., 3/Wk. x 4 Wk.)*		

13. CURRENT PLAN UPDATE, FUNCTIONAL GOALS *(Specify changes to goals and plan.)*

GOALS *(Short Term)*

PLAN

OUTCOME *(Long Term)*

I HAVE REVIEWED THIS PLAN OF TREATMENT AND RECERTIFY A CONTINUING NEED FOR SERVICES. ☐ N/A ☐ DC	14. RECERTIFICATION FROM THROUGH N/A
15. PHYSICIAN'S SIGNATURE	16. DATE	17. ON FILE *(Print/type physician's name)* ☐

18. REASON(S) FOR CONTINUING TREATMENT THIS BILLING PERIOD *(Clarify goals and necessity for continued skilled care.)*

19. SIGNATURE *(or name of professional, including prof. designation)*	20. DATE	21. ☐ CONTINUE SERVICES **OR** ☐ DC SERVICES

22. FUNCTIONAL LEVEL *(At end of billing period — Relate your documentation to functional outcomes and list problems still present.)*

22. SERVICE DATES FROM   THROUGH

Form CMS-701(11-91)

INSTRUCTIONS FOR COMPLETION OF FORM CMS-701

(Enter dates as 6 digits, month, day, year)

1. **Patient's Name** - Enter the patient's last name, first name and middle initial as shown on the health insurance Medicare card.

2. **Provider Number** - Enter the number issued by Medicare to the billing provider *(i.e., 00–7000)*.

3. **HICN** - Enter the patient's health insurance number as shown on the health insurance Medicare card, certification award, utilization notice, temporary eligibility notice, or as reported by SSO.

4. **Provider Name** - Enter the name of the Medicare billing provider.

5. **Medical Record No.** - *(optional)* Enter the patient's medical/clinical record number used by the billing provider. *(This is an item which you may enter for your own records.)*

6. **Onset Date** - Enter the date of onset for the patient's primary medical diagnosis, if it is a new diagnosis, or the date of the most recent exacerbation of a previous diagnosis. If the exact date is not known enter 01 for the day *(i.e., 120191)*. The date matches occurrence code 11 on the UB-92.

7. **SOC** *(start of care)* **Date** - Enter the date services began at the billing provider (the date of the first Medicare billable visit which **remains the same on subsequent claims** until discharge or denial corresponds to occurrence code 35 for PT, 44 for OT, 45 for SLP and 46 for CR on the UB-92).

8. **Type** - Check the type therapy billed; i.e., physical therapy (PT), occupational therapy (OT), speech-language pathology (SLP), cardiac rehabilitation (CR), respiratory therapy (RT), psychological services (PS), skilled nursing services (SN), or social services (SW).

9. **Primary Diagnosis** - Enter the pertinent written medical diagnosis resulting in the therapy disorder and relating to 50% or more of effort in the plan of treatment.

10. **Treatment Diagnosis** - Enter the written treatment diagnosis for which services are rendered. For example, for PT the primary medical diagnosis might be Degeneration of Cervical Intervertebral Disc while the PT treatment DX might be Frozen R Shoulder or, for SLP, while CVA might be the primary medical DX, the treatment DX might be Aphasia. If the same as the primary DX enter SAMPLE.

11. **Visits From Start of Care** - Enter the **cumulative total** visits *(sessions)* completed since services were started at the billing provider for the diagnosis treated, through the last visit on this bill. *(Corresponds to UB-92 value code 50 for PT, 51 for OT, 52 for SLP, or 53 for cardiac rehab.)*

12. **Current Frequency/Duration** - Enter the current frequency and duration of your treatment; e.g., 3 times per week for 4 weeks is entered 3/Wk x 4Wk.

13. **Current Plan Update, Functional Goals** - Enter the current plan of treatment goals for the patient for this billing period. *(If the same as shown on the CMS-700 or previous 701 enter "same".)* Enter the short-term goals to reach overall long-term outcome. Justify intensity if appropriate. Estimate time-frames to meet goals, when possible.

14. **Recertification** - Enter the inclusive dates when recertification is required, **even if the ON FILE box is checked in item 17.** Check the N/A box if recertification is not required for the type of service rendered.

15. **Physician's Signature** - If the form CMS-701 is used for recertification, the physician enters his/her signature. If recertification is not required for the type of service rendered, check N/A box. **If the form CMS-701 is not being used for recertification, check the ON FILE box - item 17.** If discharge is ordered, check DC box.

16. **Date** - Enter the date of the physician's signature only if the form is used for recertification.

17. **On File** *(Means certification signature and date)* - Enter the **typed/printed name of the physician** who certified the plan of treatment that is on file at the billing provider. If recertification is not required for the type of service checked in item 8, type/print the name of the physician who referred or ordered the service, **but do not check the ON FILE box.**

18. **Reason(s) For Continuing Treatment This Billing Period** - Enter the **major reasons** why the patient needs to continue skilled rehabilitation **for this billing period** (e.g., briefly state the patient's need for specific functional improvement, skilled training, reduction in complication or improvement in safety and how long you believe this will take, if possible or state your reasons for recommending discontinuance). Complete by the rehab specialist prior to physician's recertification.

19. **Signature** - Enter the signature *(or name)* and the professional designation of the individual justifying or recommending need for care *(or discontinuance)* for this billing period.

20. **Date** - Enter the date of the rehabilitation professional's signature.

21. Check the box if services are continuing or discontinuing at end of this billing period.

22. **Functional Level** *(end of billing period)* - Enter the pertinent progress made through the end of this billing period. Use objective terminology. Compare progress made to that shown on the previous CMS-701, item 22, or the CMS-700, items 20 and 21. Date progress when function can be consistently performed or when meaningful functional improvement is made or when significant regression in function occurs. Your intermediary reviews this progress compared to that on the prior CMS-701 or 700 to determine coverage for this billing period. Send a photocopy of the form covering the previous billing period.

23. **Service Dates** - Enter the From and Through dates which represent this billing period *(should be monthly)*. Match the From and Through dates in field 6 on the UB-92. DO NOT use 00 in the date. Example: 01 08 91 for January 8, 1991.

Chapter 19

Sample Occupational Therapy Assistant Supervision Grid

Using this grid, supervisors can compile all the regulatory, reimbursement, and professional standard language related to supervision from your state in one easy-to-reference page for posting in an occupational therapy department.

WISCONSIN COTA SUPERVISION GRID—2004				
Supervision document	How often provided	When close or general	Co-signature and supervision log	COTA's roles and tasks
State Licensure				
Medicare				
Medicaid				
DPI—School System				
AOTA Guidelines, Supervision Roles				

Chapter 20

Medicare SNF PPS and Consolidated Billing

The following information, which, unless otherwise noted, is reprinted verbatim from the SNF Final rule (*Federal Register,* Vol. 64, No. 146) published July 30, 1999, can be used as a guide to the PPS and consolidated billing issues most pertinent to occupational therapy practitioners. Issues have been grouped together, and section headings with *Federal Register* page references have been added to help you locate specific issues.

Recently, the Centers for Medicare and Medicaid has placed all regulations in online manuals. These contain the most up-to-date information. Consult the various providers, settings, and payment manuals at www.cms.gov.

Requirements Affecting Rehabilitation Services Under the SNF PPS

Criteria for Rehabilitation Therapy (pg. 41660(J))

Although rehabilitation therapy may begin as early as day one of the Medicare Part A SNF stay, we note that all of the rehabilitation therapy services (physical therapy, occupational therapy, and speech-language pathology) must meet each of the following criteria in order to be coded in the MDS as minutes of rehabilitation therapy:
- The service must be ordered by a physician.
- The therapy intervention must relate directly and specifically to an active written treatment regimen established by the physician after any needed consultation with the qualified rehabilitation therapy professional and must be reasonable and necessary to the treatment of the beneficiary's illness or injury (Section 230 of the *Medicare Skilled Nursing Facility Manual*, HCFA Pub. 12).
- An appropriately licensed or certified individual must provide or directly supervise the therapeutic service and coordinate the intervention with nursing services.

Physician Signature on Plan of Care (pg. 41660(J))

Medicare allows the professional therapist to develop a suggested plan of treatment and to begin providing services based on that plan prior to obtaining the physician's signature on the plan. We continue to require that the plan of treatment must be a physician's responsibility after any needed consultation with a qualified therapist, and that the requirement for physician verification of the suggested plan of treatment will be obtained within a reasonable amount of time. However, a physician signature must be obtained before the facility bills Medicare for payment for the rehabilitation therapy services provided to the beneficiary based on the plan of treatment he or she has approved. In this way, the facility can be sure that the level of therapy for which it bills Medicare is the level the physician deems to be medically necessary. We expect that the type and intensity of therapy billed will always match the type and intensity of therapy on the signed therapy plan of treatment.

We understand that many physicians use the fax to participate actively in the review of written plans of care and so believe that it is appropriate to accept physicians' faxed signatures for the plan of treatment. As always, whenever the plan of treatment is altered in any way, the modification must be made in writing. If the physician is not the person making the modification, the therapist who is making the change must notify the physician timely, and the physician must sign the change within a reasonable amount of time.

Supervision of Occupational Therapy Assistants (pg. 41661(J))

Physical and occupational therapy assistants may provide rehabilitation therapy services under the supervision of the professional therapist. A rehabilitation therapy assistant must be under the general supervision of a professional therapist who is accessible while the assistant is providing services to the beneficiary. The therapy assistant cannot supervise a therapy aide. It is up to the professional therapist to ensure that the assistant is capable of performing therapy services without the more stringent "line-of-sight" level of supervision required by therapy aides.

Supervision of Therapy Aides (pg. 41661(J))

A therapy aide must be supervised personally by the professional therapist in such a way that the therapist has visual contact with the aide at all times. Therapy aides are not to perform any services without "line-of-sight" supervision. Similarly, a therapy aide must never be responsible for provision of group therapy services, as this is well beyond the scope of services that they are qualified to provide.

Supervision of Therapy Students (pg. 41661(J) and 64 Fed. Reg. 28575 (November 4, 1999))

A therapy student who is participating in field experience must also be under the "line-of-sight" level of supervision of the professional therapist. Even though these students may become licensed therapists within months of the field training portion of their school program, they are not licensed or certified for practice in an unsupervised status. Further, the minutes of therapy services provided by the students may be recorded on the MDS as minutes of therapy received by the beneficiary. Medicare recognizes the costs associated with approved educational activities as a pass-through (see §413.85 and 64 Fed. Reg. 28575 (November 4, 1999).

Evaluation (pg. 41661(J))

The initial evaluation, performed by the licensed therapist and necessary for the development of the plan of treatment, must be performed during the beneficiary's SNF stay. It is not acceptable to use an evaluation that was performed for instance, in the acute care hospital or the rehabilitation hospital setting as the evaluation of the beneficiary in the SNF, because the beneficiary's status must be evaluated as he or she presents in the SNF setting. The evaluation, and the resultant plan of treatment, developed in the acute care hospital or rehabilitation hospital is relevant to the specific type of setting and is not interchangeable with an evaluation and plan of treatment developed for the beneficiary in the SNF setting. The time that it takes for the therapist to perform this evaluation may not be recorded as minutes of therapy received by the beneficiary.

Whether the time spent evaluating the beneficiary is counted depends on whether it is the formal initial evaluation or an evaluation performed after the course of therapy has begun. The time it takes to perform the formal initial evaluation and develop the treatment goals and the plan of treatment may not be counted as minutes of therapy received by the beneficiary. However, a reevaluation—that is, a hands-on examination of the beneficiary and not simply an update to the documentation and revision of the care plan—that is performed once a therapy regimen is underway (for example, evaluating goal achievement as part of the therapy session) may be counted as minutes of therapy received.

This policy was established because we do not wish to provide an incentive for facilities to perform initial evaluations for therapy services for patients who have no need of those

specialized services. However, we believe that the initial evaluation is an appropriate cost of doing business. Therefore, the cost of the initial assessment is included in the payment rates for all Medicare beneficiaries in covered Part A SNF stays.

Group Treatment (pg. 41662(J))

The Long-Term Care Resident Assessment Instrument Questions and Answers Version 2.0, clarifies how to account for therapy provided to an individual within a group setting. It states that if the group has four or fewer participants per supervising therapist (or therapy assistant under general supervision by the therapist) then it is appropriate to report the full time as therapy for each patient. The example used is that of a therapist working with three patients for 45 minutes on training to return to the community. Each patient's MDS would reflect receipt of 45 minutes of therapy for this session.

Although we recognize that receiving physical therapy, occupational therapy, or speech therapy as part of a group has clinical merit in select situations, we do not believe that services received within a group setting should account for more than 25 percent of the Medicare resident's therapy regimen during the SNF stay. For this reason, no more than 25 percent of the minutes reported in the MDS may be provided within a group setting. This limit is to be applied for each therapy discipline; that is, only 25 percent of the physical therapy minutes reported in the MDS may be minutes received in a group setting and, similarly, only 25 percent of the occupational therapy, or the speech therapy minutes reported may be minutes received in a group setting.

To summarize, the minutes of therapy provided by at least one supervising therapist (or therapy assistant under general supervision by the therapist) within a group of four or fewer participants, may be fully counted, provided that those minutes account for no more than 25 percent of the resident's weekly therapy in that discipline, as reported in the MDS. The supervising therapist may not be supervising any individuals other than the four or fewer individuals who are in the group at the time of the therapy session. Naturally, provision of group therapy time in excess of the 25 percent threshold is allowable, but those minutes may not be counted in section P of the MDS for purposes of RUG–III classification for Medicare Part A beneficiaries.

MDS Issues
Grace Days (pg. 41657(G1))

Days 6, 7, and 8, of the Medicare covered stay, were provided as grace days for setting the assessment reference date for the Medicare 5-day assessment. This assessment is to have an assessment reference date (MDS 2.0, Item A3a) of any

Day 1–8 of the Medicare Part A stay. Days 1–5 are optimal but Days 6–8 are also acceptable, and for some residents may actually be more appropriate; for example, to allow maximum flexibility for nurses to determine when to set the assessment reference date for the beneficiary's MDS, and thereby lessen the burden of the increased frequency of assessments that accompanied the PPS. Thus, the resident can be assessed using any one of these first eight days as the assessment reference date for the Medicare-required 5-day assessment.

However, we discourage the routine use of grace days for assessing every Medicare admission. We plan to identify patterns of inappropriate use as we gain a better understanding of what facilities' practice patterns are. When a facility routinely uses a grace day as the assessment reference date for the 5-day assessment, it loses the cushion that these days provide against performing the MDS later than day eight and, thus, risks being faced with payment at the default rate.

At this time our main interest is to encourage facilities to perform assessments timely and to recognize the grace days as a cushion and to use them as such, rather than as deadlines for setting each beneficiary's assessment reference date. The grace days are also provided to offset any incentive that facilities may have to initiate therapy services before the beneficiary is able to tolerate that level of activity.

Our discussion in the interim final rule about the possibility of audits was intended to address the possible practice of routinely using grace days for Medicare assessments. We were cognizant that the routine use of a grace day for the 5-day assessment would pose a temptation to back-date the assessment fraudulently when day eight was missed. We believed that any facility that routinely used grace days for the required assessments was liable to have assessments billed at the default rate; and that the absence of default rate billings in the facility claims might indicate that some misrepresentation of the assessment reference dates had occurred.

Unlike the routine use of grace days described above, we do expect that many beneficiaries who classify into the rehabilitation category will have 5-day assessment reference dates that fall on grace days. There are many cases in which the beneficiary is not physically able to begin therapy services until he or she has been in the facility for a few days. Thus, for a beneficiary who does not begin receiving rehabilitation therapy until the fifth, sixth, or seventh day of his or her SNF stay, the assessment reference date may be set for one of the grace days in order to capture an adequate number of days and minutes in section P of the current version of the MDS to qualify the resident for classification into one of the rehabilitation therapy RUG–III groups.

Another reason for the provision of 3 grace days for the 5-day assessment was to make it possible for beneficiaries to classify into the two highest RUG–III rehabilitation sub-categories. Classification into the Ultra High and Very High Rehabilitation sub-categories is not possible unless the beneficiary receives the sub-category's minimum level of services during the first seven days of the stay.

We also intended to minimize the incentive to facilities to provide too high a level of rehabilitation therapy to newly admitted beneficiaries. Having these extra few days allows time for those beneficiaries who need it, to stabilize from the acute care setting and be prepared for the beginning of rehabilitation in the SNF. We expect facilities will not compromise any beneficiary's health by beginning rehabilitation therapy prematurely or at a level that is too rigorous for the individual's status. In summary, use of grace days is acceptable and permitted for patients with any condition. However, a facility that uses grace days routinely may be subject to audit to determine that assessment reference dates are accurately reflected.

Counting and Recording Therapy Minutes on the MDS (pg. 41661(J))

The rehabilitation therapy time reported on the MDS is a record of the time the beneficiary spent receiving therapy services, not a record of the therapist's time. As stated in the August 1996 publication, Long Term Care Resident Assessment Instrument Questions and Answers, Version 2.0, the beneficiary's "therapy time starts when he begins the first treatment activity or task and ends when he finishes with the last apparatus and the treatment is ended."

Set-up time is included, as is time under the therapist's or therapy assistant's direct supervision. Physical therapy, occupational therapy, and speech therapy provided outside the building may be counted and recorded on the MDS, as long as the staff who provide therapy are qualified to provide the service. In the State Operations Manual (SOM, HCFA Pub. 7) Transmittal 272, pp. R64, "The therapy treatment may occur inside or outside the facility." This includes the time it takes for the therapist to take the beneficiary to his or her home for a home visit before discharge as long as the therapist uses the time in the car to teach or discuss the beneficiary's treatment or treatment goals, and for family conferences when the beneficiary is also present.

Prohibition on Limiting Services Based on MDS Minutes (pg. 41662(J))

Under section 1814(a)(2)(B) of the Act, a covered SNF level of care is defined in terms of those services that necessitate the involvement of skilled personnel, are needed and received on a daily basis and, as a practical matter, can be provided only in an SNF on an inpatient basis. Additionally, the requirements for participation at section

1819(b)(4)(A) of the Act require an SNF to furnish the full range of nursing and specialized rehabilitative services needed to attain or maintain each resident's highest practicable state of well-being, in accordance with the comprehensive plan of care. This means that there are to be no limits placed on the services to be provided to the beneficiary due to the facilities interpretations of how many minutes are "allowed" by the given RUG–III group.

The RUG–III classification system uses minimum levels of minutes per week as qualifiers for classification into the rehabilitation therapy groups. These minutes are minimums and are not to be used as upper limits for service provision. Similarly, there are instances in which beneficiaries in the so-called "clinical categories," Extensive Services, Special Care and Clinically Complex, will need some limited amounts of rehabilitation therapy services, which they should receive, even though they may not require a level that would qualify them for one of the rehabilitation groups. The SNF PPS is based on averages, and a facility that continues to provide services as they are needed by its beneficiaries should receive

payments that, in the aggregate, are adequate to pay for those services. Any policy of holding therapy to the bare minimum, regardless of beneficiary need, is inconsistent with the statutory requirements discussed above, and will result in poor outcomes, longer lengths of stay, and a degradation in the facility's quality of care.

Consolidated Billing

Consolidated billing (CB) applies only to services and supplies furnished to a SNF resident in a Part A covered stay and to physical, occupational, and speech therapy services in the Part B stay. Effective April 1, 2001, fiscal intermediaries will make payment for occupational therapy services for all Part B inpatients and outpatients based on the applicable fee schedule *(Medicare Physician Fee Schedule)*. Consequently, all services billed under Part B are to be billed using HCPCS codes, whether the beneficiary resides in a certified bed or a non-certified bed. For further information, consult www.cms.gov.

Chapter 21

State Medicaid Offices, Health Departments, and Workers' Compensation Departments

State Medicaid Offices

Administers the medical assistance program that finances medical care for income assistance recipients and other eligible medically needy persons.

Alabama
Commissioner
Medicaid Agency
PO Box 5624
Montgomery, AL 36103-5624
(334) 242-5600

Alaska
Director
Division of Medical Assistance
PO Box 110660
Juneau, AK 99811-0660
(907) 465-3355
Fax (907) 465-2204

American Samoa
State Medicaid Officer
Department of Health
LBJ Tropical Medical Center
Pago Pago, AS 96799
011-684-633-4590

Arizona
Director
Health Care Cost Containment System
801 E. Jefferson Street
Phoenix, AZ 85034
(800) 523-0231
TDD (800) 826-5140

Arkansas
Director
Department of Human Services
PO Box 1437, Slot 1100
Little Rock, AR 72203-1437
(501) 682-8292

California
Deputy Director of Programs
Department of Health Services
714 P Street, Room 1253
Sacramento, CA 95814
(916) 654-0391
TDD (916) 657-2861

Colorado
Executive Director
Department of Health Care Policy and Financing
1575 Sherman Street
Denver, CO 80203-1714
(303) 866-2993
Fax (303) 866-4411
TDD (303) 866-3883

Connecticut
Deputy Commissioner
Department of Social Services
25 Sigourney Street
Hartford, CT 06106-5033
(800) 842-1508
TDD (800) 842-4524

Delaware
Director
Medical Assistance Program
Department of Health and Social Services
1901 N. DuPont Highway
New Castle, DE 19720
(800) 372-2022

District of Columbia
Deputy Director
Medical Assistance Administration
825 North Capitol Street, NE, 5th Floor
Washington, DC 20020
(202) 442-5988
Fax (202) 442-4808

Florida
Director of Medicaid
Agency for Health Care Administration
2727 Mahan Drive
Tallahassee, FL 32308-5403
(888) 419-3456

Georgia
Director
Department of Community Health
2 Peachtree Street, NW, Suite 4043
Atlanta, GA 30303-3159
(404) 656-4507

Guam
Acting Administrator
Bureau of Health Care Financing
Department of Public Health and Social Services
PO Box 2816
Agana, GU 96910
(671) 735-7269

Hawaii
Administrator
Med QUEST Division
Department of Human Services
PO Box 399
Honolulu, HI 96809-0339
(808) 692-8056

Idaho
Administrator
Division of Medicaid
Department of Health and Welfare
PO Box 83720
Boise, ID 83720-0036
(208) 364-1802

Illinois
Administrator
Medical Operations
Department of Public Aid
201 S. Grand Avenue E., 3rd Floor
Springfield, IL 62763-0001
(800) 252-8635
TTY (800) 447-6404

Indiana
Assistant Secretary
Medicaid Policy and Planning
Family and Social Services Administration
402 W. Washington Street, Room W382
Indianapolis, IN 46204-2739
(317) 233-4455

Iowa
Director
Medical Services Division
Department of Human Services
Hoover State Office Building, 5th Floor
Des Moines, IA 50319-0114
(515) 281-8621

Kansas
Commissioner
Division of Medical Services
Adult and Medical Services
915 Harrison Street, SW
Topeka, KS 66612
(785) 296-3959
Fax (785) 296-2173
TTY (785) 296-1491

Kentucky
Deputy Commissioner
Department for Medicaid Services, 3rd Floor
275 E. Main Street
Frankfort, KY 40621
(502) 564-4321

Louisiana
Director
Bureau of Health Services Financing
PO Box 91030
Baton Rouge, LA 70821-9030
(225) 342-5774
Fax (225) 342-3893

Maine
Director
Bureau of Medical Services
Department of Human Services
11 State House Station
Augusta, ME 04333-0011
(207) 624-7539
TTY (207) 287-1828

Maryland
Deputy Secretary for Health Care Financing
Department of Health and Mental Hygiene
201 W. Preston Street
Baltimore, MD 21201
(410) 767-5800
TDD (800) 735-2258

Massachusetts
Commissioner
Division of Medical Assistance
600 Washington Street
Boston, MA 02111
(617) 628-4141

Michigan
Chief Executive Officer
Medical Services Administration
Department of Community Health
400 South Pine
Lansing, MI 48909
(517) 335-5001

Minnesota
Medicaid Director
Assistant Commissioner Health Care
Department of Human Services
444 Lafayette Road
St. Paul, MN 55155-3852
(612) 282-9921

Mississippi
Executive Director
Division of Medicaid
Office of the Governor
239 N. Lamar Street, Suite 801
Robert E. Lee Building
Jackson, MS 39201-1399
(601) 359-6050

Missouri
Director
Division of Medical Services
615 Howerton Court
PO Box 6500
Jefferson City, MO 65102-6500
(573) 751-3425
Fax (573) 751-6564
TTY (800) 735-2966

Montana
Administrator
Division of Health Policy and Services
1400 Broadway
Helena, MT 59601
(406) 444-4540
Fax (406) 444-1861

Nebraska
Acting Administrator
Medicaid Division
Department of Health and Human Services
301 Centennial Mall S., 5th Floor
Lincoln, NE 68509-5026
(402) 471-9147

Nevada
Deputy Administrator
State Welfare Division
2527 N. Carson Street
Carson City, NV 89710
(775) 687-4128

New Hampshire
Medicaid Director
Medicaid Administration Bureau
Department of Health and Human Services
6 Hazen Drive
Concord, NH 03301-6521
(603) 271-4353

New Jersey
Director
Division of Medical Assistance
    and Health Services
Department of Human Services
PO Box 712
Trenton, NJ 08625-0712
(609) 588-2600

New Mexico
Director
Medical Assistance Division
Department of Human Services
PO Box 2348
Santa Fe, NM 87504-2348
(505) 827-3100
Fax (505) 827-3185

New York
Deputy Director
Department of Health
Office of Medicaid Management
RM 1466, Corning Tower Building
Albany, NY 12237
(518) 474-3018

North Carolina
Director
Division of Medical Assistance
Department of Human Resources
1985 Umstead Drive
PO Box 29529
Raleigh, NC 27626-0529
(919) 857-4011

North Dakota
Director
Division of Medical Assistance
Department of Human Services
600 E. Boulevard Avenue
Bismarck, ND 58505-0261
(701) 328-3194
Fax (701) 328-2359
TTY (800) 366-6888

Northern Mariana Islands
Medical Administrator
Department of Public Health and
    Environmental Services
Commonwealth of Northern Mariana Islands
PO Box 409 CK
Saipan, MP 96950
(670) 234-8931

Ohio
Deputy Director
Office of Medicaid
Department of Human Services
30 E. Broad Street, 31st Floor
Columbus, OH 43215
(614) 644-0140

Oklahoma
State Medicaid Director
Health Care Authority
4545 N. Lincoln Boulevard, Suite 124
Oklahoma City, OK 73105
(405) 522-6205

Oregon
Director
Senior and Disabled Services Division
Department of Human Resources
500 Summer Street NE, E25
Salem, OR 97310-1015
(503) 945-5944
Fax (503) 378-2897
TTY (503) 947-5330

Pennsylvania
Deputy Secretary
Medical Assistance Programs
Department of Public Welfare
Health and Welfare Building, Room 515
Harrisburg, PA 17120
(717) 787-1870

Puerto Rico
Medicaid Director
Office of Economic Assistance to the
    Medically Indigent
Department of Health
GPO Box 70184
San Juan, PR 00936
(809) 765-1230

Rhode Island
Associate Director
Division of Medical Services
Department of Human Services
600 New London Avenue
Cranston, RI 02920
(401) 464-3113

South Carolina
Director
Department of Health and Human Services
PO Box 8206
Columbia, SC 29202-8206
(803) 898-2500

South Dakota
Program Administrator
Medical Services
Department of Social Services
700 Governors Drive
Pierre, SD 57501-2291
(605) 773-3165

Tennessee
Director of Operations
Department of Finance and Administration
729 Church Street
Nashville, TN 37247-6501
(615) 741-0213

Texas
State Medicaid Director
Health and Human Services Commission
701 W. 51st Street
Austin, TX 78751
(512) 424-6549

Utah
Executive Director
Division of Health Care Financing
Department of Health
PO Box 143106
Salt Lake City, UT 84114-1000
(801) 538-6155

Vermont
Director
Office of Health Access
Department of Social Welfare
103 S. Main Street
Waterbury, VT 05676
(802) 241-3985

Virgin Islands (U.S.)
Director
Bureau of Health Insurance and Medical
  Assistance
Department of Health
210-3A Altona
Suite 302, Frostco Center
Charlotte Amalie, VI 00802
(809) 774-4624

Virginia
Director
Department of Medical Assistance Services
600 E. Broad Street, Suite 1300
Richmond, VA 23219
(804) 786-4231

Washington
Assistant Secretary
Medical Assistance Administration
PO Box 45562
Olympia, WA 98504-5080
(360) 902-7855

West Virginia
Commissioner
Bureau for Medical Services
Department of Health and Human Resources
7012 MacCorkle Avenue SE
Charleston, WV 25304
(304) 926-1703

Wisconsin
Administrator
Division of Health Care Financing
Department of Health and Social Services
1 W. Wilson Street, Room 350
Madison, WI 53702
(608) 266-8922
TTY (608) 267-7371

Wyoming
Administrator
Division of Health Care Financing
Department of Health
North Building, Room 259B
6101 Yellowstone Road
Cheyenne, WY 82002
(307) 777-7531

State Health Departments

Enforces public health laws and administers health programs and services in the state.

Alabama
State Health Officer
Department of Public Health
RSA Tower
PO Box 3017
Montgomery, AL 36130-3017
(334) 206-5200

Alaska
Commissioner
Department of Health and Social Services
PO Box 110610
Juneau, AK 99811-0601
(907) 465-3030
Fax (907) 465-3068

American Samoa
Director
Medical Services Department
America Samoan Government
PO Box 4030
Pago Pago, AS 96799
(684) 633-4590

Arizona
Director
Department of Health Services
1740 W. Adams Street
Phoenix, AZ 85007
(602) 542-1001
Fax (602) 542-0883

Arkansas
Director
Department of Health
4815 W. Markham
Little Rock, AR 72205-3867
(501) 661-2000
Fax (501) 671-1450

California
Director
Department of Health Services
PO Box 942732
Sacramento, CA 94234-7320
(916) 445-4171
TDD (916) 657-2861

Colorado
Executive Director
Department of Health
1575 Sherman Street
Denver, CO 80203-1714
(303) 866-2993

Connecticut
Commissioner
Department of Public Health
410 Capitol Avenue
PO Box 340308
Hartford, CT 06134
(860) 509-8000
TDD (860) 509-7191

Delaware
Director
Department of Health and Social Services
417 Federal Street
Dover, DE 19903
(302) 739-4700

District of Columbia
Commissioner
Department of Human Services
825 North Capitol Street NE
Washington, DC 20002
(202) 442-5999

Florida
Deputy Secretary
Department of Health
4052 Bald Cypress Way, Bin A00
Tallahassee, FL 32399-0701
(850) 245-4443

Georgia
Director
Public Health Division
Two Peachtree Street NW, 7th Floor
Atlanta, GA 30303-3142
(404) 657-2700

Guam
Director
Public Health and Social Services Department
PO Box 2816
Agana, GU 96932
(617) 735-7123

Hawaii
Director
Department of Health
1250 Punchbowl Street
Honolulu, HI 96813
(808) 586-4400

Idaho
Administrator
Health Division
Department of Health and Welfare
450 W. State Street
PO Box 83720
Boise, ID 83720-0036
(208) 334-5945

Illinois
Chairman
Department of Public Health
535 W. Jefferson Street
Springfield, IL 62761
(217) 782-6187
Fax (217) 782-3987
TTY (800) 547-0466

Indiana
Commissioner
Health Department
2 N. Meridian Street
Indianapolis, IN 46204
(317) 233-7400

Iowa
Director
Department of Public Health
Lucas State Office Building
321 E. 12th Street
Des Moines, IA 50319-0075
(515) 281-7689

Kansas
Director
Health Division
Department of Health and Environment
1000 SW Jackson Street, Suite 300
Topeka, KS 66612
(785) 296-1343
Fax (785) 296-1562

Kentucky
Commissioner
Public Health Department
Cabinet for Health Services
275 E. Main Street
4th Floor West
Frankfort, KY 40621
(502) 564-3970

Louisiana
Secretary
Public Health Office
Department of Health and Hospitals
1201 Capitol Access Road
PO Box 629
Baton Rouge, LA 70821-0629
(225) 342-9500
Fax (225) 342-5568

Maine
Director
Bureau of Health
11 State House Station
Augusta, ME 04333
(207) 287-8016
Fax (207) 287-8066
TTY (207) 287-9058

Maryland

Secretary
Department of Health and Mental Hygiene
201 W. Preston Street, 5th Floor
Baltimore, MD 21201
(410) 767-6860

Massachusetts

Commissioner
Department of Public Health
250 Washington Street
Boston, MA 02108-4619
(617) 727-6000
TTY (617) 624-6001

Michigan

Director
Department of Community Health
320 S. Walnut Street, 6th Floor
Lansing, MI 48913
(517) 335-8024

Minnesota

Commissioner
Department of Health
85 E. Seventh Place
PO Box 64975
St. Paul, MN 55164
(612) 215-5800

Mississippi

State Health Officer
Department of Health
570 E. Woodrow Wilson
Jackson, MS 39215-1700
(601) 576-7951
Fax (601) 576-7823

Missouri

Director
Department of Health
PO Box 570
Jefferson City, MO 65102
(573) 751-6400
Fax (573) 751-6401

Montana

Director
Public Health and Human Services
1400 Broadway
PO Box 202951
Helena, MT 59620-2951
(406) 444-4540
Fax (406) 444-1861

Nebraska

Director
Health and Human Services
PO Box 95044
Lincoln, NE 68509-5044
(402) 471-2306

Nevada

Administrator
Health Division
Department of Human Resources
505 E. King Street, Room 201
Carson City, NV 89710
(775) 687-3876

New Hampshire

Commissioner
Department of Health and Human Services
129 Pleasant Street
Concord, NH 03301-3857
(603) 271-4331
Fax (603) 271-4912
TDD (800) 735-2964

New Jersey

Commissioner
Department of Health and Senior Services
PO Box 360
Trenton, NJ 08625-0360
(609) 292-7837
Fax (609) 292-7837

New Mexico

Secretary
Department of Health
1190 St. Francis Drive
PO Box 26110
Santa Fe, NM 87502-6110
(505) 827-2613

New York
Commissioner
Department of Health
Mayor Erastus Corning II Tower
Empire State Plaza
Albany, NY 12237-0001
(518) 474-2011

North Carolina
Secretary
Department of Health and Human Services
Adams Building, 101 Blair Drive
Raleigh, NC 27626
(919) 733-4534
Fax (919) 715-4645

North Dakota
State Health Officer
Department of Health
600 E. Boulevard Avenue
Bismarck, ND 58505-0200
(701) 328-2372
Fax (701) 328-4727

Ohio
Director
Department of Health
246 N. High Street
PO Box 118
Columbus, OH 43266-0118
(614) 466-2253

Oklahoma
Commissioner
Department of Health
1000 NE 10th Street
Oklahoma City, OK 73117-1299
(405) 271-5600

Oregon
Administrator
Health Division
Department of Human Resources
800 NE Oregon Street
Portland, OR 97232
(503) 731-4031

Pennsylvania
Secretary
Department of Health
Health and Welfare Building, Box 90
Harrisburg, PA 17108
(877) PA-HEALTH

Puerto Rico
Secretary
Department of Health
PO Box 70184
San Juan, PR 00936-0184
(809) 274-7676

Rhode Island
Director
Department of Health
3 Capitol Hill
Providence, RI 02908
(401) 277-2231
Fax (401) 222-6548

South Carolina
Commissioner
Department of Health and Human Services
PO Box 8206
Columbia, SC 29202
(803) 898-3300

South Dakota
Secretary
Department of Health
600 E. Capitol Avenue
Pierre, SD 57501-2536
(605) 773-3361

Tennessee
Commissioner
Department of Health
425 Fifth Avenue, N.
Nashville, TN 37247-0101
(615) 741-3111

Texas
Commissioner
Department of Health
1100 W. 49th Street
Austin, TX 78756-3199
(512) 458-7111
TDD (512)458-7708

The Occupational Therapy Assistant: Resources for Practice and Education

Utah
Executive Director
Department of Health
288 N. 1460 West
Salt Lake City, UT 84116-0700
(801) 538-6111

Vermont
Commissioner
Department of Health
Human Services Agency
PO Box 70
Burlington, VT 05402
(802) 863-7280

Virgin Islands (U.S.)
Commissioner
Department of Health
48 Sugar Estate
St. Thomas, VI 00802
(340) 774-0117

Virginia
Commissioner
Department of Health
PO Box 2448
Richmond, VA 23218
(804) 786-3561

Washington
Secretary
Department of Health
1112 SE Quince
PO Box 47890
Olympia, WA 98504-7890
(360) 236-4030

West Virginia
Commissioner
Bureau of Public Health
1900 Kanawha Boulevard, E.
Charleston, WV 23505
(304) 558-2971

Wisconsin
Administrator
Public Health Division
Department of Health and Family Services
PO Box 7850
Madison, WI 53707-7850
(608) 266-1251

Wyoming
Director
Department of Health
1117 Hathaway Building
2300 Capitol Avenue
Cheyenne, WY 82002
(307) 777-7656

State Workers' Compensation Departments

Administers laws providing insurance and compensation for workers for job-related illness, injury, or death.

Alabama
Administrator Workers' Compensation Division
Department of Industrial Relations
649 Monroe Street
Montgomery, AL 36131
(334) 242-2868

Alaska
Director
Division of Workers' Compensation
Department of Labor
1111 W. Eighth Street
PO Box 25512
Juneau, AK 99802-5512
(907) 465-2790

Arizona
President
State Compensation Fund
3031 N. Second Street
Phoenix, AZ 85012
(602) 631-2000

Arkansas
Chairman
Workers' Compensation Commission
324 Spring Street
PO Box 950
Little Rock, AR 72203-0950
(501) 682-3930

California
Administrator
Division of Workers' Compensation
455 Golden Gate Avenue, 9th Floor
San Francisco, CA 94102
(415) 703-4600

Colorado
Director
Division of Workers' Compensation
Department of Labor and Employment
1515 Arapahoe Street
Tower 2, Suite 500
Denver, CO 80202-2117
(303) 575-8700

Connecticut
Chairman
Workers' Compensation Commission
Capitol Place
21 Oak Street, 4th Floor
Hartford, CT 06106
(860) 493-1500

Delaware
Office of Workers' Compensation
State Office Building,
6th Floor
820 N. French Street
Wilmington, DE 19801
(302) 761-8200

District of Columbia
Director
Office of Workers' Compensation
1200 Upshur Street, NW
PO Box 56098
Washington, DC 20011
(202) 576-6265

Florida
Director
Division of Workers' Compensation
200 E. Gaines Street
Tallahassee, FL 32399
(850) 921-6966

Georgia
Chairman
Board of Workers' Compensation
270 Peachtree Street, NW
Atlanta, GA 30303-1299
(404) 656-3875

Guam
Director
Labor Department
504 E. Sunset Boulevard
Tiyan, PO Box 9970
Tamuning, GU 96931-9970
(671) 475-0160

Hawaii
Administrator
Disability Compensation Division
Department of Labor and Industrial Relations
830 Punchbowl Street
Honolulu, HI 96813
(808) 586-8600

Idaho
Chairman
Industrial Commission
317 Main Street
PO Box 83720
Boise, ID 83720-0041
(208) 334-6000

Illinois
Chairman
Industrial Commission
100 W. Randolph Street, Suite 8-200
Chicago, IL 60601
(312) 814-6611

Indiana
Chairman
Workers' Compensation Board
Government Center South
402 W. Washington Street, Room W196
Indianapolis, IN 46204
(317) 232-3808

Iowa
Director
Iowa Workforce Development
1000 E. Grand Avenue
Des Moines, IA 50319
(515) 281-5387

Kansas
Director
Division of Workers' Compensation
800 SW Jackson, Suite 600
Topeka, KS 66612
(785) 296-34410

Kentucky
Chairman
Workers' Compensation Board
Office of Workers Claims
657 Chamberlin Avenue
Frankfort, KY 40601
(502) 564-5550

Louisiana
Assistant Secretary
Office of Workers' Compensation
PO Box 94040
Baton Rouge, LA 70804
(225) 342-7555

Maine
Executive Director
Workers' Compensation Board
27 State House Station
Augusta, ME 04333-0027
(207) 287-7096

Maryland
Chairman
Workers' Compensation Commission
10 E. Baltimore Street
Baltimore, MD 21202
(410) 767-0900

Massachusetts
Chairman
Department of Industrial Accident
600 Washington Street, 7th Floor
Boston, MA 02111
(617) 727-4900

Michigan
Director
Bureau of Workers' and Unemployment Compensation
PO Box 30016
Lansing, MI 48909
(314) 456-2400

Minnesota
Commissioner
Workers' Compensation Division
443 Lafayette Road N.
St. Paul, MN 55155
(651) 284-5005

Mississippi
Chairman
Workers' Compensation Commission
PO Box 5300
Jackson, MS 39296-5300
(601) 987-4200

Missouri
Acting Director
Division of Workers' Compensation
Department of Labor and Industrial Relations
3315 W. Truman Boulevard
PO Box 58
Jefferson City, MO 65102-0504
(573) 751-4231

Montana
President
State Comp. and Mutual Insurance Fund
Department of Administration
5 S. Last Chance Gulch
Helena, MT 59620
(406) 444-6500

Nebraska
Presiding Judge
Workers' Compensation Court
State House, 13th Floor
PO Box 98908
Lincoln, NE 68509-8908
(402) 471-6468

Nevada
Northern District Manager
Business and Industry Commission
Division of Industrial Relations
400 W. King Street, Suite 400
Carson City, NV 89703
(775) 684-7260

New Hampshire
Administrator
Workmens' Compensation Division
Department of Labor
95 Pleasant Street
Concord, NH 03301
(603) 271-3174

New Jersey
Chief Judge
Division of Workers' Compensation
PO Box 381
Trenton, NJ 08625
(609) 292-2414

New Mexico
Director
Workmens' Compensation Administration
2410 Centre Avenue SE
PO Box 27198
Albuquerque, NM 87125-7198
(505) 841-6000

New York
Chair
State Workers' Compensation Board
100 Broadway-Menands
Albany, NY 12241
(518) 474-6670

North Carolina
Chairman
Industrial Commission
Dobbs Building, 6th Floor
430 N. Salisbury Street
Raleigh, NC 27603
(919) 807-2500

North Dakota
Executive Director
Workers' Compensation Bureau
500 E. Front Avenue
Bismarck, ND 58504-5685
(701) 328-3800

Ohio
Director
Bureau of Workers' Compensation
30 W. Spring Street
Columbus, OH 43215-2256
(614) 644-6292

Oklahoma
Chief Judge
Workers' Compensation Court
Denver N. Davison Court Building
1915 N. Stiles Avenue
Oklahoma City, OK 73105
(405) 522-8600

Oregon
Chair
Workers' Compensation Division
350 Winter Street, NE, Room 27
Salem, OR 97310
(503) 947-7810

Pennsylvania
Director
Bureau of Workers' Compensation
1171 South Cameron Street, Room 324
Harrisburg, PA 17104
(717) 772-4447

Puerto Rico
Administrator
Labor and Human Resources Department
505 Munoz-Rivera Avenue, 21st Floor
Hato Rey, PR 00918
(787) 754-2119

Rhode Island
Director
Workers' Compensation Division
Department of Labor
1511 Pontiac Avenue
Cranston, RI 02920
(401) 462-8100

South Carolina
Chairman
Workers' Compensation Commission
1612 Marion Street
Columbia, SC 29201
(803) 737-5768

South Dakota
Director
Division of Labor and Management
Kneip Building, 3rd Floor
700 Governors Drive
Pierre, SD 57501-2291
(605) 773-3681

Tennessee
Director
Workers' Compensation Division
Gateway Plaza, 2nd Floor
710 James Robertson Parkway
Nashville, TN 37243-0655
(615) 532-4812

Texas
Chairman
Workers' Compensation Commission
Southfield Building, 4000 S. IH-35
Austin, TX 78704
(512) 804-4100

Utah
President
Workers Compensation Fund of Utah
PO Box 57929
Murray, UT 84157-0929
(801) 288-8007

Vermont
Commissioner
Division of Workers' Compensation
National Life Building, Drawer 20
Montpelier, VT 05620-3401
(802) 828-2286

Virgin Islands (U.S.)
Commissioner
Department of Labor
21-31 Hospital Street
Christiansted
St. Croix, VI 00850
(340) 773-1994

Virginia
Chairman
VA Workers' Compensation Commission
100 DMV Drive
Richmond, VA 23220
(804) 367-8600

Washington
Director
Department of Labor amd Industries
PO Box 44001
Olympia, WA 98504-4000
(360) 902-4213

West Virginia
Executive Director
Workers' Compensation Division
PO Box 3824
Charleston, WV 25338
(304) 926-5048

Wisconsin
Administrator
Workers' Compensation Division
PO Box 7901
Madison, WI 53707
(608) 266-1340

Wyoming
Administrator
Workers' Safety and Compensation Division
Herschler Building E.
122 W. 25th Street
Cheyenne, WY 82002
(307) 777-7159

Chapter 22

Regulations for OTAs Using *CPT* Codes

Background

The profession of occupational therapy has been reporting its services using the American Medical Association (AMA) *Current Procedural Terminology (CPT)* since the beginning of CPT. Initially, most occupational therapy services were reported by physician offices, clinics, and other providers that employed occupational therapists. In 1987, Congress enacted legislation that expanded Medicare coverage for treatment by occupational therapists as independent practitioners and coverage as a Part B benefit in all outpatient settings. Payment for occupational therapy services was incorporated into the Medicare physicians' resource-based relative value system (RBRVS) fee schedule effective with 1992 legislation. The Balanced Budget Act of 1997 required that, beginning in January 1999, occupational therapy services provided to Medicare beneficiaries in all outpatient settings would be reported by *CPT* code and paid under the RBRVS fee schedule.

AMA Health Care Professionals Advisory Committee (HCPAC)

In 1993, the American Occupational Therapy Association (AOTA) was invited by the AMA to become one of the founding non-physician societies comprising the Health Care Practitioners Advisory Committee (HCPAC), a group formed to assist in future *CPT* development. Since then, AOTA advisors have served on the *CPT* HCPAC and have developed numerous new and revised codes. An AOTA representative also serves on the HCPAC Review Board, which recommends work values and practice expense data for non-physician services. Additionally, AOTA's advisor currently represents the HCPAC members on the AMA's Practice Expense Advisory Committee, which was formed to determine clinical practice expense for existing *CPT* codes. The recommendations of the HCPAC Review Board are used by the Centers for Medicare and Medicaid (CMS) in calculating payment under the Medicare RBRVS fee schedule.

CPT Code Changes Affecting Occupational Therapy

The majority of *CPT* codes used by occupational therapists are found in the Physical Medicine and Rehabilitation (PM&R) section (97XXX). Since joining the HCPAC in 1994, AOTA has initiated numerous changes to the content and structure of this section, often in conjunction with other professional societies. However, occupational therapists often report codes outside of the PM&R section, such as swallowing and oral function evaluation/treatment (92526/92610–92614), neuromuscular procedures (95XXX), neuro-cognitive testing (96XXX), health and behavior (96150–96155), and casting/splinting (29XXX).

The chart on the following page gives a brief history of some of the significant changes to *CPT* affecting occupational therapy practice that AOTA has initiated or supported since 1994.

Use of CPT Codes

Specific services provided by an occupational therapist may be limited by the applicable Occupational Therapist State Practice Act. However, the AMA does not determine which practitioners can use which codes. Most public and private insurers only stipulate that the service performed must be within a practitioner's scope of practice. Since occupational therapists treat both physical and psychosocial conditions within a number of subspecialties, a wide range of codes should be available to occupational therapy practitioners. For example, although many therapists do not use physical agent modalities (i.e., 97010–97039) in their practices, these codes would be appropriately reported by an occupational therapist with a hand subspecialty.

The Balanced Budget Act of 1997 required that all Medicare outpatient therapy services (i.e., physical therapy,

Effective Year of Change	Description of Change
1995	*CPT* Section 97001–97799 renamed *Physical Medicine and Rehabilitation* and restructured to separate physical agent modalities from procedures; new codes added and nomenclature modified to better reflect therapy practice.
1996	Activities of daily living (ADL) code split into two new and redefined codes: Self care/home management (97535) and Community/work reintegration (97537).
1997	Orthotics fitting and training (97504) and Prosthetics training (97520) codes modified.
1998	Occupational therapy (97003) and Physical therapy evaluation and re-evaluation (97004) codes added.
1999	Manipulation and mobilization services combined into one new code, Manual therapy techniques (97140).
2001	Cognitive/sensory integrative treatment code split and redefined into two new codes, Development of cognitive skills (97532) and Sensory integrative techniques (97533).
	Two new wound debridement codes, Selective debridement (97601) and Non-selective debridement (97602), added.
2002	Health and Behavior Assessment/Intervention section (96150–96155) added to describe non-psychiatric assessment and treatment of behavioral, emotional, and cognitive factors affecting physical health problems.
	Neuromuscular reeducation (97112) modified to include "sitting activities."
	Orthotics fitting and training (97504) modified to include "trunk."
	Self-care/home management training (97535) modified to reflect "assistive technology."
2003	Evaluative and Therapeutic Services subsection added to Special Otorhinolaryngologic Services section to describe evaluation and treatment related to augmentative and alternative communicating devices and evaluations of oral and laryngeal swallowing functions.
2004	Assistive technology assessment (97755) code added, and assistive technology devices/equipment terminology added to existing community/work reintegration training (97537) code.
2005	Four new wound care debridement codes (97597, 97598, 97605, 97606) added to Active Wound Care Management subsection of Medicine to report selective debridement based on total surface area of wound(s) size and new procedures to describe negative pressure wound therapy techniques.

and speech-language pathology) be reported by *CPT* codes. CMS designated a group of *CPT* codes, including all of the PM&R codes, as "rehabilitation." No restrictions were made among the therapies in regard to use of specific codes, and therapists were instructed to use those codes within their scope of practice that best describes the treatment provided.

With the increased use of *CPT* for all aspects of occupational therapy, AOTA has offered several educational opportunities, through workshops, telephone seminars, and written material, for occupational therapists to learn proper coding techniques. In 1999, AOTA received the AMA's *Award for Educational Excellence* in recognition of its series of *Practice Guidelines*, which assisted occupational therapists in "translating" commonly accepted occupational therapy interventions into *CPT* nomenclature.

AOTA's Position

AOTA supports the use of a wide range of *CPT* codes by occupational therapists to accurately reflect occupational therapy treatment. This is consistent with AOTA's *Occupational Therapy Practice Framework, Guide to Occupational Therapy Practice,* and *Practice Guidelines.* Therapists should be familiar with restrictions in state law regarding practice. In addition, therapists should understand and use correct *CPT* rules, provide documentation in patient records to substantiate correct coding, and be able to demonstrate proficiency in any specialized treatment provided for which a specific code is used.

Resources

CPT 2004 (AMA)
Occupational Therapy Practice Framework (AOTA)
Guide to Occupational Therapy Practice (AOTA) Occupational Therapy Practice Guidelines (AOTA)

Last Updated December 2004

PART IV

Ethical Jurisdiction

A code of ethics can define a profession. Occupational therapy has a strong, comprehensive code; guidelines to that code; and core values and attitudes. These documents outline the ethical guidelines of our profession and can be used by occupational therapy practitioners and students as a moral compass for safe, legal, ethical, best practice that actively seeks to do good and causes no harm.

State regulations are fairly clear laws and rules about conducting practice and can assist practitioners in preventing unlawful practice. Ethical dilemmas are often harder to define and to know how to determine a course of action or deal with gray areas. The resources in this section can help guide occupational therapists' and occupational therapy assistants' decision-making in many situations.

For occupational therapy assistants, the *Code of Ethics* can be used to ensure appropriate supervision. In the absence of a comprehensive regulatory rule in a state's language related to supervision, Principle 4.E—"Occupational therapy personnel shall protect service recipients by ensuring that duties assumed by or assigned to other occupational therapy personnel match credentials, qualifications, experience, and scope of practice"—could be used to let supervisors know that they are not following the standards of the profession. Principle 3.F—"Occupational therapy practitioners shall provide appropriate supervision to individuals for whom the practitioners have supervisory responsibility in accordance with Association policies; local, state, and federal laws; and institutional values"—also can be helpful.

Productivity requirements in many areas of practice can create ethical considerations. Clear-cut guidelines are not always identifiable in regulatory language, so guidelines to the code can assist practitioners in providing support for a stance against practicing in an unethical or fraudulent manner.

Practitioners are urged to keep these documents and the regulatory rules together and to ensure that each document has been read and integrated into everyday practice. To help with this task, the following are included in this section:

- Chapter 23. Purpose of a Professional Code of Ethics and an Overview of the Ethical Jurisdiction of the AOTA, NBCOT, and State Regulatory Boards
- Chapter 24. Guidelines for Responding to Questions About Ethical Dilemmas
- Chapter 25. Scope of the Commission on Standards and Ethics Disciplinary Action Program
- Chapter 26. *Occupational Therapy Code of Ethics* (2000)
- Chapter 27. Guidelines to the *Occupational Therapy Code of Ethics* (2000)
- Chapter 28. Enforcement Procedures for the *Occupational Therapy Code of Ethics* (2004)
- Chapter 29. Core Values and Attitudes of Occupational Therapy Practice
- Chapter 30. Standards of Practice for Occupational Therapy
- Chapter 31. Ethical Knowledge = Collaborative Power
- Chapter 32. Successful OT–OTA Partnerships: Staying Afloat in a Sea of Ethical Challenges.

Chapter 23

Purpose of a Professional Code of Ethics and an Overview of the Ethical Jurisdiction of the AOTA, NBCOT, and State Regulatory Boards

There are three specific agencies that have jurisdiction and concerns about the ethical conduct of occupational therapy personnel: the American Occupational Therapy Association (AOTA), the National Certification Board for Occupational Therapy (NBCOT), and state regulatory boards (licensure, registration, and trademark).

AOTA

AOTA is a voluntary membership organization that represents and promotes the interests of persons who choose to become members. Because membership is voluntary, AOTA has no direct authority over practitioners and students who are not members. AOTA has no direct legal mechanism for preventing nonmembers who are incompetent, unethical, or unqualified from practicing. It is important to remember that AOTA is concerned about ethical conduct across the multiple roles that occupational therapists and occupational therapy assistants can play—student, researcher, educator, manager, etc. The Commission on Standards and Ethics (SEC) is the volunteer-sector component of AOTA that is responsible for writing, revising and enforcing the *Occupational Therapy Code of Ethics* (AOTA, 2003) and the Enforcement Procedures. The SEC is also responsible for informing and educating members about current ethical issues, and for reviewing allegations of unethical conduct by AOTA members.

There are four types of disciplinary action:

1. *Reprimand* is a formal expression of disapproval of conduct communicated privately by letter from the Chairperson of SEC.
2. *Censure* is a formal expression of disapproval that is public.
3. *Suspension* requires removal of membership for a specified period of time.
4. *Revocation* prohibits a person from being a member of AOTA indefinitely (AOTA, 2000a).

NBCOT

NBCOT is the national credentialing agency that certifies (and recertifies) qualified persons as OTRs and COTAs. This organization has jurisdiction over all NBCOT certified practitioners as well as those currently eligible to sit for the next exam. Initial certification is required for all students who successfully complete occupational therapy or occupational therapy assistant programs and wish to practice occupational therapy. These individuals must successfully pass a written certification examination. Recertification is not mandatory. Only occupational therapists and occupational therapy assistants with current certification are allowed to represent themselves as OTR or COTA.

NBCOT does not use the AOTA *Code of Ethics* as their guide in reviewing complaints about incompetent or impaired practitioners, but has its own set of procedures for disciplinary action. The three main categories of violations that warrant disciplinary action are incompetence, unethical behavior, and impairment. When NBCOT receives a complaint, they initiate an intensive, confidential review process to determine whether the allegations are warranted. If so, the Disciplinary Action Committee (DAC) may select one of several sanctions depending upon the seriousness of the misconduct. Below is a listing of the available options, starting with the least severe action and progressing to most severe. All sanctions are made public except for reprimand and ineligibility (http://www.nbcot.org/revised_procedures.htm).

NBCOT has six types of disciplinary action:

1. *Reprimand* is a formal, written expression of disapproval of conduct communicated privately and retained in the individual's certification file.
2. *Censure* is a formal expression of disapproval that is publicly proclaimed.
3. *Ineligibility* to take the certification exam may be determined indefinitely or for a specific period of time.
4. *Probation* requires that the individual fulfill certain conditions such as education, supervision, or counseling for

a specified time. The individual must meet these conditions to remain certified.

5. *Suspension* is the loss of certification for a specified period of time. The DAC uses suspension when they determine that the person must complete specific amounts of public service or participate in a rehabilitation program.

6. *Revocation* means that the individual loses certification permanently.

State Regulatory Boards

State regulatory boards (SRBs) are public bodies created by state legislatures to ensure the health and safety of the citizens of that state. Their specific responsibility is to protect the public from potential harm caused by incompetent or unqualified practitioners. State regulation may be in the form of licensure or registration. The legal guidelines of each state usually specify the scope of practice for the profession and the qualifications that professionals must meet to practice. In addition, the SRB usually provides a description of ethical behavior. In most cases the SRBs have adopted the AOTA *Occupational Therapy Code of Ethics* for this purpose. The majority of states use AOTA's *Code of Ethics* as their template for reviewing complaints about harm to the public by a practitioner who is licensed in their state. However, since most states are reluctant to open their laws for review unless it is absolutely essential, states in many cases are using older versions of the Code as their point of reference.

Each state regulatory board has direct jurisdiction over those therapists practicing in that state. By the very nature of this limited jurisdiction, each state can monitor the practitioners in that state more closely than national organizations such as AOTA and NBCOT can. They have the authority by state law to discipline members of a profession practicing in that state if they have caused harm to citizens of that state. SRBs can also intervene in situations where the person has been convicted of an illegal act that directly affects professional practice (for example, the misappropriation of funds through false billing practices).

The primary concern of each state is to protect the people living in that state. They therefore limit their review of complaints to those involving such a threat. When an SRB determines that an individual has violated the law, it can elect several different sanctions as a disciplinary measure. Examples of disciplinary actions are public censure, temporary suspension of practice privileges, permanent prohibition from practice in that state, monetary fine, and imprisonment.

Where to Go First

As you can see, AOTA, NBCOT, and SRBs have specific jurisdictions over occupational therapy. Some areas of concern overlap among the three areas. Others are separate and distinct. If you need information or want to file a complaint, it is helpful to know which of the three is the most appropriate to contact. To do so you should ask the following three questions:

1. Did the alleged violation take place in a state that regulates occupational therapy practice?
2. Is the individual a member of AOTA?
3. What consequences do I consider appropriate if the complaint is determined to be justified? (Hansen, 2000b)

Certainly in some instances, you would have a choice of any of the three agencies. For example, all three have concerns if there has been harm or potential harm to a consumer. On the other hand, ethical violations of professional values that have no potential to cause harm would likely be of interest to only AOTA. For example, AOTA would be concerned about a violation of a verbal contract to provide a continuing education workshop, but NBCOT and SRBs would not.

You should also consider what disciplinary action you would consider appropriate for a particular violation. Do you want to revoke or restrict the person's state licensure? Do you want the organization to either suspend or revoke the individual's certification? Would it be more appropriate in your mind to restrict or prohibit the person's ability to be a member of AOTA? You need to seek advice before filing a complaint to be sure that you have selected the agency with the jurisdiction to achieve the consequences you consider commensurate to the violation (Hansen, 2000a, 2000c).

References

American Occupational Therapy Association. (2000a). Enforcement procedure for occupational therapy code of ethics. *American Journal of Occupational Therapy, 54,* 617–621.

American Occupational Therapy Association. (2000b). Occupational therapy code of ethics. *American Journal of Occupational Therapy, 54,* 614–616.

Hansen, R. A. (2000a). Disciplinary action: Whose responsibility? In P. Kyler (Ed.), *Reference guide to the occupational therapy code of ethics* (p. 21). Bethesda, MD: American Occupational Therapy Association.

Hansen, R. A. (2000b). Ethical jurisdiction of occupational therapy: The role of AOTA, NBCOT, and state regulatory boards. In P. Kyler (Ed.), *Reference guide to the occupational therapy code of ethics* (pp. 22–24). Bethesda, MD: American Occupational Therapy Association.

Hansen, R. A. (2000c). Guidelines for responding to questions about ethical dilemmas. In P. Kyler (Ed.), *Reference guide to the occupational therapy code of ethics* (p. 20). Bethesda, MD: American Occupational Therapy Association.

Adapted from American Occupational Therapy Association. (2003). *Reference guide to the Occupational Therapy Code of Ethics, 2003 edition* (pp. 24–26). Bethesda, MD: Author.

Chapter 24

Guidelines for Responding to Questions About Ethical Dilemmas

1. Ask the person to relay information in an anonymous fashion (without names of individuals and facilities). This enables you to remain more objective about the situation and able to provide recommendations that could not be construed as biased or prejudicial.
2. Listen carefully. Ask the person what they would like to see happen. Sometimes the individual will have a very clear idea of the action that he or she thinks should be taken; but other times, the person will not.
3. You can explain the options that are available. The first step usually is to make sure that the person has discussed this issue in some detail with the individual(s) involved and/or pursued consideration of the concern within the procedures in place within the institution or facility where the misconduct occurred. If these preliminary avenues have been attempted and no satisfactory resolution reached, then the person has several options with

other agencies that may have jurisdiction over the ethical conduct of occupational therapy personnel.
4. If the person wishes to talk with someone who is knowledgeable about such issues, tell them to call one of the following individuals:
   a. AOTA Ethics Officer
   b. Chairperson of the AOTA Commission on Standards and Ethics
   c. NBCOT Director of Regulatory Affairs
   d. Office of the state regulatory board.

Author

Ruth A. Hansen, PhD, OTR, FAOTA,
Chairperson, Commission on Standards and Ethics (SEC) (1988–1994)

Edited March 2003

Legal Options

- Contact the state attorney general's office (Medicaid or malpractice).

- Call or write to the field office of the Office of the Inspector General (Medicare).

Ethical Options

- Contact AOTA to file complaints against AOTA members.

- Contact NBCOT about any person who is currently certified by that agency (occupational therapist or occupational therapy assistant).

- Contact the state regulatory board, which has jurisdiction over all individuals practicing in that state (primary concern is protecting the public from harm).

Disciplinary Action: Whose Responsibility?

Jurisdiction

NBCOT—All certified individuals (occupational therapists and occupational therapy assistants) and persons who are currently applicants to sit for the occupational therapy and occupational therapy assistant examinations.

SRBs—All individuals regulated in that state (varies from state to state), e.g., occupational therapists, occupational therapy assistants, occupational therapy aides, and students.

AOTA—All members of AOTA. Includes all membership categories, i.e., occupational therapists, occupational therapy assistants, students, and associates.

Ruth A. Hansen, PhD, OTR, FAOTA
Chairperson, Commission on Standards and Ethics
(SEC) (1988–1994)

September 15, 1994, Revised May 1999
Edited July 2000

	NBCOT	SRB	AOTA
1. Who should I call if I have questions about			
a. Ethical violations that could cause harm or has potential to cause harm to a consumer/the public	X	X	X
b. Violations that do not cause harm or have a limited potential of causing harm to a consumer/the public			X
c. Violations of professional values that do not relate directly to potential harm to the public			X
2. Where did the alleged violation occur, and who was involved in the alleged incident?			
a. Took place in a state with rules, regulations, and disciplinary procedures in place	X	X	X
b. Took place in an unregulated state	X		X
c. Was committed by an AOTA member	X	X	X
d. Was committed by a person who is not a member of AOTA	X	X	
3. What is the disciplinary action that you wish as a consequence of filing a complaint?			
a. Restrict or revoke licensure		X	
b. Restrict or revoke certification	X		
c. Restrict or prohibit membership in AOTA			X

September 15, 1994
Edited July 2000

Adapted from American Occupational Therapy Association. (2003). *Reference guide to the occupational therapy code of ethics, 2003 edition* (pp. 22–23). Bethesda, MD: Author.

The Occupational Therapy Assistant: Resources for Practice and Education

Chapter 25

Scope of the Commission on Standards and Ethics Disciplinary Action Program

The Commission on Standards and Ethics (SEC), one of three commissions within the American Occupational Therapy Association (AOTA), serves to promote and maintain quality standards of professional conduct. The goals of the SEC are to identify ethical trends, inform and educate members about current ethical issues, uphold the practice and education standards, and review all allegations of unethical conduct.

The SEC is responsible for the *Occupational Therapy Code of Ethics (2000)* and the *Enforcement Procedures for Occupational Therapy Code of Ethics (2002)*. The *Occupational Therapy Code of Ethics (2000)* is a public statement of the values and principles that guide the behavior of members of the profession. The SEC has jurisdiction over individuals who are members of the Association, including occupational therapists, occupational therapy assistants, associates, and students. The roles of practitioner, educator, manager, researcher, and consultant are assumed. To ensure adherence by AOTA members, procedures have been developed for the investigation and adjudication of alleged violations. The *Enforcement Procedures for Occupational Therapy Code of Ethics (2002)* define the scope of disciplinary action for the Code. These procedures are intended to enable the Association to act fairly in the performance of its responsibilities as a professional organization while safeguarding the rights of members against whom complaints have been made.

Many cases that are brought to the SEC are the same as or similar to those cases brought to the National Board for Certification in Occupational Therapy (NBCOT) and state regulatory boards. These cases include fraudulent documentation, sexual misconduct, non-adherence to contracts, and professional incompetence in providing direct service. However, some ethical issues are more likely to concern only the SEC. Examples of such issues are plagiarism, supervision of students or staff, misrepresentation of research findings, or incompetence in teaching.

The SEC's disciplinary actions are independent of disciplinary actions by NBCOT or state regulatory agencies. However, the SEC routinely notifies NBCOT and the state regulatory board when the SEC makes a final decision concerning a complaint. When a complaint is under active consideration by the Disciplinary Action Committee of the NBCOT or the state regulatory board, the SEC may choose to defer action until the NBCOT or state board acts on the case. This is done to protect the rights of the individuals involved in the complaint.

This document was approved by the Commission on Standards and Ethics, August 27, 1994.

Edited July 2000
Edited March 2003

Adapted from American Occupational Therapy Association. (2003). *Reference guide to the Occupational Therapy Code of Ethics, 2003 edition* (p. 27). Bethesda, MD: Author.

Chapter 26

Occupational Therapy Code of Ethics—2000

PREAMBLE

The American Occupational Therapy Association's (AOTA's) Code of Ethics is a public statement of the common set of values and principles used to promote and maintain high standards of behavior in occupational therapy. The American Occupational Therapy Association and its members are committed to furthering the ability of individuals, groups, and systems to function within their total environment. To this end, occupational therapy personnel (including all staff and personnel who work and assist in providing occupational therapy services, (e.g., aides, orderlies, secretaries, technicians) have a responsibility to provide services to recipients in any stage of health and illness who are individuals, research participants, institutions and businesses, other professionals and colleagues, students, and to the general public.

The *Occupational Therapy Code of Ethics* is a set of principles that applies to occupational therapy personnel at all levels. These principles to which occupational therapists and occupational therapy assistants aspire are part of a lifelong effort to act in an ethical manner. The various roles of practitioner (occupational therapist and occupational therapy assistant), educator, fieldwork educator, clinical supervisor, manager, administrator, consultant, fieldwork coordinator, faculty program director, researcher/scholar, private practice owner, entrepreneur, and student are assumed.

Any action in violation of the spirit and purpose of this Code shall be considered unethical. To ensure compliance with the Code, the Commission on Standards and Ethics (SEC) establishes and maintains the enforcement procedures. Acceptance of membership in the American Occupational Therapy Association commits members to adherence to the Code of Ethics and its enforcement procedures. The Code of Ethics, *Core Values and Attitudes of Occupational Therapy Practice* (AOTA, 1993), and the *Guidelines to the Occupational Therapy Code of Ethics* (AOTA, 1998) are aspirational documents designed to be used together to guide occupational therapy personnel.

Principle 1. Occupational therapy personnel shall demonstrate a concern for the well-being of the recipients of their services. (beneficence)

A. Occupational therapy personnel shall provide services in a fair and equitable manner. They shall recognize and appreciate the cultural components of economics, geography, race, ethnicity, religious and political factors, marital status, sexual orientation, and disability of all recipients of their services.

B. Occupational therapy practitioners shall strive to ensure that fees are fair and reasonable and commensurate with services performed. When occupational therapy practitioners set fees, they shall set fees considering institutional, local, state, and federal requirements, and with due regard for the service recipient's ability to pay.

C. Occupational therapy personnel shall make every effort to advocate for recipients to obtain needed services through available means.

Principle 2. Occupational therapy personnel shall take reasonable precautions to avoid imposing or inflicting harm upon the recipient of services or to his or her property. (nonmaleficence)

A. Occupational therapy personnel shall maintain relationships that do not exploit the recipient of services sexually, physically, emotionally, financially, socially, or in any other manner.

B. Occupational therapy practitioners shall avoid relationships or activities that interfere with professional judgment and objectivity.

Principle 3. Occupational therapy personnel shall respect the recipient and/or their surrogate(s) as well as the recipient's rights. (autonomy, privacy, confidentiality)

A. Occupational therapy practitioners shall collaborate with service recipients or their surrogate(s) in setting goals and priorities throughout the intervention process.

B. Occupational therapy practitioners shall fully inform the service recipients of the nature, risks, and potential outcomes of any interventions.

C. Occupational therapy practitioners shall obtain informed consent from participants involved in research activities and indicate that they have fully informed and advised the participants of potential risks and outcomes. Occupational therapy practitioners shall endeavor to ensure that the participant(s) comprehend these risks and outcomes.

D. Occupational therapy personnel shall respect the individual's right to refuse professional services or involvement in research or educational activities.

E. Occupational therapy personnel shall protect all privileged confidential forms of written, verbal, and electronic communication gained from educational, practice, research, and investigational activities unless otherwise mandated by local, state, or federal regulations.

Principle 4. Occupational therapy personnel shall achieve and continually maintain high standards of competence. (duties)

A. Occupational therapy practitioners shall hold the appropriate national and state credentials for the services they provide.

B. Occupational therapy practitioners shall use procedures that conform to the standards of practice and other appropriate AOTA documents relevant to practice.

C. Occupational therapy practitioners shall take responsibility for maintaining and documenting competence by participating in professional development and educational activities.

D. Occupational therapy practitioners shall critically examine and keep current with emerging knowledge relevant to their practice so they may perform their duties on the basis of accurate information.

E. Occupational therapy practitioners shall protect service recipients by ensuring that duties assumed by or assigned to other occupational therapy personnel match credentials, qualifications, experience, and scope of practice.

F. Occupational therapy practitioners shall provide appropriate supervision to individuals for whom the practitioners have supervisory responsibility in accordance with Association policies, local, state and federal laws, and institutional values.

G. Occupational therapy practitioners shall refer to or consult with other service providers whenever such a referral or consultation would be helpful to the care of the recipient of service. The referral or consultation process should be done in collaboration with the recipient of service.

Principle 5. Occupational therapy personnel shall comply with laws and Association policies guiding the profession of occupational therapy. (justice)

A. Occupational therapy personnel shall familiarize themselves with and seek to understand and abide by applicable Association policies; local, state, and federal laws; and institutional rules.

B. Occupational therapy practitioners shall remain abreast of revisions in those laws and Association policies that apply to the profession of occupational therapy and shall inform employers, employees, and colleagues of those changes.

C. Occupational therapy practitioners shall require those they supervise in occupational therapy-related activities to adhere to the Code of Ethics.

D. Occupational therapy practitioners shall take reasonable steps to ensure employers are aware of occupational therapy's ethical obligations, as set forth in this Code of Ethics, and of the implications of those obligations for occupational therapy practice, education, and research.

E. Occupational therapy practitioners shall record and report in an accurate and timely manner all information related to professional activities.

Principle 6. Occupational therapy personnel shall provide accurate information about occupational therapy services. (veracity)

A. Occupational therapy personnel shall accurately represent their credentials, qualifications, education, experience, training, and competence. This is of particular importance for those to whom occupational therapy personnel provide their services or with whom occupational therapy practitioners have a professional relationship.

B. Occupational therapy personnel shall disclose any professional, personal, financial, business, or volunteer affiliations that may pose a conflict of interest to those with whom they may establish a professional, contractual, or other working relationship.

C. Occupational therapy personnel shall refrain from using or participating in the use of any form of communication that contains false, fraudulent, deceptive, or unfair statements or claims.

D. Occupational therapy practitioners shall accept the responsibility for their professional actions which reduce the public's trust in occupational therapy services and those that perform those services.

Principle 7. Occupational therapy personnel shall treat colleagues and other professionals with fairness, discretion, and integrity. (fidelity)

A. Occupational therapy personnel shall preserve, respect, and safeguard confidential information about colleagues and staff, unless otherwise mandated by national, state, or local laws.

B. Occupational therapy practitioners shall accurately represent the qualifications, views, contributions, and findings of colleagues.

C. Occupational therapy personnel shall take adequate measures to discourage, prevent, expose, and correct any breaches of the Code of Ethics and report any breaches of the Code of Ethics to the appropriate authority.

D. Occupational therapy personnel shall familiarize themselves with established policies and procedures for handling concerns about this Code of Ethics, including familiarity with national, state, local, district, and territorial procedures for handling ethics complaints. These include policies and procedures created by the American Occupational Therapy Association, licensing and regulatory bodies, employers, agencies, certification boards, and other organizations who have jurisdiction over occupational therapy practice.

References

American Occupational Therapy Association. (1993). Core values and attitudes of occupational therapy practice. *American Journal of Occupational Therapy, 47,* 1085–1086.

American Occupational Therapy Association. (1998). Guidelines to the occupational therapy code of ethics. *American Journal of Occupational Therapy, 52,* 881–884.

Authors

THE COMMISSION ON STANDARDS AND ETHICS (SEC):
Barbara L. Kornblau, JD, OTR, FAOTA, Chairperson
Melba Arnold, MS, OTR/L
Nancy Nashiro, PhD, OTR, FAOTA
Diane Hill, COTA/L, AP
Deborah Y. Slater, MS, OTR/L
John Morris, PhD
Linda Withers, CNHA, FACHCA
Penny Kyler, MA, OTR/L, FAOTA, Staff Liaison

April 2000

Adopted by the Representative Assembly 2000M15

Note. This document replaces the 1994 document, *Occupational Therapy Code of Ethics (American Journal of Occupational Therapy, 48,* 1037–1038).

Prepared 4/7/2000

Previously published and copyrighted in 2000 by the American Occupational Therapy Association, Inc. in the *American Journal of Occupational Therapy, 54,* 614–616.

Adapted from American Occupational Therapy Association. (2003). *Reference guide to the Occupational Therapy Code of Ethics, 2003 edition.* (pp. 10–12). Bethesda, MD: Author.

Chapter 27

Guidelines to the *Occupational Therapy Code of Ethics* (2000)

Introduction

The Guidelines to the Occupational Therapy Code of Ethics (2000) are organized under main topics that reflect the issues that members of the American Occupational Therapy Association (AOTA) most frequently raise. The topic headings are honesty, communication, ensuring the common good, competence, confidentiality, conflict of interest, the impaired practitioner, sexual relationships, and payment for services. Following each heading is a brief description of the topic and a general description of the desired behaviors. Several statements that are examples of desired action in more specific situations follow these descriptions. The final section of the paper describes steps that can be taken to resolve ethical issues.

The Guidelines to the Occupational Therapy Code of Ethics (2000) are overarching statements of morally correct action. The Guidelines also indicate a level of expected professional behavior. The Guidelines can be used to provide clarification when a perplexing problem arises, can be used as educational or supervisory tools, and can be used to educate the public. The *Guidelines, Core Values and Attitudes of Occupational Therapy Practice* (AOTA, 1993), and the *Occupational Therapy Code of Ethics* (AOTA, 2000) are all aspirational rather than legal documents. These documents are designed to be used together in the deliberation of ethical concerns. The Guidelines are moral and philosophical statements that encourage occupational therapy practitioners to attain a high level of professional behavior. They also bind the profession to the singular purpose of assuring the public of high quality occupational therapy services. The following terms are used throughout this document and are defined as follows:

- *Occupational Therapist*—Any individual initially certified to practice as an occupational therapist or licensed or regulated by a state, district, commonwealth or territory of the United States to practice as an occupational therapist.

- *Occupational Therapy Assistant*—Any individual certified to practice as an occupational therapy assistant or licensed or regulated by a state, district, commonwealth, or territory of the United States to practice as an occupational therapy assistant.

- *Occupational Therapy Practitioner*—A term that is inclusive of both occupational therapists and occupational therapy assistants.

- *Occupational Therapy Personnel*—For the purposes of this paper, this term includes all staff and personnel who work and assist in providing occupational therapy services (e.g., aides, orderlies, secretaries, technicians).

1. **Honesty:** *Be honest with yourself, be honest with all you come in contact with. Know your strengths and limitations.*

   1.1 In education, research, and clinical practice, individuals must be honest in receiving and disseminating information by providing opportunities for informed consent and for discussion of available options.

   1.2 Occupational therapy practitioners must be certain that informed consent has been obtained prior to the initiation of services, including evaluation. If the service recipient cannot give informed consent, the practitioner must be sure that consent has been obtained from the person who is legally responsible for the service recipient.

   1.3 Occupational therapy practitioners must be truthful about their individual competencies as well as the competence of those under their supervision. In some cases the therapist may need to refer the client to another professional to assure that the best possible services are provided.

   1.4 Referrals to other health care specialists shall be based exclusively on the other provider's competence and ability to provide the needed service.

   1.5 All documentation must accurately reflect the nature and quantity of services provided.

1.6 Occupational therapy practitioners terminate services when the services do not meet the needs and goals of the service recipient, or when services no longer produce a measurable outcome.

1.7 All marketing and advertising must be truthful and carefully presented to avoid misleading the consumer.

2. **Communication:** *Communication is important in all aspects of occupational therapy. Individuals must be conscientious and truthful in all facets of written, verbal, and electronic communication.*

2.1 Occupational therapy personnel do not make deceptive, fraudulent, or misleading statements about the nature of the services they provide or the outcomes that can be expected.

2.2 Occupational therapy personnel shall not divulge confidential information or information that may cause harm to the consumer. Caution must be taken to assure that confidentiality is maintained in verbal, written, or electronically transmitted communications.

2.3 Professional contracts for occupational therapy services shall explicitly describe the type and duration of services as well as the duties and responsibilities of all involved parties.

2.4 Documentation for reimbursement purposes shall be done in accordance with applicable laws and regulations.

2.5 Documentation shall accurately reflect the service delivered and the outcomes. It shall be of the kind and quality that satisfies the scrutiny of peer reviews, legal proceedings, and accrediting agencies.

2.6 Occupational therapy personnel must be honest in gathering and giving fact-based information regarding job performance and fieldwork performance. Information given shall be timely and truthful, accurate, and respectful of all parties involved.

2.7 Documentation for supervisory purposes shall accurately reflect the factual components of the interactions and the expected outcomes.

2.8 Occupational therapy personnel must give credit and recognition when using the work of others.

2.9 Occupational therapy personnel do not fabricate data, falsify information, or plagiarize.

2.10 Occupational therapy personnel refrain from using biased or derogatory language in written, verbal, and electronic communication about patients, clients, students, research subjects, and colleagues.

2.11 Occupational therapy personnel who provide information through oral and written means shall emphasize that service delivery for individual problems cannot be treated without proper individualized evaluations and plans of care.

3. **Ensuring the Common Good:** *Individuals are expected to increase everyone's awareness of the profession's social responsibilities to help ensure the common good.*

3.1 Occupational therapy practitioners take steps to make sure that employers are aware of the ethical concepts of the profession and occupational therapy personnel's adherence to those ethical concepts.

3.2 Occupational therapy personnel shall be diligent stewards of human, financial, and material resources of their employers. They shall refrain from exploiting these resources for personal gain.

3.3 Occupational therapy personnel shall never use funds for unintended purposes or misappropriate funds.

3.4 Occupational therapy personnel should actively work with their employer to prevent discrimination and unfair labor practices. They should also advocate for employees with disabilities to ensure the provision of reasonable accommodations.

3.5 Occupational therapy personnel should actively participate with their employer in the formulation of policies and procedures. They should do this to ensure that these policies and procedures are legal and that they are consistent with the Occupational Therapy Code of Ethics (2000).

3.6 Occupational therapy personnel who participate in a business arrangement as owner, stockholder, partner, or employee have an obligation to maintain the ethical principles and standards of the profession. They also shall refrain from working for or doing business with organizations that engage in illegal business practices (e.g., fraudulent billing).

3.7 Occupational therapy personnel in educational settings are responsible for promoting ethical conduct by students and by both academic and clinical colleagues.

3.8 Occupational therapy personnel involved in or preparing to be involved in research (educational or clinical) need to obtain formal institutional approval prior to initiating that research.

3.9 Occupational therapy personnel shall respect the right of the individual to decline to receive occupational therapy interventions or to be involved in research.

4. **Competence:** *Individuals are expected to work within their areas of competence and to pursue opportunities to update, increase, and expand their competence.*

4.1 Occupational therapy personnel developing new areas of competence (skills, techniques, approaches) must engage in appropriate study and training, under appropriate supervision, before incorporating new areas into their practice.

4.2 When generally recognized standards do not exist in emerging areas of practice, occupational therapy personnel must take responsible steps to ensure their own competence.

4.3 When conducting research, occupational therapists must know the profession's standards and guidelines and the state and federal laws governing research.

4.4 Occupational therapy personnel shall develop an understanding and appreciation for different cultures in order to be able to provide culturally competent service. Culturally competent practitioners are aware of how service delivery can be affected by economic, ethnic, racial, geographic, gender, religious, and political factors as well as marital status, sexual orientation, and disability.

4.5 In areas where the ability to communicate with the client is limited (aphasia, different language, literacy), occupational therapy personnel shall take appropriate steps to ensure comprehension and meaningful communication.

4.6 Occupational therapy personnel do not encourage or facilitate the use of skilled occupational therapy interventions or techniques by unqualified persons.

5. **Confidentiality:** *Information that is confidential must remain confidential. This information cannot be shared either verbally, electronically, or in writing without appropriate consent. Information must be shared on a need-to-know basis only with those having primary responsibilities for decision making.*

5.1 All occupational therapy personnel shall respect the confidential nature of information gained in any occupational therapy interaction. The only exceptions are when a practitioner or staff member believes that an individual is in serious, foreseeable, or imminent harm. In this instance, laws and regulations require disclosure to appropriate authorities without consent.

5.2 Occupational therapy personnel shall respect the individual's right to privacy.

5.3 Occupational therapy personnel shall take all due precautions to maintain the confidentiality of all verbal, written, and electronic communications that are confidential.

5.4 Occupational therapy personnel shall maintain as confidential information derived from working relationships with other occupational therapy practitioners. Peer review information is held as confidential unless written permission is obtained from the individual receiving the review.

6. **Conflict of Interest:** *Avoidance of real or perceived conflict of interest is imperative to maintaining the integrity of interactions.*

6.1 Occupational therapy personnel shall be alert to and avoid any action that would interfere with the exercise of impartial professional judgment during the delivery of occupational therapy services.

6.2 Occupational therapy personnel shall not take advantage of or exploit anyone to further their own personal interests.

6.3 Gifts and remuneration from individuals, agencies, or companies must be reported in accordance with employer policies as well as state and federal guidelines. Many institutions have a "zero tolerance" policy that absolutely prohibits an employee from accepting gifts, favors, or additional payment from clients, vendors, and outside agencies.

6.4 Occupational therapy personnel shall not accept obligations or duties that may compete with or be in conflict with their duties to their employers.

6.5 Occupational therapy personnel shall not use their position or the knowledge gained from their position in such a way that knowingly gives rise to real or perceived conflict of interest between themselves and their employers or other organizations.

7. **Impaired Practitioner:** *Occupational therapy personnel who cannot competently perform their duties after reasonable accommodation are considered to be impaired. The occupational therapy practitioner's basic duty to students, patients, colleagues, and research subjects is to ensure that no harm is done. It is difficult to report a professional colleague who is impaired. The motive for this action must be to provide for the protection and safety of all, including the person who is impaired.*

7.1 It is the individual responsibility of occupational therapy personnel to be aware of their own personal problems and limitations that may interfere with their ability to perform their job competently. They should know when these problems have the potential of causing harm to patients, colleagues, students, research subjects, and others.

7.2 The individual should seek the appropriate professional help and take steps to remedy personal problems and limitations that interfere with job performance.

7.3 Occupational therapy personnel who believe that a colleague's impairment interferes with safe and effective practice should, when possible, discuss their questions and concerns with the individual and assist their colleague in seeking appropriate help or treatment.

7.4 When efforts to assist an impaired colleague fail, the occupational therapy practitioner is responsible for reporting the individual to the appropriate authority (employer, agency, licensing or regulatory board, certification body, professional organization).

8. **Sexual Relationships:** *Sexual relationships that occur during any professional interaction are forms of misconduct.*

8.1 Because of potential coercion or harm to former patients, clients, consumers, students, or research subjects, occupational therapy practitioners are responsible for ensuring that the individual with whom they enter into a romantic/sexual relationship has not been coerced or exploited in any way.

8.2 Sexual relationships with current patients, clients, employees, consumers, students, or research subjects are not permissible, even if the relationship is consensual.

8.3 Occupational therapy personnel must not sexually harass any persons, including, but not limited to, students, employees, patient, clients, trainees, colleagues, or research subjects. Sexual harassment is defined as unwanted verbal or physical conduct of a sexual nature. It includes sexual advances or sexual solicitations that interfere with the work or academic performance of the individual and that create a hostile, offensive, or intimidating environment.

8.4 Occupational therapy personnel have full responsibility to set clear and appropriate boundaries in their professional interactions.

9. **Payment for Services:** *Occupational therapy personnel shall not guarantee or promise specific outcomes for occupational therapy services. Payment for occupational therapy services shall not be contingent on successful outcomes.*

9.1 Occupational therapy personnel shall not collect illegal fees. Fees shall be fair and reasonable and commensurate with services delivered.

9.2 Occupational therapy personnel do not ordinarily participate in bartering for services because of potential exploitation and conflict of interest. However, such an arrangement may be appropriate if it is not clinically contraindicated, if the relationship is not exploitative, and if bartering is a culturally appropriate custom.

9.3 Although it is not universally possible, occupational therapy practitioners can render pro bono ("for the good," free of charge) or reduced fee occupational therapy services for selected individuals with limited financial resources. Occupational therapy personnel may also provide pro bono services by engaging in activities to improve access to occupational therapy or by providing individual service and expertise to charitable organizations.

10. **Resolving Ethical Issues**

10.1 Occupational therapy personnel are obligated to be familiar with the Occupational Therapy Code of Ethics (2000) and its application to their respective work environments. Occupational therapy practitioners are expected to share the Occupational Therapy Code of Ethics (2000) with their employer and other employees and colleagues. Lack of familiarity and awareness of the Occupational Therapy Code of Ethics (2000) is not an excuse or a defense against a charge of ethical misconduct.

10.2 Occupational therapy personnel who are uncertain of whether a specific action would violate the Occupational Therapy Code of Ethics (2000) have a responsibility to consult with knowledgeable individuals, ethics committees, or other appropriate authorities. All consulting shall be done within recognized proscriptions of confidentiality.

10.3 Conflicts between personal and organizational ethics do occur. However, the occupational therapy practitioners must clarify the nature of the conflict, make known their commitment to the Occupational Therapy Code of Ethics (2000), and, where possible, seek to resolve the conflict in a way that permits the fullest adherence to the Occupational Therapy Code of Ethics (2000).

10.4 The occupational therapy practitioner shall attempt to resolve violations informally by bringing them to the attention of the person or persons responsible.

10.5 If the informal resolution is not appropriate or is not effective, the next step is to take action by consultation or referral to institutional, local, district, territorial, state, or national groups who have jurisdiction over occupational therapy practice.

10.6 Occupational therapy personnel shall cooperate with ethics committee proceedings and comply with resulting requirements. Failure to cooperate is, in itself, an ethical violation.

10.7 Occupational therapy personnel shall not file frivolous ethics complaints aimed at harming a colleague rather than protecting the public.

References

American Occupational Therapy Association. (1993). Core values and attitudes of occupational therapy practice. *American Journal of Occupational Therapy, 47,* 1085–1086.

American Occupational Therapy Association. (1994). Occupational therapy code of ethics. *American Journal of Occupational Therapy, 48,* 1037–1038.

American Occupational Therapy Association. (1996). Bylaws. In *Reference manual of the official documents of the American Occupational Therapy Association, Inc.* (6th ed.). Bethesda, MD: Author.

Author

Ruth A. Hansen, PhD, FAOTA
For Mary P. Taugher, PhD, OT, FAOTA, Chairperson,
Commission on Standards and Ethics (1995–1998)

Approved SEC March 1998

Edited July 2000

Adapted from American Occupational Therapy Association. (2003). *Reference guide to the Occupational Therapy Code of Ethics, 2003 edition.* (pp. 16–20). Bethesda, MD: Author.

Chapter 28

Enforcement Procedures for the *Occupational Therapy Code of Ethics* (2004)

1. Introduction

The American Occupational Therapy Association (AOTA) and its members are committed to furthering each individual's ability to function fully within his or her total environment. To this end, the occupational therapist and occupational therapy assistant render services to clients in all phases of health and illness, to institutions, to organizations to other professionals and colleagues, to students, and to the public.

The AOTA's Occupational Therapy Code of Ethics, its Guidelines and Core Values (hereinafter jointly referred to as "Ethics Standards") are public statements of values and principles to use as a guide in promoting and maintaining high standards of behavior in occupational therapy.

The Ethics Standards apply to occupational therapy personnel at all levels. They apply to professional roles such as those of practitioner, educator, fieldwork educator or coordinator, clinical supervisor, manager, administrator, consultant, faculty, program director, researcher/scholar, private practice owner, entrepreneur, student, and other professional roles, including elective and appointed volunteer roles within the AOTA. More broadly, these Ethics Standards apply not only to conduct within occupational therapy roles, but also to conduct that may affect the performance of occupational therapy or the reputation of the profession. The principal purposes of the Ethics Standards are to help protect the public and to reinforce its confidence in the occupational therapy profession rather than to resolve private business, legal, or other disputes for which there are other more appropriate forums.

To ensure compliance with the Ethics Standards, these Enforcement Procedures are established and maintained by the Commission on Standards and Ethics (hereinafter referred to as the "SEC"). Acceptance of membership in the AOTA commits members to adherence to the Ethics Standards and cooperation with its Enforcement Procedures. The SEC urges particular attention to the following issues:

1.1 *Professional Responsibility, Other Processes*—All occupational therapy personnel have an obligation to maintain the standards of ethics of their profession and to promote and support these standards among their colleagues. Each member must be alert to practices that undermine these standards and is obligated to take action that is appropriate in the circumstances. At the same time, members must carefully weigh their judgments as to potentially unethical practice to ensure that they are based on objective evaluation and not on personal bias or prejudice, inadequate information, or simply differences of professional viewpoint. It is recognized that individual occupational therapy personnel may not have the authority or ability to address or correct all situations of concern. Whenever feasible and appropriate, members should first pursue other corrective steps within the relevant institution or setting before resorting to the AOTA ethics complaint process.

1.2 *Jurisdiction*—The Code of Ethics (hereinafter referred to as the "Code") applies to persons who are or were members of the AOTA at the time of the conduct in question. Later non-renewal or relinquishment of membership does not affect AOTA jurisdiction. The Code that is applicable to any complaint shall be the Code in force at the time the alleged act or omission occurred, unless the date of the alleged act or omission cannot be precisely determined. In that case, the conduct shall be judged by the Code in force on the date of the complaint.

1.3 *Disciplinary Actions/Sanctions (Pursuing a Complaint)*—If the SEC determines that unethical conduct has occurred, it may impose sanctions including reprimand, censure, probation, suspension, or permanent revocation of membership in the AOTA. In all cases except those involving only reprimand, the AOTA will report the conclusions and sanctions in its official publications and will also communicate to any appropriate persons or entities. The potential sanctions are defined as follows:

1.3.1 *Reprimand*—A formal expression of disapproval of conduct communicated privately by letter from the Chairperson of the SEC that is non-disclosable and noncommunicative to other bodies (e.g., State Regulatory Boards, National Board for Certification in Occupational Therapy, hereinafter known as NBCOT).

1.3.2 *Censure*—A formal expression of disapproval that is public.

1.3.3 *Probation of membership subject to terms*—Failure to meet terms will subject a member to any of the disciplinary actions or sanctions.

1.3.4 *Suspension*—Removal of membership for a specified period of time.

1.3.5 *Revocation*—Permanent denial of membership.

1.4 *Educative Letters*—If the SEC determines that the alleged conduct, even if proven, does not appear to be unethical, but may not be completely in keeping with the aspirational nature of the Code or within the prevailing standards of practice or good professionalism, the SEC may send a letter to educate the Respondent only regarding standards of practice and/or good professionalism. In addition, a different educative letter, if appropriate, may be sent to the Complainant.

1.5 *Advisory Opinions*—The SEC may issue general advisory opinions on ethical issues to inform and educate the membership. These opinions shall be publicized to the membership.

1.6 *Rules of Evidence*—The SEC proceedings shall be conducted in accordance with fundamental fairness. However, formal rules of evidence that are employed in legal proceedings do not apply to these Enforcement Procedures. The Judicial Council and the Appeal Panel can consider any evidence that they deem appropriate and pertinent.

1.7 *Confidentiality and Disclosure*—In order to address the legitimate interests of the Respondent, Complainant, witnesses, and others involved in the investigation and processing of an ethics complaint, the ethics enforcement proceedings including findings are confidential. Appropriate confidentiality shall be maintained by all who are involved in reporting and processing ethics matters, including witnesses and complainant. The only exception to this would be in terms of reporting public sanction or disciplinary action.

1.7.1 *Disclosure*—The SEC may seek information and documentation from state licensing agencies, academic councils, courts, employers, and other persons and entities. Except as necessary to obtain relevant evidence or administer the ethics process, or for other good cause, or when the SEC takes a public action in a case, the SEC shall not disclose to clients, colleagues, support personnel of the Respondent, or others, information or documentation developed in the course of the proceedings under these Procedures. The SEC may determine what disclosures are appropriate for particular parties. Final decisions of the Judicial Council and the Appeal Panel will be publicized as provided in these Procedures.

2. Complaints

2.1 *Interested Party Complaints*

2.1.1 Complaints stating an alleged violation of the Code may originate from any individual, group, or entity within or outside the Association. All complaints must be in writing, signed by the Complainant(s), and submitted to the Chairperson of the SEC at the address of the AOTA's Headquarters. All complaints shall identify the person against whom the complaint is directed (the Respondent), the ethical principles that the Complainant believes have been violated, and the key facts of the alleged violations. If lawfully available, supporting documentation should be attached.

2.1.2 Within 90 days of receipt of a complaint, the SEC shall make a preliminary assessment of the complaint and decide whether it presents sufficient questions as to a potential ethics violation that an investigation is warranted. Commencing an investigation does not imply a conclusion that an ethical violation has in fact occurred, or any judgment as to the ultimate sanction, if any, that may be appropriate.

2.2 *Complaints Initiated by the SEC*

2.2.1 The SEC itself may initiate a complaint (a "sua sponte" complaint) when it receives information from a governmental body, certification or similar body, public media, or other source indicating that a person subject to its jurisdiction may have committed acts which violate the Code. The AOTA will ordinarily act promptly after learning of the basis of a sua sponte complaint, but there is no specified time limit.

If the SEC passes a motion to initiate a sua sponte complaint, the members of the SEC will complete the Formal Statement of Complaint Form (attached at end of this document) and will describe the nature of the factual allegations that led to the complaint and the manner in which the SEC learned of the matter. The Complaint Form will be signed by the Chairperson of the SEC on behalf of the SEC, and will serve in lieu of the Claimant Questionnaire. The form will be given to the SEC staff liaison.

Sua Sponte complaints fall into two broad categories:

- *de jure* (by law) complaints are those arising from the findings of a governmental or a credentialing body recognized by the AOTA (e.g., state or federal courts, NBCOT, state licensure boards); and

- *de facto* (by facts) complaints are those arising from information coming to the attention of the SEC in any other fashion that suggests a possible violation of the Code (e.g., information gathered during the investigation of another complaint, newspaper articles, or evidence arising in civil suits).

2.2.2 *De Jure* Complaints—*de jure* sua sponte complaints will proceed as follows:

a. The SEC staff liaison will present to the SEC any findings from external sources (as described above) pertaining to members of the AOTA that come to his or her attention and that may warrant sua sponte complaints.

b. Since *de jure* complaints are based upon the findings of fact or conclusions of another official body, the SEC will decide whether or not to act based on such findings or conclusions, and will not initiate another investigation, absent clear and convincing evidence that such findings and conclusions were erroneous. Based upon the information presented by the SEC staff liaison, the SEC will determine whether the findings of the public body also are sufficient to demonstrate a violation of the Code and therefore warrant an ethics charge.

c. If the SEC decides that a formal charge is warranted, the Chairperson of the SEC will notify the Respondent in writing of the formal charge and the proposed disciplinary action. In response to the *de jure* sua sponte charge by the SEC, the Respondent may either

1. Accept the decision of the SEC (as to both the ethics violation and the sanction) based solely upon the findings of fact and conclusions of the SEC or the public body; or,

2. Accept the charge that the Respondent committed unethical conduct, but within 30 days submit to the SEC a statement

setting forth the reasons why any sanction should not be imposed, or reasons why the sanction should be mitigated or reduced; or,

3. Within 30 days, present information showing the findings of fact of the official body relied upon by the SEC to initiate the charge are clearly erroneous and request reconsideration by the SEC. The SEC may have the option of opening an investigation or modifying the sanction in the event they find clear and convincing evidence that the findings and the conclusions of the other body are erroneous.

d. In cases of *de jure* complaints, a Judicial Council hearing can later be requested (pursuant to Section 5 below) only if the Respondent has first exercised option 2 or 3.

2.2.3 *De Facto* Complaints—A *de facto* sua sponte complaint may be filed if the AOTA learns through a public source (such as a newspaper article) that there may be a substantial basis for finding an ethics violation. The AOTA does not, however, undertake systematically to canvass all public media; it may or may not learn of events that warrant a *de facto* sua sponte complaint. *De facto* sua sponte cases will proceed as follows:

a. The SEC staff liaison will present the material to the SEC.

b. At this point, the SEC has two ways it can proceed:

1. If the SEC chooses to do an investigation, the regular procedures for Investigation (Section 3) will be followed; or,

2. If the SEC determines that there is sufficient information to support a violation of the Code and no further investigation is warranted, the respondent will be notified. The complaint form and supporting documentation, charge, and proposed sanction will be submitted to the Respondent, who will be afforded the opportunity to respond in any of the following 3 ways:

- Accept the charge of the SEC (as to both the ethics violation and the sanction) based solely upon the findings of fact and conclusions of the SEC and the information submitted; or,

- Accept the charge that the Respondent committed unethical conduct, but within 30 days submit to the SEC any new information relating to the charge that the Respondent would like the SEC to consider in connection with deciding upon a different sanction; or, the Respondent may submit a statement setting forth the reasons why any sanction should not be imposed or reasons why the sanction should be mitigated or reduced; or,

- Within 30 days advise the SEC that he or she contests the charge and request the SEC do a formal investigation to allow new or additional information to be presented that may alter the decision to find an ethical violation.

2.3 *Continuation of Complaint Process*—If a member relinquishes membership, fails to renew membership, or fails to cooperate with the ethics investigation, the SEC shall nevertheless continue to process the complaint, noting in its report the circumstances of the Respondent's action. Such actions shall not deprive the SEC of jurisdiction.

3. SEC Review and Investigations

3.1 *Initial Action*—The purpose of the preliminary review is to decide whether or not the information submitted with the complaint warrants opening the case. If in its preliminary review of the complaint, the SEC determines that an investigation is not warranted, the Complainant will be so notified.

3.2 *Dismissal of Complaints*—The SEC may at any time dismiss a complaint for any of the following reasons:

    3.2.1 *Lack of Jurisdiction*—The SEC determines that it has no jurisdiction over the Respondent (e.g., a complaint against a person who is or was not a member at the time of the alleged incident or who has never been a member).

    3.2.2 *Absolute Time Limit/Not Timely Filed*—The SEC determines that the violation of the Code is alleged to have occurred more than 7 years prior to the filing of the complaint.

    3.2.3 *Subject to Jurisdiction of Another Authority*—The SEC determines that the complaint is based on matters that are within the authority of, and are more properly dealt with by, another governmental or nongovernmental body, such as a state regulatory board, NBCOT, an AOTA component other than the SEC, an employer, or a court (e.g., accusing a superior of sexual harassment at work, accusing someone of anticompetitive practices subject to the antitrust laws).

    3.2.4 *No Ethics Violation*—The SEC finds that the complaint, even if proven, does not state a basis for action under the Code (e.g., simply accusing someone of being unpleasant or rude on an occasion).

    3.2.5 *Insufficient Evidence*—The SEC determines that there clearly would not be sufficient factual evidence to support a finding of an ethics violation.

    3.2.6 *Corrected Violation*—The SEC determines that any violation it might find already has been or is being corrected, and that this is an adequate result in the given case.

    3.2.7 *Other good cause.*

3.3 *Investigator (Avoidance of Conflict of Interest)*—The Investigator chosen shall not have a conflict of interest (i.e., shall never have had a substantial professional, personal, financial, business, or volunteer relationship with either the Complainant or the Respondent). In the event that the SEC staff liaison has such a conflict, the SEC Chairperson in collaboration with the AOTA Ethics Officer shall appoint an alternate Investigator who has no conflict of interest.

3.4 *Investigation*—If an investigation is deemed warranted, the SEC Chairperson shall do the following within 15 days:

Appoint the SEC staff liaison at the AOTA Headquarters to investigate the complaint and notify the Respondent (by certified, return receipt mail) that a complaint has been received and an investigation is being conducted. A copy of the complaint and supporting documentation shall be enclosed with this notification. The Complainant will also receive notification by certified, return receipt mail that the complaint is being investigated.

    3.4.1 Ordinarily, the Investigator will send questions to be answered by the Complainant and the Respondent.

    3.4.2 The Complainant shall be given 30 days from receipt of the questions to respond in writing to the Investigator.

    3.4.3 The Respondent shall be given 30 days from receipt of the questions to respond in writing to the Investigator.

    3.4.4 The SEC ordinarily will notify the Complainant of any substantive new evidence adverse to the Complainant's initial complaint that is discovered in the course of the ethics investigation and allow the Complainant to respond to such adverse evidence. In such cases, the Complainant will be given a copy of such evidence and will have 14 days in which to submit a written response. If the new evidence clearly shows that there has been no ethics violation, the SEC may terminate the proceeding.

    3.4.5 The Investigator may obtain evidence directly from third parties.

3.5 *Investigation Timeline*—The investigation will be completed within 90 days of the appointment of the Investigator, unless the SEC determines that special circumstances warrant additional time for the investigation. All timelines noted here can be tolled or extended for good cause at the discretion of the SEC, including the SEC's schedule and additional requests of the Respondent. The Respondent and the Complainant shall be notified in writing if a delay occurs or if the investigational process requires more time.

3.6 *Report*—The Investigator's report shall include the complaint and any documentation on which the SEC relied in initiating the investigation, and shall state findings without recommendations.

3.7 *Cooperation by Member*—Every AOTA member has a duty to cooperate reasonably with enforcement processes under the Code. Failure of the Respondent to participate and/or cooperate with the investigative process of the SEC shall not prevent continuation of the ethics process, and this behavior itself may constitute a violation of the Code.

3.8 *Referral of Complaint*—The SEC may at any time refer a matter to NBCOT, state regulatory boards, or other recognized authorities for appropriate action. Despite such referral to an appropriate authority, the SEC shall retain jurisdiction. SEC action may be stayed for a reasonable period pending notification of a decision by that authority, at the discretion of the SEC (and such delays will extend the time periods under these Procedures). A stay in conducting an investigation shall not constitute a waiver by the SEC of jurisdiction over the matters. The SEC shall provide written notice by mail (requiring signature and proof of date of receipt) to the Respondent and the Complainant of any such stay of action.

4. Commission on Standards and Ethics Review and Decision

4.1 *Charges*—The SEC shall review the Investigator's report and shall render a decision on whether a charge by the SEC is warranted within 90 days of receipt of the report. The SEC may, in the conduct of its review, take whatever further investigatory actions it deems

necessary. If the SEC determines that an ethics complaint warrants a charge, the SEC shall proceed with a disciplinary proceeding by promptly sending a notice of the charge(s) to the Respondent and Complainant by mail with signature and proof of date received. The notice of the charge(s) shall describe the alleged conduct that, if proven, would constitute a violation of the Code. The notice of charge(s) shall describe the conduct in sufficient detail to inform the Respondent of the nature of the unethical behavior that is alleged. The SEC may indicate in the notice its preliminary view (absent contrary facts or mitigating circumstances) as to what sanction would be warranted if the violation is proven.

4.2 *Respondent's Response*—Within 30 days of notification of the SEC's decision to charge, and proposed sanction, if any, the Respondent shall either

    4.2.1 Advise the SEC Chairperson in writing that he or she accepts the SEC's charge of an ethics violation and the proposed sanction and waives any right to a Judicial Council hearing; or,

    4.2.2 Advise the SEC Chairperson in writing that he or she accepts the SEC's charge of an ethics violation, but believes the sanction is not justified and requests a hearing before the Judicial Council on that matter alone; or,

    4.2.3 Advise the SEC Chairperson in writing that he or she contests the SEC's charge and the proposed sanction and requests a hearing before the Judicial Council.

    Failure of the Respondent to take one of these actions within the time specified will be deemed to constitute acceptance of the charge and proposed sanction. If the Respondent requests a Judicial Council hearing, it will be scheduled. If the Respondent does not request a Judicial Council hearing, but accepts the decision, the SEC will notify all relevant parties and implement the sanction.

5. The Judicial Council

5.1 *Purpose*—The purpose of the Judicial Council (hereinafter to be known as "the Council") hearing is to provide the Respondent an opportunity to present evidence and witnesses to answer and refute the charge and/or the proposed sanction and to permit the SEC Chairperson or designee (the "SEC Chair") to present evidence and witnesses in support of his or her charge. The Council shall consider the matters alleged in the complaint, the matters raised in defense, and other relevant facts, ethical principles, and law. The Council may question the parties concerning, and determine ethical issues arising from, the factual matters in the case even if those specific ethical issues were not raised by the Complainant. The Council may reverse or modify the decision of the SEC if it finds that the decision was clearly erroneous or a material departure from its written procedure.

5.2 *Parties*—The parties to a Council Hearing are the Respondent and the SEC Chairperson.

5.3 *Panel Selection*—The Council is comprised of three members in good standing of the AOTA, and one public member with knowledge of the profession and ethical issues. The Council shall be drawn from a pool of qualified individuals/ members who have been identified as meeting the criteria for selection outlined in the *Judicial Council General Procedures* (2002) and who are available for a period of 3 years. The Council shall be appointed by the liaison to the SEC within 30 days of the notification, to hear the formal charge(s) against the Respondent and decide the merits of the case. Members appointed shall not have any conflict of interest, (i.e., shall never have had a substantial professional, personal, financial, business, or volunteer relationship with either the Complainant or the Respondent or other persons indicated in the record as material to the matter).

5.4 *Hearing*—Not less than 45 days in advance of the hearing, the Council shall notify in writing all appropriate parties of the date, time, and place for the hearing. Case material will be sent to all parties and the Council members by national delivery service or mail with signature required and proof of date received with return receipt. Within 30 days of notification of the hearing, the Respondent shall submit to the Council a written response to the charges, including a detailed statement as to the reasons that he or she is appealing the decision and a list of potential witnesses (if any) with a statement indicating the subject matter they will be addressing. The SEC Chairperson, as the Complainant before the Council, will also submit a list of potential witnesses (if any) to the Council with a statement indicating the subject matter they will be addressing. Only under limited circumstances may the Council consider additional material evidence from the Respondent or the SEC not presented or available to the SEC prior to the issuance of their proposed sanction. Such new or additional evidence may be considered by the Council if the Council is satisfied that the Respondent or the SEC has demonstrated the new evidence was previously unavail-

able and provided it is submitted to all parties in writing no later than 15 days prior to the hearing. The Chair of the Council (in consultation with the other members) may permit testimony by conference call, limit participation of witnesses in order to curtail repetitive testimony, or prescribe other reasonable arrangements or limitations. The Respondent may elect to appear (at Respondent's own expense) and present testimony. An oral affirmation of truthfulness will be requested from each participant in the Council hearing. The total hearing shall be limited to 2 hours. A transcript, videotape, or audiotape record shall be maintained of the Council hearing, as determined by the discretion of the Council.

5.5 *Counsel*—The Respondent may be represented by legal counsel at his or her own expense. The SEC Chairperson and the Association Legal Counsel shall advise and represent the Association at the hearing. The Association Legal Counsel also advises the Council. All parties shall have the opportunity to confront and cross-examine witnesses.

5.6 *Decision*—The Council shall submit its decision in writing to the AOTA President (or his or her designee) within 30 days of receiving the written transcription of the hearing, unless special circumstances warrant additional time.

5.7 *Notification*—Promptly after the report has been transmitted to the President, the Council shall notify all parties of its decision within 15 working days via mail (with signature and proof of date received) addressed to the Respondent, the SEC Chairperson, and other appropriate parties.

5.8 *Appeal*—Within 30 days after notification of the Council's decision, a Respondent upon whom a sanction was imposed may appeal the decision as provided in Section 6. Within 30 days after notification of the Council's decision, the SEC may also appeal the decision as provided in Section 6. If no appeal is filed within that time, the President shall notify appropriate bodies within the Association and make any other notifications deemed necessary.

6. Appeal Process

6.1 *Appeals*—Either the SEC or the Respondent may appeal. Appeals shall be written, signed by the appealing party, and sent by certified mail to the President c/o the Ethics Office of AOTA. The grounds for the appeal shall be fully explained in this document. When an appeal is requested, the other party will be notified.

6.2 *Grounds for Appeal*—Appeals shall generally address only the issues, procedures, or sanctions that are part of the record before the Judicial Council. However, in the interests of fairness, the Appeal Panel may consider newly available evidence relating to the original charge only under extraordinary circumstances. The Vice-President, Secretary, and Treasurer of the AOTA shall constitute the Appeal Panel. In the event of vacancies in these positions or the existence of a conflict of interest, the Vice President shall appoint replacements drawn from among the other Board members. If the entire Board of Directors has a conflict of interest (e.g., the Complainant or Respondent is or was recently a member of the Board of Directors), the Board Appeal process shall be followed. The President shall not serve on the Appeal Panel.

6.3 *Appeal Process*—The President shall forward any letter of appeal to the Appeal Panel within 15 days of receipt. Within 45 days after the Appeal Panel receives the appeal, the Panel shall determine whether a hearing is warranted according to the Board of Directors policy on appeals (unless it is an SEC appeal). If the Panel decides that a hearing is warranted, timely notice for such hearing shall be given to the parties. Participants at the hearing shall be limited to the Respondent and legal counsel (if so desired), the SEC Chairperson, Judicial Council Chair, Legal Counsel for the Association, or others approved in advance by the Appeal Panel as necessary to the proceedings.

6.4 *Decision*

    6.4.1 The Appeal Panel shall have the power to (a) affirm the decision, or (b) modify the decision, or (c) reverse or remand to the SEC, but only if there were procedural errors materially prejudicial to the outcome of the proceeding or if the Judicial Council decision was against the clear weight of the evidence.

    6.4.2 Within 45 days after receipt of the appeal if no hearing was granted, or within 30 days after the appeal hearing, the Appeal Panel shall notify the President of the Association of its decision. The President shall promptly notify the Respondent, the original Complainant, appropriate bodies of the Association and any other parties deemed appropriate. For Association purposes, the decision of the Appeal Panel shall be final.

7. Notifications

All notifications referred to in these Procedures shall be in writing and shall be delivered by national delivery service or mail with signature and proof of date of receipt required.

8. Records and Reports

At the completion of the Ethics process, the written records and reports that state the initial basis for the complaint, material evidence, and the disposition of the complaint shall be retained in the Ethics Office for a period of 5 years. Electronic files will be kept indefinitely.

9. Publication

Final decisions will be publicized only after any Appeal Panel process has been completed.

10. Modification

AOTA reserves the right to (a) modify the time periods, procedures, or application of these Procedures for good cause consistent with fundamental fairness in a given case, and (b) modify its Code of Ethics and/or these Procedures, with such modifications to be applied only prospectively.

Adopted by the Representative Assembly 2004C49 as Attachment B of the Standard Operating Procedures (SOP) of the Commission on Standards and Ethics (SEC)

Revised by BPPC 1/04
Adopted by RA 4/96, 5/04
Revised by SEC 4/98, 4/00, 1/02, 1/04

Originally published as American Occupational Therapy Association. (2004). Enforcement procedures for the *Occupational Therapy Code of Ethics. American Journal of Occupational Therapy, 58,* 653–661.

AMERICAN OCCUPATIONAL THERAPY ASSOCIATION
COMMISSION ON STANDARDS AND ETHICS

*Statement of Formal Complaint of Alleged Violation
of the Occupational Therapy Code of Ethics*

If an investigation is deemed necessary, a copy of this form will be provided to the individual against whom the complaint is filed.

DATE _____

COMPLAINANT: (Information regarding individual filing the complaint)

_____   _____
NAME   SIGNATURE

_____   _____
ADDRESS   TELEPHONE

_____   _____
                                                                E-MAIL ADDRESS

RESPONDENT: (Information regarding individual against whom the complaint is directed)

_____   _____
NAME   TELEPHONE

_____   _____
ADDRESS   E-MAIL ADDRESS

Indicate the Ethical Principle(s) you believe have been violated:

_____

Summarize in an attachment **the facts and circumstances, including dates and events, warranting the complaint**. Attach documentation that you think would help the Commission on Standards and Ethics in its assessment of this complaint. *Please sign and date all documents you have written and are submitting.* **Do not include confidential documents such as patient or employment records.** (Statements from witnesses are not necessary at this time.)

If you have filed a complaint about this same matter to any other agency (e.g., NBCOT, state regulatory board; academic institution; any federal, state, or local official), indicate to whom it was submitted and the approximate date(s).

What steps have been taken to resolve this complaint?

I certify that the statements/information within this complaint are correct and truthful to the best of my knowledge.

_____
SIGNATURE

Send completed form, with accompanying documentation, **IN AN ENVELOPE MARKED** *CONFIDENTIAL* **to:**

Commission on Standards and Ethics
American Occupational Therapy
**   Association, Inc.**
Attn: Staff Liaison to the SEC/Ethics Office
4720 Montgomery Lane, PO Box 31220
Bethesda, MD 20824-1220

Sec/forms/complaint form, Revised: 12/7/00

Office Use Only:
Membership Verified? Yes No
BY _____

Chapter 29

Core Values and Attitudes of Occupational Therapy Practice

Introduction

In 1985, the American Occupational Therapy Association (AOTA) funded the Professional and Technical Role Analysis Study (PATRA). This study had two purposes: to delineate the entry-level practice of OTRs and COTAs through a role analysis and to conduct a task inventory of what practitioners actually do. Knowledge, skills, and attitude statements were to be developed to provide a basis for the role analysis. The PATRA study completed the knowledge and skills statements. The Executive Board subsequently charged the Standards and Ethics Commission (SEC) to develop a statement that would describe the attitudes and values that undergird the profession of occupational therapy. The SEC wrote this document for use by AOTA members.

The list of terms used in this statement was originally constructed by the American Association of Colleges of Nursing (AACN) (1986). The PATRA committee analyzed the knowledge statements that the committee had written and selected those terms from the AACN list that best identified the values and attitudes of our profession. This list of terms was then forwarded to SEC by the PATRA Committee to use as the basis for the Core Values and Attitudes paper.

The development of this document is predicated on the assumption that the values of occupational therapy are evident in the official documents of the American Occupational Therapy Association. The official documents that were examined are: (a) *Dictionary Definition of Occupational Therapy* (AOTA, 1986), (b) *The Philosophical Base of Occupational Therapy* (AOTA, 1979), (c) *Essentials and Guidelines for an Accredited Educational Program for the Occupational Therapist* (AOTA, 1991a), (d) *Essentials and Guidelines for an Accredited Educational Program for the Occupational Therapy Assistant* (AOTA, 1991b), and (e) *Occupational Therapy Code of Ethics* (AOTA, 1988). It is further assumed that these documents are representative of the values and beliefs reflected in other occupational therapy literature.

A *value* is defined as a belief or an ideal to which an individual is committed. Values are an important part of the base or foundation of a profession. Ideally, these values are embraced by all members of the profession and are reflected in the members' interactions with those persons receiving services, colleagues, and the society at large. Values have a central role in a profession, and are developed and reinforced throughout an individual's life as a student and as a professional.

Actions and attitudes reflect the values of the individual. An attitude is the disposition to respond positively or negatively toward an object, person, concept, or situation. Thus, there is an assumption that all professional actions and interactions are rooted in certain core values and beliefs.

Seven Core Concepts

In this document, the *core values and attitudes* of occupational therapy are organized around seven basic concepts—altruism, equality, freedom, justice, dignity, truth, and prudence. How these core values and attitudes are expressed and implemented by occupational therapy practitioners may vary depending upon the environments and situations in which professional activity occurs.

Altruism is the unselfish concern for the welfare of others. This concept is reflected in actions and attitudes of commitment, caring, dedication, responsiveness, and understanding.

Equality requires that all individuals be perceived as having the same fundamental human rights and opportunities. This value is demonstrated by an attitude of fairness and impartiality. We believe that we should respect all individuals, keeping in mind that they may have values, beliefs, or lifestyles that are different from our own. Equality is practiced in the broad professional arena, but is particularly important in day-to-day interactions with those individuals receiving occupational therapy services.

Freedom allows the individual to exercise choice and to demonstrate independence, initiative, and self-direction. There is a need for all individuals to find a balance between autonomy and societal membership that is reflected in the choice of various patterns of interdependence with the human and nonhuman environment. We believe that individuals are internally and externally motivated toward action in a continuous process of adaptation throughout the life span. Purposeful activity plays a major role in developing and exercising self-direction, initiative, interdependence, and relatedness to the world. Activities verify the individual's ability to adapt, and they establish a satisfying balance between autonomy and societal membership. As professionals, we affirm the freedom of choice for each individual to pursue goals that have personal and social meaning.

Justice places value on the upholding of such moral and legal principles as fairness, equity, truthfulness, and objectivity. This means we aspire to provide occupational therapy services for all individuals who are in need of these services and that we will maintain a goal-directed and objective relationship with all those served. Practitioners must be knowledgeable about and have respect for the legal rights of individuals receiving occupational therapy services. In addition, the occupational therapy practitioner must understand and abide by the local, state, and federal laws governing professional practice.

Dignity emphasizes the importance of valuing the inherent worth and uniqueness of each person. This value is demonstrated by an attitude of empathy and respect for self and others. We believe that each individual is a unique combination of biologic endowment, sociocultural heritage, and life experiences. We view human beings holistically, respecting the unique interaction of the mind, body, and physical and social environment. We believe that dignity is nurtured and grows from the sense of competence and self-worth that is integrally linked to the person's ability to perform valued and relevant activities. In occupational therapy we emphasize the importance of dignity by helping the individual build on his or her unique attributes and resources.

Truth requires that we be faithful to facts and reality. Truthfulness or veracity is demonstrated by being accountable, honest, forthright, accurate, and authentic in our attitudes and actions. There is an obligation to be truthful with ourselves, those who receive services, colleagues, and society. One way that this is exhibited is through maintaining and upgrading professional competence. This happens, in part, through an unfaltering commitment to inquiry and learning, to self-understanding, and to the development of an interpersonal competence.

Prudence is the ability to govern and discipline oneself through the use of reason. To be prudent is to value judiciousness, discretion, vigilance, moderation, care, and circumspection in the management of one's affairs, to temper extremes, make judgments, and respond on the basis of intelligent reflection and rational thought.

Summary

Beliefs and values are those intrinsic concepts that underlie the core of the profession and the professional interactions of each practitioner. These values describe the profession's philosophy and provide the basis for defining purpose. The emphasis or priority that is given to each value may change as one's professional career evolves and as the unique characteristics of a situation unfold. This evolution of values is developmental in nature. Although we have basic values that cannot be violated, the degree to which certain values will take priority at a given time is influenced by the specifics of a situation and the environment in which it occurs. In one instance dignity may be a higher priority than truth; in another prudence may be chosen over freedom. As we process information and make decisions, the weight of the values that we hold may change. The practitioner faces dilemmas because of conflicting values and is required to engage in thoughtful deliberation to determine where the priority lies in a given situation.

The challenge for us all is to know our values, be able to make reasoned choices in situations of conflict, and be able to clearly articulate and defend our choices. At the same time, it is important that all members of the profession be committed to a set of common values. This mutual commitment to a set of beliefs and principles that govern our practice can provide a basis for clarifying expectations between the recipient and the provider of services. Shared values empower the profession and, in addition, builds trust among ourselves and with others.

References

American Association of Colleges of Nursing. (1986). *Essentials of College and University Education for Professional Nursing. Final report.* Washington, DC: Author.

American Occupational Therapy Association. (1979). Resolution C, 531–79. The philosophical base of occupational therapy. *American Journal of Occupational Therapy, 33,* 785.

American Occupational Therapy Association. (1986, April). *Dictionary definition of occupational therapy.* Adopted and approved by the Representative Assembly to fulfill Resolution #596-83. (Available from AOTA, 4720 Montgomery Lane, PO Box 31220, Bethesda, MD 20824.)

American Occupational Therapy Association. (1988). Occupational therapy code of ethics. *American Journal of Occupational Therapy, 42,* 795–796.

American Occupational Therapy Association. (1991a). Essentials and guidelines for an accredited educational program for the occupational therapist. *American Journal of Occupational Therapy, 45,* 1077–1084.

American Occupational Therapy Association. (1991b). Essentials and guidelines for an accredited educational program for the occupational therapy assistant. *American Journal of Occupational Therapy, 45,* 1085–1092.

Prepared by Elizabeth Kanny, MA, OTR, Education Representative (1990–1996) for the Standards and Ethics Commission
Ruth A. Hansen, PhD, OTR, FAOTA, Chairperson (1988–1994)

Approved by the Representative Assembly June 1993

Previously published and copyrighted by the American Occupational Therapy Association in the *American Journal of Occupational Therapy, 47,* 1085–1086.

Adopted from American Occupational Therapy Association. (2003). *Reference guide to the Occupational Therapy Code of Ethics, 2003 edition.* (pp. 13–15). Bethesda, MD: Author.

Chapter 30

Standards of Practice for Occupational Therapy

Preface

The Standards of Practice for Occupational Therapy are requirements for the occupational therapy practitioner (registered occupational therapist and certified occupational therapy assistant) for the delivery of occupational therapy services that are client centered and interactive in nature (American Occupational Therapy Association [AOTA], 1995). The registered occupational therapist supervises the certified occupational therapy assistant, and both work together in a collaborative manner to meet the needs of the client. However, the registered occupational therapist is ultimately responsible and accountable for the delivery of occupational therapy services. This document identities minimum standards for occupational therapy practice.

The minimum educational requirements for the registered occupational therapist are described in the current *Essentials and Guidelines of an Accredited Educational Program for the Occupational Therapist* (AOTA, 1991a). The minimum educational requirements for the certified occupational therapy assistant are described in the current *Essentials and Guidelines of an Accredited Educational Program for the Occupational Therapy Assistant* (AOTA, 1991b).

Definitions

Assessment. Specific tools, instruments, or interactions used during the evaluation process. An assessment is a component part of the evaluation process (Hinojosa & Kramer, 1998).

Client. A person, group, program, organization, or community for whom the occupational therapy practitioner is providing services (AOTA, 1995).

Evaluation. The process of obtaining and interpreting data necessary for understanding the individual, system, or situation. This includes planning for and documenting the evaluation process, results, and recommendations, including the need for intervention and/or potential change in the intervention plan (Hinojosa & Kramer, 1998).

Occupational therapy practitioner. Any individual initially certified to practice as an occupational therapist or occupational therapy assistant or licensed or regulated by a state, district, commonwealth, or territory of the United States to practice as an occupational therapist or occupational therapy assistant (AOTA, 1997).

Performance areas. Broad categories of human activity that are typically part of daily life. They are activities of daily living, work and productive activities, and play or leisure activities (AOTA, 1994c).

Performance components. Elements of performance required for successful engagement in performance areas, including sensorimotor, cognitive, psychosocial, and psychological aspects (AOTA, 1994c).

Performance contexts. Situations or factors that influence an individual's engagement in desired and/or required performance areas. Performance contexts consist of temporal aspects (chronological, developmental, life cycle, disability status) and environmental aspects (physical, social, political, cultural) (AOTA, 1994c).

Screening. Obtaining and reviewing data relevant to a potential client to determine the need for further evaluation and intervention.

Transition. Process involving actions coordinated to prepare for or facilitate change, such as from one functional level to another, from one life stage to another, from one program to another, or from one environment to another.

Standard I: Professional Standing and Responsibility

1. An occupational therapy practitioner delivers occupational therapy services that reflect the philosophical base of occupational therapy (AOTA, 1979) and are consistent with the established principles and concepts of theory and practice.

2. An occupational therapy practitioner delivers occupational therapy services in accordance with AOTA's standards and policies. The nature and scope of occupational therapy services provided must be in accordance with laws and regulations.

3. An occupational therapy practitioner maintains current licensure, registration, or certification as required by laws or regulations.

4. An occupational therapy practitioner abides by AOTA's *Occupational Therapy Code of Ethics* (AOTA, 1994a).

5. An occupational therapy practitioner assures continued competency by establishing, maintaining, and updating professional performance, knowledge, and skills.

6. A registered occupational therapist provides supervision for a certified occupational therapy assistant in a collaborative manner as defined by official AOTA documents and in accordance with laws or regulations.

7. A certified occupational therapy assistant seeks and follows supervision from a registered occupational therapist in the delivery of occupational therapy services.

8. An occupational therapy practitioner is knowledgeable about AOTA's *Standards of Practice for Occupational Therapy;* the *Philosophical Base of Occupational Therapy* (AOTA, 1979); and other AOTA, state, and federal documents relevant to practice and service delivery.

9. An occupational therapy practitioner maintains current knowledge of legislative, political, social, cultural, and reimbursement issues that affect clients and the practice of occupational therapy.

10. A registered occupational therapist is knowledgeable about research in the practitioner's areas of practice. A registered occupational therapist applies timely research findings ethically and appropriately to evaluation and intervention processes and discusses applicable research findings with the certified occupational therapy assistant.

11. A registered occupational therapist systematically assesses the efficiency and effectiveness of occupational therapy services and designs and implements processes to support quality service delivery.

12. A certified occupational therapy assistant collaborates with the registered occupational therapist in assessing the efficiency and effectiveness of occupational therapy services and assists in designing and implementing processes to support quality service delivery.

Standard II: Referral

1. A registered occupational therapist accepts and responds to referrals in accordance with AOTA's *Statement of Occupational Therapy Referral* (AOTA, 1994b) and in compliance with laws or regulations.

2. A registered occupational therapist accepts and responds to referrals for evaluation or evaluation with intervention in performance areas, performance components, or performance contexts when clients may have a functional limitation or disability or may be at risk for a disabling condition.

3. A registered occupational therapist refers clients to appropriate resources when the needs of the client can best be served by the expertise of other professionals or services.

4. An occupational therapy practitioner educates current and potential referral sources about the scope of occupational therapy services and the process of initiating occupational therapy services.

Standard III: Screening

1. A registered occupational therapist screens independently or as a member of a team in accordance with laws and regulations. A certified occupational therapy assistant may contribute to the screening process under the supervision of a registered occupational therapist.

2. A registered occupational therapist selects screening methods appropriate to the client's performance context.

3. A registered occupational therapist communicates screening results and recommendations to the appropriate person, group, or organization. A certified occupational therapy assistant may contribute to this process under the supervision of a registered occupational therapist.

Standard IV: Evaluation

1. A registered occupational therapist evaluates performance areas, performance components, and performance contexts. A certified occupational therapy assistant may contribute to the evaluation process under the supervision of a registered occupational therapist.

2. An occupational therapy practitioner educates clients and appropriate others about the purposes and procedures of the occupational therapy evaluation.

3. A registered occupational therapist selects assessments to evaluate the client's level of function related to performance areas, performance components, and performance contexts.

4. An occupational therapy practitioner follows defined protocols when standardized assessments are used.

5. A registered occupational therapist analyzes, interprets, and summarizes assessment data to determine the client's current functional status and to develop an appropriate intervention plan. The certified occupational therapy assistant may contribute to this process under the supervision of a registered occupational therapist.

6. A registered occupational therapist completes and documents occupational therapy evaluation results within the time frames, formats, and standards established by practice settings, government agencies, external accreditation programs, and payers. A certified occupational therapy assistant may contribute to documentation of evaluation results under the supervision of a registered occupational therapist and in accordance with laws or regulations.

7. A registered occupational therapist communicates evaluation results, within the boundaries of client confidentiality, to the appropriate person, group, or organization. A certified occupational therapy assistant may contribute to this process under the supervision of a registered occupational therapist.

8. A registered occupational therapist recommends additional consultations when the results of the evaluation indicate that intervention by other professionals would be beneficial.

Standard V: Intervention Plan

1. A registered occupational therapist develops and documents an intervention plan that is based on the results of the occupational therapy evaluation and the desires and expectations of the client and appropriate others about the outcome of service. A certified occupational therapy assistant may contribute to the intervention plan under the supervision of a registered occupational therapist.

2. A registered occupational therapist ensures that the intervention plan is documented within time frames, formats, and standards established by the practice settings, agencies, external accreditation programs, and payers.

3. A registered occupational therapist includes in the intervention plan client-centered goals that are clear, measurable, behavioral, functional, contextually relevant, and appropriate to the client's needs, desires, and expected outcomes. A certified occupational therapy assistant may contribute to this process.

4. A registered occupational therapist includes in the intervention plan the scope, frequency, duration of services, and the needs of the client.

5. A registered occupational therapist reviews the intervention plan with the client and appropriate others. A certified occupational therapy assistant may contribute to this process.

Standard VI: Intervention

1. A registered occupational therapist implements the intervention plan through the use of specified purposeful activities or therapeutic methods that are meaningful to the client and are effective methods for enhancing occupational performance. A certified occupational therapy assistant may implement the intervention plan under the supervision of a registered occupational therapist.

2. An occupational therapy practitioner informs clients and appropriate others regarding the relative benefits and risks of the intervention.

3. An occupational therapy practitioner maintains or seeks current information on resources relevant to the client's needs.

4. A registered occupational therapist reevaluates during the intervention process and documents changes in the client's goals, performance, and needs. A certified occupational therapy assistant may contribute to the reevaluation process.

5. A registered occupational therapist modifies the intervention process to reflect changes in client status, desires, and response to intervention. A certified occupational therapy assistant may identify the need for modifications and may contribute to the intervention modifications under the supervision of a registered occupational therapist.

6. An occupational therapy practitioner documents the occupational therapy services provided within the time frames, formats, and standards established by the practice settings, agencies, external accreditation programs, and payers.

Standard VII: Transition Services

1. A registered occupational therapist prepares a formal transition plan that is based on identified needs. A certified occupational therapy assistant may contribute to the preparation of a formal transition plan.

2. An occupational therapy practitioner facilitates the transition process in cooperation with the client, family members, significant others, team, and community resources and individuals, when appropriate.

Standard VIII: Discontinuation

1. A registered occupational therapist discontinues services when the client has achieved predetermined goals, has achieved maximum benefit from occupational therapy services, or does not desire to continue services. A certified occupational therapy assistant may recommend discontinuation of occupational therapy services to the supervising registered occupational therapist.

2. A registered occupational therapist prepares and implements a discontinuation plan that addresses appropriate follow-up resources. A certified occupational therapy assistant may contribute to the implementation of a dis-

continuation plan under the supervision of a registered occupational therapist.

3. A registered occupational therapist documents changes in the client's status between the initial evaluation and discontinuation of services. A certified occupational therapy assistant may contribute to the process under the supervision of a registered occupational therapist.

4. A registered occupational therapist documents recommendations for follow-up or reevaluation, when applicable.

References

American Occupational Therapy Association. (1979). The philosophical base of occupational therapy. *American Journal of Occupational Therapy, 33,* 785.

American Occupational Therapy Association. (1991a). Essentials and guidelines of an accredited educational program for the occupational therapist. *American Journal of Occupational Therapy, 45,* 1077–1084.

American Occupational Therapy Association. (1991b). Essentials and guidelines of an accredited educational program for the occupational therapy assistant. *American Journal of Occupational Therapy, 45,* 1085–1092.

American Occupational Therapy Association. (1994a). Occupational therapy code of ethics. *American Journal of Occupational Therapy, 48,* 1037–1038.

American Occupational Therapy Association. (1994b). Statement of occupational therapy referral. *American Journal of Occupational Therapy, 48,* 1034.

American Occupational Therapy Association. (1994c). Uniform terminology for occupational therapy–Third edition. *American Journal of Occupational Therapy, 49,* 1047–1054.

American Occupational Therapy Association. (1995). Concept paper: Service delivery in occupational therapy. *American Journal of Occupational Therapy, 49,* 1029–1031.

American Occupational Therapy Association. (1997). Bylaws. Article III, Section 1. Bethesda, MD: Author.

Hinojosa, J., & Kramer, P. (Eds.). (1998). *Occupational therapy evaluation of clients: Obtaining and interpreting data.* Bethesda, MD: American Occupational Therapy Association.

COMMISSION ON PRACTICE
Linda Kohlman Thomson, MOT, OT(C), FAOTA, Chairperson

Adopted by the Representative Assembly 1998M15

Note: This document replaces the *1994 Standards of Practice for Occupational Therapy.* These standards are intended as recommended guidelines to assist occupational therapy practitioners in the provision of occupational therapy services. These standards serve as a minimum standard for occupational therapy practice and are applicable to all individual populations and the programs in which these individuals are served.

Previously published and copyrighted in 1998 by the American Occupational Therapy Association in the *American Journal of Occupational Therapy, 52,* 866–869.

Chapter 31

Ethical Knowledge = Collaborative Power

David A. Leary and Jacalyn Mardirossian

Note. The term occupational therapy practitioner *refers to both occupational therapists and occupational therapy assistants.*

We have worked together at the University of Southern California for several years and have introduced students to the American Occupational Therapy Association's (AOTA's) official documents. We have also collaborated on a module on supervision and role delineation for the occupational therapist and occupational therapy assistant. It has been really surprising to us that our students are often better informed about AOTA's official documents than some of our practicing colleagues, since the answers to so many practice questions are found in these documents.

The key element of our basis for applying all of our professional knowledge is the *Occupational Therapy Code of Ethics* (2000).[1] This is the foundation for all of the other official documents of our profession.

Here are just four principles from the *Code of Ethics* (2000)[1] that are relevant to role delineation:

- *Principle 4E:* Occupational therapy practitioners shall protect service recipients by ensuring that duties assumed by or assigned to other occupational therapy personnel match credentials, qualifications, experience, and scope of practice.
- *Principle 4F:* Occupational therapy practitioners shall provide appropriate supervision to individuals for whom the practitioners have supervisory responsibility in accordance with Association policies; local, state, and federal laws; and institutional values.
- *Principle 5C:* Occupational therapy practitioners shall require those they supervise in occupational therapy-related activities to adhere to the *Code of Ethics.*
- *Principle 5E:* Occupational therapy practitioners shall record and report in an accurate and timely manner all information related to professional activities.

An occupational therapy practitioner familiar with the *Code of Ethics* and its application to practice will be able to relate its principles to AOTA's *Guide for Supervision of* *Occupational Therapy Personnel in the Delivery of Occupational Therapy Services.*[2] This ability is especially important in the current health care climate because changes in practice are occurring very quickly, and funding issues can conflict with quality service.

For example, a recent graduate who had started a new job called one day to ask for some advice. "Joan" was hired as the only occupational therapist (OT) in her practice setting and was told that an occupational therapy assistant (OTA) would be interviewed shortly. She was then told that she would be traveling to several satellite clinics throughout the week to do evaluations. When Joan expressed concern about how to treat her clients after the evaluations while traveling to different sites, she was offered the support of a rehabilitation aide.

Joan's supervisor, who was not an occupational therapist, told her that the aide would deliver her treatments throughout the week. Joan believed that this service delivery would not be ethical, so she reviewed the *Guidelines for the Use of Aides in Occupational Therapy Practice.*[3] This document states that "Only carefully selected, specific aspects of service delivery can be safely and ethically delegated to aides" (p. 595). It also says that "Aides are primarily used to support the delivery of occupational therapy by assuming responsibility for non-client-related tasks" (p. 595). Most importantly for Joan, it says that "For best practice, tasks delegated to aides should receive continuous supervision.... Continuous supervision means that the occupational therapy supervisor is in sight of the aide who is performing delegated client-related tasks" (p. 596).

Joan's supervisor had also been under the impression that an occupational therapy assistant would not require any supervision from Joan. Joan referred to the *Occupational Therapy Roles*[4] document, which states "COTAs at all levels require at least general supervision by an OTR. The level of supervision is related to the ability of the COTA to safely and effectively provide those interventions delegated by an OTR.... COTAs will require closer supervision for interventions that are more complex or evaluative in nature and for areas in which service competencies have not been developed. Service competency is the ability to use the identified intervention in a safe and effective manner" (p. 1090).

After relaying this information to her supervisor and explaining the supervisory requirements of the occupational therapist/occupational therapy assistant team, Joan became involved in the interview process for the occupational therapy assistant. She was able to ask insightful questions regarding service competency and previous supervision experiences with the candidates to determine their skill levels. By educating her supervisor and taking on additional responsibilities, she had followed Principle 5D of AOTA's *Code of Ethics* (2000)[1]: "Occupational therapy practitioners shall take reasonable steps to ensure employers are aware of occupational therapy's ethical obligations, as set forth in this *Code of Ethics,* and of the implications of those obligations for occupational therapy practice, education, and research."

Myth or Reality?

Many occupational therapy practitioners who leave the medical model and begin community-based practice have questioned the continued applicability of the OT/OTA supervisory guidelines. This relationship is not based on setting, but on whether each person is functioning in an occupational therapy role. By determining whether the following statements are a myth or reality, practitioners may better understand how the OT/OTA team can work together ethically and effectively, regardless of practice setting.

Statement: None of AOTA's official documents indicate the requirement of a cosignature, so notes written by an OTA do not have to be cosigned.

Myth: Although AOTA's official documents do not stipulate the requirement of a cosignature, state law or third-party reimbursers may, and they are the ruling authority. Often, this cosignature on documentation is seen as evidence of collaboration between the OT and the OTA. Check with your state regulatory board and reimbursers to determine whether OTA notes must be cosigned by an OT.

Statement: The OT has full responsibility for supervising all of the occupational therapy treatment that the OTA administers.

Reality: The OT is indeed responsible for all OTA treatment. However, according to the *Guide for Supervision,*[2] the level of supervision varies, based on "an assessment of the OTA's skills, the demands of the job, the needs of the service recipients, and the service setting requirements" (p. 593). "In all cases, it is the occupational therapy practition-

er's ethical responsibility to ensure that the amount, degree, and pattern of supervision are consistent with the service competency demonstrated" (p. 594).

Statement: The OT has all the responsibility of delegating every task in an occupational therapy department that consists of an OT, two OTAs, and one OT aide.

Myth: The *Occupational Therapy Roles*[4] document and the *Guide for Supervision*[2] support supervisory roles for both the OT and the OTA. Although an OTA always requires at least a general level of supervision from an OT, the OTA can provide supervision to a less experienced OTA or an OT aide. This supervision would always involve collaboration with an OT.

For example, if the OT has 3 years' experience and one of the OTAs has 5 years' experience, the OT will provide routine or general supervision. After service competency has been established, it is likely that treatment collaboration would take place less frequently and for a shorter amount of time than it would with a less experienced OTA.

If the other OTA has only 6 months of practice experience, he or she will require close supervision. The more experienced OTA, working in collaboration with the OT, may provide some of this supervision. After the OTA's service competency is established by the OT, delegating appropriate tasks might include the OTA selecting and delegating appropriate tasks to the OT aide, in collaboration with the OT.

Statement: The OT has to know how to do everything an OTA does in order to supervise.

Myth: This statement refers to the idea of *service competency.* If an OTA has 10 years of experience in making splints and the OT who is partnered with this OTA has 1 year of experience but is knowledgeable about the theory, rationale, contraindications, and other issues regarding splinting, the OT can still establish service competency. If the OT has evaluated the OTA's ability and skills in splinting and believes that he or she is competent, and there are collaborative discussions addressing which clients receive splints, the types of splints to use, and other related questions, then supervision may look more like a professional dialogue and interaction.[2]

AOTA describes supervision as a "mutual undertaking between the supervisor and the supervisee that fosters growth and development..." (p. 592).[2] This collaboration benefits service recipients by enhancing the education and clinical skills of both the OT and the OTA.

Statement: There is little value in demonstrating to OT students how to provide supervision to OTAs because they will learn it on the job.

Myth: Many OT/OTA teams don't work well because they don't understand each other's roles, responsibilities, and skills. Establishing the basics of this relationship during their education will help practitioners work together, particularly in settings where good models for this relationship do not exist.

Statement: The decision regarding who should do a specific assessment should be based on experience, theory base, and regulatory requirements.

Reality: According to AOTA's Commission on Practice, *evaluation* refers to the process of obtaining and interpreting data necessary for intervention, and *assessment* refers to specific tools or instruments used during the evaluation process.[6] The OT is responsible for completing the comprehensive evaluation of a client's occupational performance issues. This evaluation may require specific, detailed assessments. An OTA can assist with the data collection, provided the OT has established his or her service competency. The OT must be confident that the assessments will be administered in the standardized manner by the OTA, and that the results will be gathered safely and effectively. During this process, the OTA will always require some level of supervision, based on experience. The decision regarding which assessments may be helpful would be determined solely by the OT or collaboratively with the OTA. The OTA role does not include independently evaluating a client's occupational performance.[4]

Statement: Theory base and the ability to interpret evaluation results are good definers of the difference between an OT's and an OTA's education.

Reality: According to "Standard IV: Evaluation" in the *Standards of Practice for Occupational Therapy,*[5] "A registered occupational therapist analyzes, interprets, and summarizes assessment data to determine the client's current functional status and to develop an appropriate intervention plan. The certified occupational therapy assistant may contribute to this process under the supervision of a registered occupational therapist" (p. 867).

Statement: Good communication involves the occupational therapist telling the occupational therapy assistant what to do clearly and precisely.

Myth: According to "Standard I: Professional Standing and Responsibility" in the *Standards of Practice for Occupational Therapy,*[5] "A registered occupational therapist provides supervision for a certified occupational therapy assistant in a collaborative manner...." (p. 866) In cases where the OTA has more experience than the OT, the OT has an ethical responsibility to take advantage of this

knowledge. Principle 4G of the *Code of Ethics* (2000)[1] states that "Occupational therapy practitioners shall refer to or consult with other service providers whenever such a referral or consultation would be helpful to the care of the recipient of service...."

Statement: Occupational therapists do not do activities of daily living assessments.

Myth: The Occupational Therapy Roles[4] document states that the OT "screens individuals to determine the need for intervention" and "evaluates individuals to obtain and interpret data necessary for planning intervention and for intervention" (p. 1088).

Statement: If you do not create an effective team immediately, it is too late.

Myth: The most effective way to begin creating an effective team of occupational therapy practitioners is to look at the experiences and skills of each person. The OT and OTA will have different education and skills. Both will be responsible for following our profession's official documents. The *Code of Ethics* (2000)[1] states that this is the responsibility of *both* the OT and the OTA. If a third party is needed to facilitate effective communication and agreement, then both the OT and OTA must seek this support. Knowledge of the roles of each member of the profession will enhance our ability to collaborate, which is why knowledge = power.

Conclusion

The *Occupational Therapy Code of Ethics* (2000)[1] guides the collaboration between occupational therapists and occupational therapy assistants, as well as our practice decisions. The ability to think clearly and incorporate accurate, current resources into our professional problem solving is critical to our success as occupational therapy practitioners. We have a valuable resource in all of our official documents, which guide us, support us, and empower us.

References

1. American Occupational Therapy Association. (2003). *Reference guide to the occupational therapy code of ethics, 2003 edition.* Bethesda, MD: Author.
2. American Occupational Therapy Association. (1999). Guide for supervision of occupational therapy personnel in the delivery of occupational therapy services. *American Journal of Occupational Therapy, 53,* 592–594.
3. American Occupational Therapy Association. (1999). Guidelines for the use of aides in occupational therapy practice. *American Journal of Occupational Therapy, 53,* 595–597.

4. American Occupational Therapy Association. (1993). Occupational therapy roles. *American Journal of Occupational Therapy, 47,* 1087–1099.
5. American Occupational Therapy Association. (1998). Standards of practice for occupational therapy. *American Journal of Occupational Therapy, 52,* 866–869.
6. American Occupational Therapy Association. (1995, July 13). Commission on Practice clarifies terms. *OT Week,* p 10.

David A. Leary, MS, OTR, is an occupational therapist with more than 10 years' experience in the field of physical disabilities, geriatrics, and management. He has taught part time in the OTA program at Mount St. Mary's College and is currently a faculty member at the University of Southern California. He has extensive teaching experience in the academic and clinical settings and has a strong commitment to implementation of professional guidelines regarding role delineation and supervision. He has served on the OTAC Education Committee in 1994 and has been an active member of OTAC and AOTA since 1988.

Jackie Mardirossian, BS, COTA, AP, is a certified occupational therapy assistant with more than 15 years' experience in the field of physical disabilities, mental health, pediatrics, and education. She was academic fieldwork coordinator and lecturer at Mount St. Mary's College and is currently Clinical Administrator of the Occupational Therapy Faculty Practice for the Department of Occupational Science and Occupational Therapy at the University of Southern California. She is the AOTA COTA State Contact Person for the state of California and on the AOTA Education SIS Nominating Committee. Locally, she is the associate director of the San Gabriel Valley Chapter of OTAC.

Originally published in *OT Practice,* December 20, 2004.

Chapter 32

Successful OT–OTA Partnerships: Staying Afloat in a Sea of Ethical Challenges

Pam Toto and Diane M. Hill

Your employer reduces the occupational therapist's hours to part-time status for "evaluations only" while increasing the use of occupational therapy assistants to provide all direct patient treatment in efforts to reduce costs.

The occupational therapist, who also serves as the department head, regularly reduces the hours of the occupational therapy assistant when productivity and census are low so that she can maintain her own full-time status.

Your employer no longer reimburses you for time not spent providing direct patient care; OT–OTA supervision must be completed on your own time and at your own expense. Do any of these scenarios sound familiar? If so, you are not alone. Dramatic changes in our health care system, especially those related to reduced reimbursement, have perpetuated unanticipated conflicts and issues among teams at all levels in the health care field. Since the surge of practitioners entering the profession, and perhaps even earlier, occupational therapy leaders have struggled to define specific roles for occupational therapists and occupational therapy assistants in traditional health care models. Emerging and expanding practice areas, as well as new holistic approaches to existing health care programs, further challenge one's ability to define this unique partnership. For many occupational therapy practitioners, these changes in practice have affected relationships, communication, and even ethics. In her book *Occupational Therapy Leadership*, Grace Gilkeson, EdD, OTR, FAOTA, wrote, "Change is inevitable, but how you handle it makes all the difference between success and failure, satisfaction and disappointment" (p. 158).[1]

OT–OTA collaboration can be powerful when both parties embrace ethical and legal decision-making and problem-solving processes. This affirmative partnership can be successful as long as all practitioners have a common set of values in their therapeutic relationships and use of self. The American Occupational Therapy Association (AOTA) provides practitioners with guidelines for ethical practice through the AOTA *Occupational Therapy Code of Ethics* (2000).[2] This document, combined with specific state regulations, provides a framework through which effective OT–OTA partnerships can be established and maintained. The following examples are common situations that may challenge professional ethics and the relationship of OT–OTA teams in practice. Solutions and strategies for maintaining strong and healthy OT–OTA partnerships also are offered.

Supervision Challenges

An occupational therapist has regularly been traveling among her company's inpatient, outpatient, and home health departments to complete evaluations and discharges. In each of these settings, occupational therapy assistants regularly provide all treatment. Because of limited time and scheduling conflicts, the occupational therapist rarely performs her supervisory role; she frequently cosigns notes without reading them, does not provide input on changes to the treatment plan, and relies on the occupational therapy assistants to determine independently when discharge is appropriate.

This situation addresses ethical and legal supervision issues, role delineation, and whether current practice patterns facilitate the best and most efficient patient care (*Occupational Therapy Code of Ethics*, Principle 5). Overriding these issues is the certainty that this OT–OTA team lacks, at the very least, effective communication.

Communication is one of the most critical variables for effective OT–OTA relationships, yet current practice trends offer significantly reduced opportunities for traditional methods of sharing information. One of the simplest ways for occupational therapists and occupational therapy assistants to communicate efficiently is through hands-on client care opportunities. If a picture is worth a thousand words, a treatment session is worth a million words!

Establish systems to ensure that the occupational therapist provides hands-on treatment at least once a week or on a regular basis for each client. In environments where the clients do not change quickly, such as long-term-care settings, consider switching caseloads 1 day per week or rotating workdays or work times for part-time employees. If the occupational therapist has time constraints that prohibit caseload changes, consider splitting the client's treatment session between the occupational therapist and the occupational therapy assistant, with the occupational therapist addressing those issues that most significantly affect goal changes and treatment plan upgrades. Providing opportunities for the occupational therapist to actually observe changes in function instead of relying on second-hand information for documentation and discharge planning can foster efficient communication between team members.

The pressure to maintain productivity standards sometimes seems to "force" practitioners to choose between direct client care and indirect, yet vital, communication. Practitioners should try to maintain more constant productivity percentages by managing and monitoring treatment caseloads throughout the week, thus allowing consistent productivity with adequate time for nonbillable necessities. It is also prudent to explore the many different modes of communication readily available as alternatives to face-to-face discussion. For example, storing information in a central, secure area or a communication book allows efficient access by all team members. Checklist notes and communication boards further increase efficiency by providing easy visual status of both direct and indirect client information. OT–OTA teams may also choose to create checklist forms to manage documentation and billing details or to ensure that all goals and performance areas and components are being addressed. (Not doing so is a common error when multiple clinicians are managing caseloads.) Laminated, wall-mounted communication boards can provide interdisciplinary team members with valuable information regarding evaluation and discharge dates, day and treatment minutes, and caseload assignments. E-mail and voicemail allow clinicians to exchange clinical information at their convenience. These alternatives, as well as regularly scheduled telephone conferences, reduce wasted time from playing "telephone tag" and interruptions during valuable direct client care.

Scope of Practice Challenges

The occupational therapy assistant is the only full-time therapy practitioner providing services in one specific school-based setting. As such, he serves as the occupational therapy representative at family meetings and interdisciplinary team conferences. Often, due to their lack of knowledge, parents and faculty members refer to the assistant as the "occupational therapist" and seek his judgment on

issues that affect the entire operation of occupational therapy services at the school. Because of time factors and the need for others to have immediate information, the occupational therapy assistant feels obligated to address all issues as they arise. As a result, the occupational therapist, who travels to several schools and, thus, spends limited time in any single setting, feels as though she is "out of the loop" and is angry that the assistant is assuming roles that she believes are beyond the scope of practice for an occupational therapy assistant.

Ethics can be challenged when practitioners assume roles not representative of their credentials (*Occupational Therapy Code of Ethics,* Principle 6A). Conversely, practitioners must acknowledge and permit fellow team members to explore all opportunities that are within their scope of practice as defined by AOTA[3] and state regulations.

The complex elements required for effective teamwork can challenge even the strongest OT–OTA partnerships. The best way to resolve conflict is to anticipate issues and avoid problems through clearly established roles and responsibilities. In a 1999 *OT Practice* article, Barbara Hanft, MA, OTR, FAOTA, and Barbara Banks, COTA, identified expectations of occupational therapists and occupational therapy assistants that must be met for success in teamwork.[4] Occupational therapy assistants expected occupational therapists to share professional knowledge, help link interventions to meaningful outcomes, provide feedback that the occupational therapy assistant has value, be dependable, and provide tangible supervision. Conversely, the occupational therapist requested that the occupational therapy assistant ask questions, follow the treatment plan, and provide feedback for modifications. It is critical that OT–OTA teams take the time to recognize and address each other's needs.

If conflict arises, assertive communication and negotiation are generally the most effective way of addressing it. Both parties should attempt to keep an open mind, remain relaxed, and agree at the outset to seek a resolution. According to Pat Crist, PhD, OTR, FAOTA, conflict is first noted as a *trigger*—any action or word that causes a negative response. "Triggers can include body language or gestures (rolling of eyes); a loud stressed voice; physical actions; or even not taking action when it is expected" (p. 5).[5] Passive or aggressive behavior can result from triggers or from any situation that causes one to perceive a threat of rejection or disapproval. When dealing with conflict, remain aware of others' trigger points and focus on the issues at hand rather than on negative emotions. Along with respect and active listening, Crist noted that using summary and reflection, incorporating "I" statements to describe the situation (e.g., "I feel..."), expressing your feelings, and noting the change you desire and the expected consequence are advantageous. Conflict is resolved in one of three ways—through authority, compromise, or consensual integration of the disagreeing parties' ideas. Consensus is the best choice in terms of team satisfaction but, unfortunately, is also the most difficult and time consuming. The sooner conflicts are managed, the easier the resolution. In this example, the occupational therapist and occupational therapy assistant should work together to identify the various job responsibilities crucial to success in this setting. Keeping their respective scopes of practice in mind, they should determine which roles are best suited for each. They will need to communicate this information to the school administrators and establish strategies to meet the needs of parents, students, and fellow professionals in a timely fashion. Lastly, the occupational therapist and occupational therapy assistant should establish a system to improve communication within their department, with an additional commitment to remain open-minded and address issues as they arise.

Novice Practitioner Challenges

An occupational therapy department in an acute care hospital recently increased service availability from 5 days per week to 7 days per week. The department supervisor has left the task of determining work schedules up to the staff. Occupational therapists and occupational therapy assistants with the most seniority have exerted their influence in this decision-making process, and as a consequence, the new graduate therapist and entry-level assistant regularly are left to work alone on the weekends. Although these novice clinicians have expressed their concern over a lack of guidance and mentorship, as well as frustration with permanent weekend duties, their complaints have not been answered.

This situation presents several concerns. From an ethical standpoint, the practitioners who are forced to work weekends regularly do not believe that they are receiving adequate supervision (*Occupational Therapy Code of Ethics,* Principle 4F). Additionally, respect for fellow team members has been replaced by personal working preferences. For OT–OTA teams and departments to develop and maintain healthy relationships, a commitment to flexibility is crucial. At a minimum, flexibility must be examined from the two key aspects of scheduling and work hours. Scheduling considerations include seeing clients at the best time of the day to meet the client's goals (e.g., seeing a client in the morning for activities of daily living [ADL] retraining) and allowing opportunities to share caseloads. Depending on the work setting, opportunities may arise to develop creative schedules that meet clients' needs more effectively. For example, when providing therapy in a skilled nursing facil-

ity, the most valuable treatment interventions may require practitioners to alternate disciplines and treatment days, save their minutes, or barter for minutes with other disciplines to provide a complete occupation-based treatment session. One comprehensive session that addresses a specific performance area in an appropriate context may meet client-centered goals more effectively than several short sessions that only allow enough time to focus on limited performance components.

Often, the distribution of duties is lopsided, with the occupational therapy assistant performing most or all of the direct client care. By caseload sharing, an OT–OTA team commits to establishing a balance of duties involved with daily practice at a given site. This balance results in improved communication and enables both the occupational therapist and the occupational therapy assistant to enjoy other aspects of the job, such as program development, interdisciplinary team participation, and administrative functions.

For many veteran clinicians, the end of the traditional work schedule has been one of the hardest new trends to accept. OT–OTA teams must continuously analyze admission patterns and schedule workdays and hours to provide the best treatment at the best time to meet their clients' goals. Some facilities may regularly schedule admissions in late afternoon, which might mean that the occupational therapist needs to start the workday later. A caseload may be heavy with clients who require ADL retraining, and thus, the occupational therapy assistant may need to start work earlier than usual. Weekend and evening services should be rotated, or positions should be established and marketed as permanent off-hours assignments. Occupational therapy practitioners should also remain cognizant of legal and ethical obligations regarding entry-level practitioners. Teaming new clinicians with more experienced therapists and assistants not only will minimize supervision issues but will also facilitate learning opportunities for both parties. As new graduates "learn the ropes" from their counterparts, senior clinicians may gain exposure to the current theories, new assessment techniques, and emerging trends in occupational therapy education. Flexibility demonstrates commitment to the profession and respect for colleagues. Remember, it is better to bend than to break.

Maintaining Competency Challenges

The occupational therapy department staff in a local skilled nursing facility has been reduced from six practitioners to one full-time occupational therapist and one full-time occupational therapy assistant. They consider themselves to be "survivors," having maintained employment and a commitment to their profession in spite of the many changes in reimbursement, documentation, supervision, and service delivery as a result of implementation of the prospective payment system (PPS). After the turmoil associated with PPS, they welcomed the renewed sense of normalcy and routine. However, this OT–OTA team now finds itself in somewhat of a rut. Each day seems remarkably the same as the pattern of meetings, documentation procedures, and treatment regimes is repeated; the budget no longer provides for continuing education; the employer does not reimburse for membership in professional associations; and there never seems to be time for program development. A profession that once offered novelty and excitement to these practitioners now seems monotonous.

As with an optimist who sees the glass half-full, so too can practitioners embrace change as an opportunity for improvement. In the March 1999 issue of the AOTA *Gerontology Special Interest Section Quarterly*, Pamela Lindstrom, MS, OTR/L, and Jennifer Westropp, MS, OTR/L, provided an explicit example of using change as a catalyst for revitalization.[6] They challenged practitioners to change their work environment to make it easier to engage in meaningful occupation-based treatment interventions. As part of their transformation, they rearranged supplies and physical space for activities and secured items such as clothing, horticulture materials, golfing equipment, and board games to help clients participate in meaningful tasks. They also created kits with supplies already assembled for occupation-based activities, such as grooming. These kits greatly reduced the time needed to set up activities. By facilitating a more occupation-based work environment, these authors improved service delivery and job satisfaction.

A commitment to excellence in occupational therapy requires us to examine our skills, practice patterns, and relationships continuously to define ways to maintain competency (*Occupational Therapy Code of Ethics*, Principles 4C and 4D). The value of new learning through continuing education or networking opportunities through membership in professional organizations may far outweigh their financial costs. OT–OTA teamwork presents an advantage to those seeking meaning and excellence in their practice through the sharing of knowledge and ideas. As the saying goes, "Two heads are better than one!"

Conclusion

Despite the challenges, OT–OTA teamwork is more critical than ever for advocacy and success in today's health care environment. As scrutiny increases over the efficacy of rehabilitation, including occupational therapy, occupational therapists and occupational therapy assistants must maintain healthy partnerships that enable the team to demonstrate the necessity of occupation to well-being. As our state and national professional associations work to improve OT–OTA role delineations and guides to practice, so too must we commit to engaging in team practice patterns that promote excellence in care and ensure viability of this essential partnership.

References

1. Gilkeson, G. (1997). *Occupational therapy leadership*. Philadelphia: F. A. Davis.
2. American Occupational Therapy Association. (2000). Occupational therapy code of ethics (2000). *American Journal of Occupational Therapy, 54,* 614–616.
3. American Occupational Therapy Association. (1993). Occupational therapy roles. *American Journal of Occupational Therapy, 47,* 1087–1099.
4. Hanft, B., & Banks, B. (1999). Competent supervision: A collaborative process. *OT Practice, 4*(5), 31–34.
5. Crist, P. (1998, February 16). Hearing, understanding, resolving. *Advance for Occupational Therapists*, p. 5.
6. Lindstrom, P. R., & Westropp, J. (1999). Renewed energy following an epiphany at Annual Conference. *Gerontology Special Interest Section Quarterly, 22*(1), 1–3.

Pam Toto, MS, OTR/L, BCG, is an adjunct instructor at the University of Pittsburgh and Philadelphia University. She also provides occupational therapy services as a direct care provider in home health care and completes functional assessments as part of a National Institutes of Health–funded research project through the Mind–Body Research Center at the University of Pittsburgh Medical Center. Pam has been editor of the *Gerontology Special Interest Section Quarterly* and the state secretary of the Pennsylvania Occupational Therapy Association.

Diane M. Hill, COTA/L, AP, is a direct care provider at an adult living community, Longwood at Oakmont, in a suburb of Pittsburgh, Pennsylvania. She is a member of the AOTA Standards and Ethics Commission and Advance Practice Program Committee. She has 14 years of experience as a practitioner and has earned the AOTA AP (advanced practitioner) credential in geriatrics.

This chapter was originally published in *OT Practice,* July 2, 2001.

PART V

Resources

One challenge facing occupational therapy assistants throughout their careers is being able to readily access the most up-to-date resources and information. This manual contains frequently used resources directed to the major themes of state and professional regulations; supervision, roles, and responsibilities; reimbursement; and ethical jurisdiction. Part V is a compilation of additional resources that will support occupational therapy assistants in their practice.

The current information climate is characterized by continuous change. Official documents get revised, rosters are updated, policies are enacted, new practice areas emerge, and ethical challenges materialize. Therefore, practitioners need to familiarize themselves with the available resources for keeping up with these changes as a part of their professional development and lifelong learning.

AOTA's Web Site—*www.aota.org*

By far the most current source of information for occupational therapy assistants is the American Occupational Therapy Association's (AOTA's) Web site. Cruising around the site will link you to valuable information, and areas that are of particular interest include "OTA Area," "Membership," "Continuing Education," "Career Information," "Professional Development Tool," "OTJobLink" (students and professionals can review job postings from top employers across the country and around the world; apply online; receive messages about job matches), and "Student Area." Set this site as your home page when you log on to the Internet.

The Reference Manual of the Official Documents of the American Occupational Therapy Association, Inc.

This compilation of official documents as approved by the AOTA Representative Assembly (RA) is fully revised biennially in even-numbered years. In odd-numbered years, an addendum is published. Both publications include the latest AOTA guidelines, standards, position papers, and statements—items that occupational therapy assistants need to stay current in their practice.

Becoming a Resource

Although it is important to stay current on issues related to occupational therapy assistants, the most important task is to become a resource yourself. For example, occupational therapy assistants can influence policy by holding the position as OTA representative to the AOTA RA, and they can serve on the AOTA Board of Directors. Occupational therapy assistant educators can help shape education by volunteering on the Commission on Education or the Accreditation Council for Occupational Therapy Education, and those in clinical practice can volunteer on the Commission on Practice or on the Commission on Standards and Ethics.

Additional resources in this section include
- Chapter 33. List of Acronyms and Terms
- Chapter 34. Standards for an Accredited Educational Program for the Occupational Therapy Assistant
- Chapter 35. Position Paper: Broadening the Construct of Independence
- Chapter 36. Occupation: A Position Paper
- Chapter 37. Statement—The Philosophical Base of Occupational Therapy
- Chapter 38. Statement—Fundamental Concepts of Occupational Therapy: Occupation, Purposeful Activity, and Function
- Chapter 39. Commission on Education Position Paper: The Viability of Occupational Therapy Assistant Education
- Chapter 40. The Need for OTA Involvement in the AOTA: "Now Is the Time."

Chapter 33

List of Acronyms and Terms

1. ACOTE®: Accreditation Council for Occupational Therapy Education
2. AOTF: American Occupational Therapy Foundation
3. ASAP: Affiliated State Association Presidents
4. ASD: Assembly of Student Delegates
5. Assembly: Representative Assembly of the Association
6. Association: The American Occupational Therapy Association, Inc.
7. Board: The Board of Directors
8. BPPC: Bylaws, Policies, and Procedures Committee
9. CCCPD: Commission on Continuing Competence and Professional Development
10. COE: Commission on Education
11. COP: Commission on Practice
12. CRAC: Credentials Review and Accountability Committee
13. NBCOT: National Board for Certification in Occupational Therapy®
14. OT: Occupational Therapist
15. OTA: Occupational Therapy Assistant
16. OTFC: OTs in Foreign Countries
17. RA: Representative Assembly of the Association
18. RACC: Representative Assembly Coordinating Council
19. SCB: Specialty Certification Board
20. SEC: Commission on Standards and Ethics
21. SISs: Special Interest Sections
22. SISSC: Special Interest Sections Steering Committee
23. WFOT: World Federation of Occupational Therapists

Chapter 34

Standards for an Accredited Educational Program for the Occupational Therapy Assistant

Adopted December 1998 by the

Accreditation Council for Occupational Therapy Education

of

The American Occupational Therapy Association, Inc.

The Accreditation Council for Occupational Therapy Education (ACOTE) of the American Occupational Therapy Association (AOTA) accredits educational programs for the occupational therapy assistant. The Standards comply with the U.S. Department of Education (USDE) criteria for recognition of accrediting agencies.

These Standards are the requirements used in accrediting educational programs that prepare individuals to become occupational therapy assistants. The extent to which a program complies with these Standards determines its accreditation status.

Sections A and C contain general standards, while Section B delineates standards specific to curriculum. The specific standards in Section B are stated as outcome-based criteria.

Preamble

The rapidly changing and dynamic nature of contemporary health and human service delivery systems requires the entry-level occupational therapy assistant to possess basic skills as a direct care provider, educator, and advocate for the profession and the consumer.

A contemporary entry-level occupational therapy assistant must

- Have acquired an educational foundation in the liberal arts and sciences, including a focus on issues related to diversity;

- Be educated as a generalist, with a broad exposure to the delivery models and systems utilized in settings where occupational therapy is currently practiced and where it is emerging as a service;
- Have achieved entry-level competence through a combination of academic and fieldwork education;
- Be prepared to work under the supervision of and in cooperation with the occupational therapist;
- Be prepared to articulate and apply occupational therapy principles, intervention approaches and rationales, and expected outcomes as these relate to occupation;
- Be prepared to be a lifelong learner and keep current with best practice;
- Uphold the ethical standards, values, and attitudes of the occupational therapy profession.

A. General Requirements for Accreditation

1.0 Sponsorship

1.1 The sponsoring institution(s) and affiliates, if any, must be accredited by recognized national, regional, or state agencies with accrediting authority.

1.2 Sponsoring institutions must be authorized under applicable law or other acceptable authority to provide a program of postsecondary education, must have degree-granting authority, or be a program offered within the military services.

1.3 For programs in which the academic and fieldwork components of the curriculum are provided by two or more institutions, responsibilities of each sponsoring institution and fieldwork site must be clearly documented in a memorandum of understanding.

1.4 Documentation must be provided that each memorandum of understanding between institutions and fieldwork sites is reviewed at least every 5 years by both parties.

1.5 Accredited occupational therapy assistant educational programs may only be established in community, technical, junior and senior colleges, universities, medical schools, vocational schools/institutions, or military services.

1.6 The sponsoring institution shall assume primary responsibility for appointment of faculty; admission of students; curriculum planning, including selection of course content; and granting the certificate or degree documenting satisfactory completion of the educational program. The sponsoring institution shall also be responsible for the coordination of classroom teaching and supervised fieldwork practice and for providing assurance that the practice activities assigned to students in a fieldwork setting are appropriate to the program.

2.0 Academic Resources

2.1 The program must have a director who is assigned to the occupational therapy assistant program on a full-time basis.

2.2 The program director shall be an occupational therapist, initially certified nationally, and credentialed according to state requirements. The director shall have a minimum of 5 years of professional experience in areas related to clinical practice, administration, and teaching. At least 1 of these years must be a full-time academic appointment with teaching responsibilities.

2.3 The program director shall have academic qualifications comparable to other administrators who manage similar programs within the institution and relevant experience in higher education requisite for providing effective leadership for the program, its faculty, and its students.

2.4 The program director must have an understanding of and experience with occupational therapy assistants, which includes clinical supervision.

2.5 The program director shall be responsible for the management and administration of the program, including planning, evaluation, budgeting, selection of faculty and staff, maintenance of accreditation, and commitment to strategies for professional development.

2.6 The program must have at least 1 additional full-time-equivalent faculty member.

2.7 The program director and faculty must possess the necessary academic and experiential qualifications and backgrounds, identified in documented descriptions of roles and responsibilities, appropriate to meet program objectives.

2.8 The occupational therapy assistant faculty will assume responsibility for development, implementation, and evaluation of fieldwork education. There will be an individual specifically identified with fieldwork coordination responsibilities.

2.9 The faculty shall include occupational therapy practitioners who have been initially certified nationally and who have documented expertise in their area(s) of teaching responsibility.

2.10 The occupational therapy assistant faculty must be sufficient in number and must possess the expertise necessary to ensure appropriate curriculum design, content delivery, and program evaluation.

2.11 Faculty responsibilities shall be consistent with the mission of the institution.

2.12 Each full-time faculty member shall have a written continuing professional growth and development plan to ensure effectiveness and currency as an academic educator consistent with the structure of the program's strategic plan.

2.13 The program shall develop a strategic plan congruent with the mission of the institution and the curriculum design. This plan shall incorporate professional development plans of the faculty and the program objectives.

2.14 The faculty/student ratio shall permit the achievement of the purpose and stated objectives of the program, be compatible with accepted practices of the institution for similar programs, promote quality education in laboratory and fieldwork experiences, and ensure student and/or consumer safety.

2.15 Clerical and support staff shall be provided to the program, consistent with institutional practice, to meet programmatic and administrative requirements.

2.16 The program shall be allocated a budget of regular institutional funds, not including grants, gifts, and other restricted sources, sufficient to implement and maintain the objectives of the program and to fulfill the program's obligation to matriculated and entering students.

2.17 Classrooms and laboratories shall be provided consistent with the program's educational objectives, teaching methods, number of students, and safety/health standards of the institution, and shall allow for efficient operation of the program.

2.18 Laboratory space shall be assigned to the occupational therapy assistant program on a priority basis.

2.19 Space shall be provided to store and secure equipment and supplies.

2.20 The program director and faculty shall have office space consistent with institutional practice.

2.21 Space shall be provided for the private advising of students.

2.22 Appropriate and sufficient equipment and supplies shall be provided for student use and for the didactic and supervised fieldwork components of the curriculum.

2.23 Students shall be given access to the evaluative and treatment technologies that reflect current practice.

2.24 Students shall have ready access to a supply of current books, journals, periodicals, computers, software, and other reference materials needed to meet the requirements of the curriculum. This may include, but is not limited to, libraries, on-line services, interlibrary loan, and resource centers.

2.25 Instructional aids and technology shall be available in sufficient quantity and quality to be consistent with the program objectives and teaching methods.

3.0 Students

3.1 Admission of students to the occupational therapy assistant program shall be made in accordance with the practices of the institution. There shall be stated admission criteria that are clearly defined and published, and reflective of the demands of the program.

3.2 Policies pertaining to standards for admission, advanced placement, transfer of credit, credit for experiential learning (if applicable), and prerequisite educational or work experience requirements shall be readily accessible to prospective students and the public.

3.3 Criteria for successful completion of each segment of the educational program and for graduation shall be given in advance to each student.

3.4 Evaluation content and methods shall be consistent with the objectives and competencies of the didactic and supervised fieldwork components of the program.

3.5 Evaluation shall be employed on a regular basis to provide students and program officials with timely indications of the students' progress and academic standing.

3.6 Students must be informed of and have access to the health services provided to other students in the institution.

3.7 Advising related to coursework in the occupational therapy assistant program and fieldwork education shall be the responsibility of the occupational therapy assistant faculty.

3.8 A mechanism shall be in place to ensure collaboration between the fieldwork educator and representatives of the academic program during fieldwork experiences.

3.9 The program faculty shall have access to institutional and community resources and make them available to students in situations that could interfere with student progress through the program.

4.0 Operational Policies

4.1 All program publications and advertising (including academic calendars, announcements, catalogs, handbooks, and Internet descriptions) must accurately reflect the program offered.

4.2 The program's accreditation status and the name, address, and telephone number of ACOTE shall be published in the catalog, program brochures for prospective students and, if available, Internet sites.

4.3 Faculty recruitment and employment practices as well as student recruitment and admission procedures shall be non-discriminatory.

4.4 Graduation requirements, tuition, and fees shall be accurately stated, published, and made known to all applicants.

4.5 The program or sponsoring institution shall have a defined and published policy and procedure for processing student and faculty grievances.

4.6 Policies and processes for student withdrawal and for refunds of tuition and fees shall be published and made known to all applicants.

4.7 Policies and procedures for student probation, suspension, and dismissal shall be published and made known.

4.8 Policies and procedures shall be published and made known for human subject research protocol; appropriate use of equipment and supplies; and for all educational activities that have implications for the health and safety of clients, students, and faculty (including infection control and evacuation procedures).

4.9 A program admitting students on the basis of ability to benefit must publicize its objectives, assessment measures, and means of evaluating ability to benefit.

4.10 Documentation of all progression and retention, graduation and credentialing requirements, including certification/licensure, shall be published and made known to applicants.

4.11 The program shall have a documented and published policy to ensure that students complete all graduation and fieldwork requirements in a timely manner.

4.12 Records regarding student admission, enrollment, and achievement shall be maintained and kept in a secure setting. Grades and credits for courses shall be recorded on students' transcripts and permanently maintained by the sponsoring institution.

5.0 Curriculum Framework

This is a description of the program that includes the mission, philosophy, and curriculum design.

5.1 The statement of the mission of the occupational therapy assistant program shall be consistent with that of the sponsoring institution.

5.2 The statement of philosophy of the occupational therapy assistant program shall reflect the current published philosophy of the profession and shall include a statement of the program's fundamental beliefs about human beings and how they learn.

5.3 The curriculum design shall reflect the mission and philosophy of both the occupational therapy assistant program and the institution and shall provide the basis for program planning, implementation, and evaluation. The design shall identify educational goals and describe the selection of the content, scope, and sequencing of coursework.

5.4 Didactic instruction and supervised practice shall follow a plan documenting learning experiences appropriate for the development of the competencies required for graduation; the plan shall also delineate the instructional methods (e.g., presentations, demonstrations, discussions) and materials that shall be used to develop these competencies.

5.5 Instruction must follow a plan that documents clearly written course syllabi that are consistent with the curriculum design and describe learning objectives and competencies to be achieved for both didactic and fieldwork education components.

5.6 Instruction must follow a plan that documents evaluation of students on a regular basis to assess their acquisition of knowledge, skills, and attitudes and their ability to apply them to occupational therapy practice.

6.0 Program Evaluation

The program must have a continuing system for reviewing the effectiveness of the educational program, especially as measured by student achievement, faculty performance, and the ability to meet program goals. Timely self-study reports must be prepared to aid the faculty and staff, the sponsoring institution, and the accrediting agencies in assessing program qualities and needs.

6.1 Programs shall routinely secure and systematically analyze sufficient qualitative and quantitative information about the extent to which the program is meeting its stated goals and objectives. This must include, but need not be limited to,
- Faculty effectiveness in their assigned teaching responsibilities;
- Students' progression through the program;
- Graduates' performance on the National Board for Certification in Occupational Therapy (NBCOT) exam; and
- Graduate job placement and performance based on employer satisfaction.

The manner in which programs seek to comply with this criterion may vary; however, timely efforts should be made to document the data and analysis provided. These sources of data may include, but should not be limited to, surveys covering type and scope of practice, salary, job satisfaction, and adequacy of the educational program in addressing education and skills, and interviews or surveys with program graduates and employers of graduates.

6.2 The results of ongoing evaluation must be appropriately reflected in the program's strategic plan, curriculum design, and other dimensions of the program.

Program evaluation should be a continuing systematic process with internal and external curriculum validation in consultation with employers, faculty, preceptors, fieldwork educators, students, and graduates, with follow-up studies of their employment and national examination performance. Other dimensions of the program merit consideration as well, such as the mission and philosophy of the program, admission criteria and process, and the purpose and productivity of all advisory bodies.

B. Specific Requirements for Accreditation

1.0 Foundational Content Requirements

Program content shall be based on a broad foundation of the liberal arts and sciences. A foundation in the biological, physical, social, and behavioral sciences supports an understanding of occupation across the life span. Coursework in these areas may be prerequisite to or concurrent with occupational therapy assistant education and shall facilitate development of the performance criteria listed below. The student will

1.1 Demonstrate oral and written communication skills.

1.2 Employ logical thinking, critical analysis, problem solving, and creativity.

1.3 Demonstrate competence in basic computer use.

1.4 Demonstrate knowledge and understanding of the structure and function of the human body to include the biological and physical sciences.

1.5 Demonstrate knowledge and understanding of human development throughout the life span.

1.6 Demonstrate knowledge and understanding of the concepts of human behavior to include the behavioral and social sciences.

1.7 Demonstrate knowledge and appreciation of the role of sociocultural, socioeconomic, diversity factors, and lifestyle choices in contemporary society.

1.8 Appreciate the influence of social conditions and the ethical context in which humans choose and engage in occupations.

2.0 Basic Tenets of Occupational Therapy

These shall facilitate development of the performance criteria listed below. The student will

2.1 Acknowledge and understand the importance of the history and philosophical base of the profession of occupational therapy.

2.2 Be able to differentiate among occupation, activity, and purposeful activity.

2.3 Understand the meaning and dynamics of occupation and purposeful activity including the interaction of performance areas, performance components, and performance contexts.

2.4 Be able to articulate to the consumer, potential employers, and the general public the unique nature of occupation as viewed by the profession of occupational therapy.

2.5 Acknowledge and understand the importance of the balance of performance areas to the achievement of health and wellness.

2.6 Understand and appreciate the role of occupation in the promotion of health and the prevention of disease and disability for the individual, family, and society.

2.7 Understand the effects of health, disability, disease processes, and traumatic injury to the individual within the context of family and society.

2.8 Exhibit the ability to analyze tasks relative to performance areas, performance components, and performance contexts.

2.9 Demonstrate appreciation for the individual's perception of quality of life, well-being, and occupation to promote health and prevention of injury and disease.

2.10 Understand the need for and use of compensatory strategies when desired life tasks cannot be performed.

2.11 Be familiar with the theories, models of practice, and frames of reference that underlie the practice of occupational therapy.

3.0 Screening and Evaluation

The process of screening and evaluation shall be done under the supervision of and in cooperation with the occupational therapist and shall be based on theoretical perspectives, models of practice, and frames of reference that facilitate development of the performance criteria listed below. The student will

3.1 Gather and share data for the purpose of screening and evaluation including, but not limited to, specified screening assessments, skilled observation, checklists, histories, interviews with the client/family/significant others, and consultations with other professionals.

3.2 Administer selected assessments and use occupation for the purpose of assessment.

3.3 Demonstrate the ability to use safety precautions with clients during the screening and evaluation process, such as standards for infection control that include, but are not limited to, universal precautions.

3.4 Document occupational therapy services to ensure accountability of service provision and to meet standards for reimbursement of services. Documentation shall effectively communicate the need and rationale for occupational therapy services.

4.0 Intervention and Implementation

The process of intervention shall be done under the supervision of and in cooperation with the occupational therapist and shall facilitate development of the performance criteria listed below. The student will

4.1 Select, adapt, and sequence relevant occupations and purposeful activities that support the intervention goals and plan as written by the occupational therapist. These occupations and purposeful activities shall be directly related to performance areas, performance components, and performance contexts. They shall be meaningful to the client, maximizing participation and independence.

4.2 Use individual and group interaction and therapeutic use of self as a means of achieving therapeutic goals.

4.3 Adapt the environment, tools, materials, and occupations to the needs of clients and their sociocultural context.

4.4 Develop and promote the use of appropriate home and community programming to support performance in the client's natural environment.

4.5 Demonstrate the ability to educate and train client/family/significant others to facilitate skills in performance areas as well as prevention, health maintenance, and safety.

4.6 Demonstrate the ability to interact through written, oral and nonverbal communication with client/family/significant others, colleagues, other health providers, and the public.

4.7 Use therapeutic adaptation with occupations pertinent to the needs of the client. This shall include, but not be limited to, family/care provider training, environmental and behavioral modifications, orthotics, prosthetics, assistive devices, equipment, and other technologies.

4.8 Exhibit the ability to use the teaching–learning process with client/family/significant others, colleagues, other health providers, and the public. This includes assisting learners to identify their needs and objectives and using educational methods that will support those needs and objectives.

4.9 Demonstrate the ability to use safety precautions with the client during therapeutic intervention, such as contraindications and use of infection control standards that include, but are not limited to, universal precautions.

4.10 Modify intervention approaches to reflect the changing needs of the client.

4.11 Demonstrate the ability to refer to specialists, internal and external to the profession, for consultation and intervention.

4.12 Monitor and reassess the effect of occupational therapy intervention and the need for continued and/or modified intervention.

4.13 Facilitate discharge planning by reviewing the needs of client/family/significant others, resources, and discharge environment. This includes, but is not limited to, identification of community, human, and fiscal resources; recommendations for environmental adaptations; and home programming.

4.14 Recommend the need for termination of occupational therapy services when stated outcomes have been achieved. This includes a summary of occupational therapy outcomes, appropriate recommendations and referrals, and discussion with the client of post-discharge needs.

4.15 Document occupational therapy services to ensure accountability of service provision and to meet standards for reimbursement of services. Documentation shall effectively communicate the need and rationale for occupational therapy services and must be appropriate to the system in which the service is delivered.

5.0 Context of Service Delivery

The knowledge and understanding of the various contexts in which occupational therapy services are provided shall facilitate development of the performance criteria listed below. The student will

5.1 Understand the models of health care, education, community, and social systems as they relate to the practice of occupational therapy.

5.2 Understand the role and responsibility of the practitioner to address changes in service delivery policies and to effect changes in the system.

6.0 Assist in Management of Occupational Therapy Services

Application of principles of management and systems in the provision of occupational therapy services to individuals and organizations shall facilitate development of the performance criteria listed below. The student will

6.1 Understand a variety of systems and service models, including, but not limited to, health care, education, community, and social models, and how these models may effect service provision.

6.2 Understand the implications and effects of federal and state regulatory and legislative bodies on practice.

6.3 Demonstrate knowledge of applicable national and state requirements for credentialing.

6.4 Demonstrate knowledge of and ability to comply with the various reimbursement mechanisms that affect the practice of occupational therapy, including, but not limited to, federal and state reimbursement practices and third-party and private payers.

6.5 Advocate for the profession and the consumer and demonstrate an understanding of the due process and appeals systems when reimbursement is not approved for occupational therapy services.

6.6 Use principles of time management, including being able to schedule and prioritize workloads.

6.7 Maintain and organize treatment areas, equipment, and supply inventory.

6.8 Maintain records as required by practice setting, third-party payers, and regulatory agencies.

6.9 Demonstrate program evaluation using predetermined criteria.

6.10 Understand the ongoing professional responsibility for providing fieldwork education and supervision.

7.0 Use of Professional Literature

The ability to read and understand professional literature and recognize its implications for practice and the provision of occupational therapy services shall facilitate development of the performance criteria listed below. The student will

7.1 Articulate the importance of professional literature for practice and the continued development of the profession.

7.2 Be able to use professional literature to make informed practice decisions, in cooperation with the occupational therapist.

7.3 Know when and how to find and use informational resources, including appropriate literature within and outside of occupational therapy.

8.0 Professional Ethics, Values, and Responsibilities

An understanding and appreciation of ethics and values of the profession of occupational therapy shall facilitate development of the performance criteria listed below. The student will

8.1 Demonstrate a knowledge and understanding of the AOTA *Code of Ethics, Core Values and Attitudes of Occupational Therapy,* and AOTA *Standards of Practice* as a guide for professional interactions and in client treatment and employment settings.

8.2 Understand the functions and influence of national, state, and local occupational therapy associations and other related professional associations.

8.3 Promote occupational therapy by educating other professionals, consumers, third-party payers, and the public.

8.4 Acknowledge the personal responsibility for planning ongoing professional development to ensure a level of practice consistent with current and accepted standards.

8.5 Demonstrate an understanding of professional responsibilities related to liability concerns under current models of service provision.

8.6 Develop an understanding of personal and professional abilities and competencies as they relate to job responsibilities.

8.7 Understand and appreciate the varied roles of the occupational therapy assistant as a practitioner and educator.

8.8 Articulate the importance of professional relationships between the occupational therapist and the occupational therapy assistant.

8.9 Understand professional responsibilities when service provision is on a contractual basis in the current system.

8.10 Demonstrate an understanding of approaches to use in resolving personal and organizational ethical conflicts.

8.11 Demonstrate an understanding of the variety of informal and formal ethical dispute resolution systems that have jurisdiction over occupational therapy practice.

8.12 Be able to assist the consumer in gaining access to occupational therapy services.

8.13 Demonstrate knowledge of advocacy for the benefit of the consumer and the profession.

9.0 Fieldwork Education

Fieldwork education is a crucial part of the preparation of the occupational therapy assistant and is best integrated as a component of the curriculum design. Fieldwork experiences should be implemented and evaluated for their effectiveness by the educational institution. The experience should provide the student with the opportunity to carry out professional responsibilities under supervision and for role modeling. The program will

9.1 Document a plan to ensure collaboration between academic and fieldwork representatives. The plan shall include agreed-upon fieldwork objectives that are documented and made known to the student.

The Occupational Therapy Assistant: Resources for Practice and Education

9.2 Ensure that the ratio of fieldwork educators to student(s) enables proper supervision and frequent assessment of the progress in achieving stated fieldwork objectives.

9.3 Ensure that fieldwork agreements shall be sufficient in scope and number to allow completion of graduation requirements in a timely manner in accordance with the policy adopted by the program.

9.4 Conduct fieldwork in settings equipped to provide application of principles learned in the academic program and appropriate to the learning needs of the student.

9.5 Require that all aspects of the fieldwork program be consistent with the curriculum design of the program.

The goal of Level I fieldwork is to introduce students to the fieldwork experience and develop a basic comfort level with and understanding of the needs of clients. Level I fieldwork shall be integral to the program's curriculum design and include experiences designed to enrich didactic coursework through directed observation and participation in selected aspects of the occupational therapy process. The focus of these experiences is not intended to be independent performance. Qualified personnel for supervised Level I fieldwork include, but are not limited to, occupational therapy practitioners initially certified nationally, psychologists, physician assistants, teachers, social workers, nurses, and physical therapists. The program will

9.6 Ensure that Level I fieldwork shall not be substituted for any part of Level II fieldwork.

9.7 Document all Level I fieldwork experiences that are provided to students.

9.8 Document mechanisms for formal evaluation of student performance on Level I fieldwork.

The goal of Level II fieldwork is to develop competent, entry-level, generalist occupational therapy assistants. Level II fieldwork shall be integral to the program's curriculum design and shall include an in-depth experience in delivering occupational therapy services to clients, focusing on the application of purposeful and meaningful occupation. It is recommended that the student be exposed to a variety of clients across the life span and to a variety of settings. The fieldwork experience shall be designed to promote clinical reasoning, appropriate to the occupational therapy assistant role; to transmit the values and beliefs that enable ethical practice; and to develop professionalism and competence as career responsibilities. The program will

9.9 Recognize that Level II fieldwork can take place in a variety of traditional settings and emerging areas of practice. The student can complete Level II fieldwork in a minimum of one setting and maximum of three different settings.

9.10 Require a minimum of the equivalent of 16 weeks of full-time Level II fieldwork. This may be completed on a full-time or part-time basis but may not be less than half-time as defined by the fieldwork site.

9.11 Ensure that the student shall be supervised by an occupational therapy practitioner, who meets state regulations and has a minimum of 1 year of practice experience, subsequent to the requisite initial certification. The supervisor may be engaged by the fieldwork site or by the educational program.

9.12 Ensure that supervision provides protection of consumers and opportunities for appropriate role modeling of occupational therapy practice. Initially, supervision should be direct, then decrease to less direct supervision as is appropriate for the setting, the severity of the client's condition, and the ability of the student.

9.13 In a setting where there is no occupational therapy practitioner on site, the program must document that there is a plan for the provision of occupational therapy services. On-site supervision must be provided in accordance with the plan and state credentialing requirements. The student must receive a minimum of 6 hours of occupational therapy supervision per week, including direct observation of client interaction. Additionally, the occupational therapy supervisor must be readily available for communication and consultation during work hours. Such fieldwork shall not exceed 8 weeks.

C. Maintaining and Administering Accreditation

1.0 Program and Sponsoring Institution Responsibilities

1.1 The accreditation review process conducted by ACOTE can be initiated only at the written request of the chief executive officer or an officially designated representative of the sponsoring institution and the occupational therapy assistant program director or dean overseeing the proposed program.

1.2 This process is initiated by submitting a letter of intent to seek accreditation to the

Accreditation Department
American Occupational Therapy Association, Inc.
4720 Montgomery Lane
P.O. Box 31220
Bethesda, MD 20824-1220

1.3 At any time before the final accreditation action is made by ACOTE, a program or sponsoring institution may withdraw its request for initial or continuing accreditation.

1.4 To maintain accreditation, the following actions are required: The program must submit a Report of Self-Study and other required reports within a period of time determined by ACOTE. The program must agree to a site visit date before the end of the period for which accreditation was previously awarded. In accordance with stated policy, the program must inform ACOTE within 90 days of a change in program director. The sponsoring institution must inform ACOTE of the transfer of program sponsorship.

1.5 The program and the sponsoring institution must pay accreditation fees within a time period specified in the ACOTE Accreditation Manual.

Failure to meet these administrative requirements for maintaining accreditation may lead to being placed on Administrative Probation and ultimately to having accreditation withdrawn.

2.0 ACOTE Responsibilities

2.1 All policies and procedures relating to the accreditation process are found in the AOTA Accreditation Council for Occupational Therapy Education (ACOTE) Accreditation Manual.

2.2 ACOTE will follow fair practice procedures when complaints are received by ACOTE indicating that accredited programs or programs seeking accreditation may not be in substantial compliance with the *Standards for an Accredited Educational Program for the Occupational Therapy Assistant* or may not be following established accreditation policies. A record of complaints is maintained by the AOTA Accreditation Department. The policy and procedure for complaints are found in the AOTA *Accreditation Council for Occupational Therapy Education (ACOTE) Accreditation Manual.*

Chapter 35

Position Paper: Broadening the Construct of Independence

We, the members of the occupational therapy profession, support the following expanded definition of *independence:* Independence is a self-directed state of being characterized by an individual's ability to participate in necessary and preferred occupations in a satisfying manner, irrespective of the amount or kind of external assistance desired or required.

We submit this Position Paper to embrace this broad definition and to support the view that

- Self-determination is essential to achieving and maintaining independence;
- An individual's independence is unrelated to whether he or she performs the activities related to an occupation himself or herself, performs the activities in an adapted or modified environment, makes use of various devices or alternative strategies, or oversees activity completion by others;
- Independence is defined by the individual's culture and values, support systems, and ability to direct his or her life; and
- An individual's independence should not be based on preestablished criteria, perception of outside observers, or how independence is accomplished.

The occupational therapy profession is committed to a broad definition of independence for all members of society. We believe that an individual's self-directed state of independence strengthens the inclusion of all people into society as functional members, regardless of how they perform their chosen endeavors. In support of this view, occupational therapy practitioners are committed to supporting and training individuals in the use of a variety of strategies to increase their independent participation in their chosen occupations. Occupational therapy practitioners support a society that embraces an expanded definition of independence and that provides reasonable accommodations that allow individuals to have access to social, educational, recreational, and vocational opportunities.

Author

Jim Hinojosa, PhD, OT, FAOTA

for

THE COMMISSION ON PRACTICE
Mary Jane Youngstrom, MS, OTR, FAOTA—Chairperson

Adopted by the Representative Assembly 2002M40

Note. This document replaces the 1995 Position Paper, *Broadening the Construct of Independence.*

Previously published and copyrighted in 2002 by the American Occupational Therapy Association in the *American Journal of Occupational Therapy, 56,* 660.

Chapter 36

Occupation: A Position Paper

Concern with the occupational nature of human beings was fundamental to the establishment of occupational therapy. Since the time of occupational therapy's founding, the term *occupation* has been used to refer to an individual's active participation in self-maintenance, work, leisure, and play (AOTA, 1993; Bing, 1981; Levine, 1991; Meyer, 1922). Within the literature of the field, however, the meaning of occupation has been ambiguous because the term has been used interchangeably with other concepts. This paper's intent is to distinguish the term occupation from other terms, to summarize traditional beliefs about its nature and its therapeutic value, and to identify factors that have impeded the study and discussion of occupation.

The Dynamic, Multidimensional Nature of Occupations

Occupations are the ordinary and familiar things that people do every day. This simple description reflects, but understates, the multidimensional and complex nature of daily occupation.

Occupations can be broadly explained as having both performance and contextual dimensions because they involve acts within defined settings (Christiansen, 1991; Nelson, 1988; Rogers, 1982). In that they frequently extend over time, occupations have a temporal dimension (Kielhofner, 1977; Meyer, 1922). Further, in that engagement in occupation is seen to be driven by an intrinsic need for mastery, competence, self-identity, and group acceptance, occupations have a psychological dimension (Brown, 1986; Burke, 1977; Christiansen, 1994; DiMatteo, 1991; Fidler, 1981; Fidler & Fidler, 1979; White, 1971). Since occupations are often associated with a social or occupational role and are therefore identifiable in the culture, they have social and symbolic dimensions (Fidler & Fidler, 1983; Frank, 1994; Mosey, 1986). Finally, because they are infused with meaning within the lives of individuals, occupations have spiritual dimensions (Clark, 1993; Mattingly

& Fleming, 1993). The term *spiritual* is used here to refer to the nonphysical and nonmaterial aspects of existence. In this sense, it is postulated that daily pursuits contribute insight into the nature and meaning of a person's life.

This multidimensional view of occupations and their central place in the experience of living was recognized early in the profession's history. Influenced by the pragmatic philosophies of John Dewey and William James (as cited in Breines, 1987), which related well-being to an individual's participation in the world around him or her, early theorists such as Tracy (1910), Dunton (1918), and Slagle (1922) contended that doing things favorably influenced interest and attention, provided relaxation, promoted moral development, reenergized the individual, normalized habits, and conferred a physical benefit (Upham, 1918). Adolph Meyer (1922) asserted that, for healthy people, daily living unfolds in a natural and balanced pattern of occupational pursuits that bring both satisfaction and fulfillment. He noted that occupations have a performance or doing component, as well as a spiritual or personal meaning component. Meyer recognized that, through daily occupations, people organized their lives in terms of time and made meaning of their existence as human beings. Meyer believed that the organizing, self-fulfilling characteristics of occupations could make them an important mechanism of adaptation. He postulated that the individual could affect his or her state of health through occupations selected and performed each day. This view has been a principle of many conceptual frames of reference developed by occupational therapy scholars since that time (Christiansen, 1991; Kielhofner, 1993; Reilly, 1962).

In summary, occupational therapy scholars agree that human occupations have emotional, cognitive, physical, spiritual, and contextual dimensions, all of which are related to general well-being. However, occupational therapy scholars have not been able to agree on the specific concepts regarding these dimensions, or on specific terms to name them.

Distinguishing Between *Occupation* and Related Terms

The physical and mental abilities and skills required for satisfactory engagement in a given occupational pursuit constitute the performance dimension of human occupation, often referred to in the occupational therapy literature as *occupational performance*. The performance dimension of occupations is that aspect which has received the most study and attention in the history of the field. This may explain why the terms *function* and *purposeful activity* have been used as synonyms for engagement in occupation (Henderson et al., 1991).

Occupations, because of their intentional nature, always involve mental abilities and skills, and typically, but not always, have an observable physical or active dimension. Whether one is laying bricks or practicing meditation exercises, one can be said to be "doing" something. Only one of these occupations, however, requires observable physical action. Whether physical or mental in nature, the behaviors necessary for completion of tasks in daily occupations can be analyzed according to specific components related to moving, perceiving, thinking, and feeling. Various occupational performance components have been described and defined within the *Uniform Terminology for Occupational Therapy—Third Edition* (AOTA, 1994).

Position papers on function and purposeful activity have been developed by the American Occupational Therapy Association (AOTA), and it is important to clarify the differences in meaning between these terms and the term *occupation*. The AOTA has proposed that when occupational therapists use the term *function,* they refer to an individual's *performance* of activities, tasks, and roles during daily occupations (occupational performance) (AOTA, 1995). *Purposeful activity* has also been recognized as a term to describe engagement in the tasks of daily living, with the use of this term emphasizing the intentional, goal-directed nature of such engagement (AOTA, 1993). In this paper, it is proposed that reference to human occupation necessarily encompasses the required human capacities to act on the environment with intentionality in a given pursuit, as well as the unique organization of these pursuits over time and the meanings attributed to them by doers as well as those observing them.

In summary, *occupations* have performance, contextual, temporal, psychological, social, symbolic, and spiritual dimensions, whereas, *function* in its specific use denotes primarily the performance dimension. While the term *purposeful activity* recognizes multiple dimensions and emphasizes intentionality, it is viewed as a term that does not capture the richness of human enterprise embodied in the word *occupation*. It is asserted that while all occupations constitute purposeful activity, not all purposeful activities can be described as occupations.

Therapeutic Benefits of Occupations

Since Adolph Meyer's (1922) philosophical essay, many scholarly papers have been written about the therapeutic value of occupations (Clark, 1993; Cynkin & Robinson, 1990; Englehardt, 1977; Reilly, 1962; Yerxa, 1967). These have identified a broad scope of benefits, ranging from the facilitation of habilitation, adaptation, and self-actualization to improvements in motor control and sensory processing. While there is growing evidence to support some of these claims, additional research is needed before it can be demonstrated that other benefits are likely valid.

Because occupation is an extremely complex phenomenon and has not been subjected to rigorous research until recently, many questions about its nature and its relationship to health and well-being remain unanswered. This emphasizes the need for further study. Current beliefs and theories about occupation should be regarded as incomplete and evolving.

Forces Advancing and Impeding the Study and Discussion of Occupation

One of the problems inhibiting the study of occupations is how to clearly, logically, and consistently describe different levels and types of occupations. Used here, the term *levels* refers to the complexity of a given occupation. For example, while getting dressed and driving to work are readily interpretable as organized sets of actions that may partially comprise a typical day, each of these involves a variety of specific and definable behaviors, such as buttoning a shirt or turning an ignition key, which are less complex. Even occupational behaviors of greater complexity, such as dressing or driving, are nested within clusters of activity that comprise and are recognized as part of larger sets of organized behavior within cultures, such as pursuing a career. This phenomenon of nesting, where simple acts can be identified as parts of more complex sets of acts, is a dimension of occupations that relates to their organization over time and can be viewed as reflecting varying levels of complexity.

The English language has words associated with occupations, such as *actions, tasks,* and *projects,* which imply differences in complexity. Evans (1987) and Kielhofner (1993) have been among those who have described the hierarchical nature of occupations, and others (Christiansen, 1991; Nelson, 1988) have suggested that it would be useful if specific terms for human enterprise denoted different levels of this hierarchy. However, there is little agreement among scholars in occupational therapy or in the social sciences for how these terms ought to be used to describe varying levels of complexity in occupational behavior.

Similar difficulties exist in describing types or categories of occupations. Certain categories of occupations have gained conventional usage by occupational therapists and are recognized in contemporary culture. These include work, self-care (or self-maintenance), play, and leisure.

Studies of human beings in different cultures have shown similarities in time use according to these general categories (Christiansen, in press). However, while general categories of occupations are recognized across cultures, the specific tasks that constitute each category and the delineation of categories vary across individuals. The classification of a given task within a larger category seems to be dependent upon the context in which it is performed. For example, sewing may be viewed as work by some and classified as leisure by others. Similarly, most occupational pursuits seem to have both a general or cultural meaning attributed by participants and observers as well as a specific and personal meaning known only to the performer (Nelson, 1988; Rommetveit, 1980). Consider, for example, that getting dressed is viewed as a necessary and practical aspect of daily life in most cultures but assumes symbolic importance when it is performed without assistance for the first time by the 3-year-old child or by an adult mastering use of a new prosthetic arm. Dressing in anticipation of a ceremony or developmental milestone, such as high school graduation or a wedding, imbues the act with special significance. Over time, the experiences embedded in daily occupations assume collective meaning and are interpreted as essential parts of a person's self-narrative or life story (Bruner, 1990; Clark, 1993; Mattingly & Fleming, 1993).

Research on Occupations and Research in Occupational Therapy

It is useful to recognize that research on occupations should be distinguished from research in occupational therapy (Mosey, 1992). In the first instance, inquiry is directed toward understanding the nature of the typical daily occupations in which people engage; that is, what people do, how they do it, and why they do it. The study of occupational therapy, conversely, concerns itself with the effect of occupation on health, development of frames of reference that facilitate the identification and remediation of occupational dysfunction, and other topical issues of significance to this science-based profession.

Research for both areas has been impeded by the lack of conventional definitions for terms related to occupation. This, in turn, has contributed to disagreements about the proper concern of practice and the appropriate focus of research (Christiansen, 1981, 1991; Kielhofner & Burke, 1977; Mosey, 1985, 1989; Rogers, 1982; Shannon, 1977). Recently, occupational science has emerged as an area of study concerned with understanding humans as occupational beings (Clark et al., 1991; Yerxa et al., 1989). As additional research enables us to learn more about the nature of occupations and their potential as a means for promoting and restoring health and well-being, it is likely that there will be continued discussion on the use of terminology to describe specific concepts.

This paper has attempted to identify distinctions among current terms relating to human occupation. As our understanding of occupations advances, more concepts and terms will evolve. It is important to continue to develop knowledge about occupations to facilitate our further understanding of an important, complex, and rich aspect of human life. In this way, the profession of occupational therapy will better appreciate the vision of its founders, more clearly understand its current state, and more likely realize the potential embodied in occupations as touchstones of human existence.

References

American Occupational Therapy Association. (1993). Position paper: Purposeful activity. *American Journal of Occupational Therapy, 47*, 1081–1082.

American Occupational Therapy Association. (1994). Uniform terminology for occupational therapy—third edition. *American Journal of Occupational Therapy, 48*, 1047–1059.

American Occupational Therapy Association. (1995). Occupational performance: Occupational therapy's definition of function. *American Journal of Occupational Therapy, 49*, 1019–1020.

Bing, R. (1981). Occupational therapy revisited: A paraphrastic journey. *American Journal of Occupational Therapy, 35*, 499–518.

Breines, E. (1987). Pragmatism as a foundation for occupational therapy. *American Journal of Occupational Therapy, 41*, 522–525.

Brown, R. (1986). *Social psychology* (2nd ed.). New York: Free Press.

Bruner, J. (1990). *Acts of meaning.* Cambridge, MA: Harvard University Press.

Burke, J. P. (1977). A clinical perspective on motivation: Pawn versus origin. *American Journal of Occupational Therapy, 31*, 254–258.

Christiansen, C. (1981). Toward resolution of crisis: Research requisites in occupational therapy. *Occupational Therapy Journal of Research, 1*, 115–124.

Christiansen, C. (1991). Occupational therapy: Intervention for life performance. In C. Christiansen & C. Baum (Eds.), *Occupational therapy: Overcoming human performance deficits* (p. 143). Thorofare, NJ: Slack.

Christiansen, C. (1994). A social framework for understanding self-care intervention. In C. Christiansen (Ed.), *Ways of liv-*

ing: *Self-care strategies for special needs* (pp. 1–26). Bethesda, MD: American Occupational Therapy Association.

Christiansen, C. (in press). Three perspectives on balance in occupation. In F. Clark & R. Zemke (Eds.), *Occupational science: The first five years*. Philadelphia: F. A. Davis.

Clark, F. A. (1993). Occupation embedded in a real life: Interweaving occupational science and occupational therapy. *American Journal of Occupational Therapy, 47*, 1067–1078.

Clark, F. A., Parham, D., Carlson, M. E., Frank, G., Jackson, J., Pierce, D., Wolfe, R. J., & Zemke, R. (1991). Occupational science: Academic innovation in the service of occupational therapy's future. *American Journal of Occupational Therapy, 45*, 300–310.

Cynkin S., & Robinson, A. M. (1990). *Occupational therapy and activities health: Toward health through activities*. Boston: Little, Brown.

DiMatteo, M. R. (1991). *The psychology of health, illness, and medical care: An individual perspective*. Pacific Grove, CA: Brooks-Cole.

Dunton, W. R. (1918). The principles of occupational therapy. *Public Health Nurse, 10*, 316–321.

Englehardt, H. T. (1977). Defining occupational therapy: The meaning of therapy and the virtues of occupation. *American Journal of Occupational Therapy, 31*, 666–672.

Evans, A. K. (1987). National Speaking: Definition of occupation as the core concept of occupational therapy. *American Journal of Occupational Therapy, 41*, 627–628.

Fidler, G. S. (1981). From crafts to competence. *American Journal of Occupational Therapy, 35*, 567–573.

Fidler, G. S., & Fidler, J. W. (1979). Doing and becoming: Purposeful action and self-actualization. *American Journal of Occupational Therapy, 32*, 305–310.

Fidler, G. S., & Fidler, J. W. (1983). Doing and becoming: The occupational therapy experience. In G. Kielhofner (Ed.), *Health through occupation* (pp. 267–280). Philadelphia: F. A. Davis.

Frank, G. (1994). The personal meaning of self-care. In C. Christiansen (Ed.), *Ways of living: Self-care strategies for special needs* (pp. 27–49). Bethesda, MD: American Occupational Therapy Association.

Henderson, A., Cermak, S., Coster, W., Murray, E., Trombly, C., & Tickle-Degnen, L. (1991). The Issue Is: Occupational science is multidimensional. *American Journal of Occupational Therapy, 45*, 370–372.

Kielhofner, G. (1977). Temporal adaptation: A conceptual framework for occupational therapy. *American Journal of Occupational Therapy, 31*, 235–242.

Kielhofner, G. (1993). *Conceptual foundations of occupational therapy*. Philadelphia: F. A. Davis.

Kielhofner, G., & Burke, J. P. (1977). Occupational therapy after sixty years: An account of changing identity and knowledge. *American Journal of Occupational Therapy, 31*, 675–689.

Levine, R. (1991). Occupation as a therapeutic medium. In C. Christiansen & C. Baum (Eds.), *Occupational therapy: Overcoming human performance deficits* (pp. 592–631). Thorofare, NJ: Slack.

Mattingly, C., & Fleming, M. (1993). *Clinical reasoning*. Philadelphia: F. A. Davis.

Meyer, A. (1922). The philosophy of occupational therapy. *Archives of Occupational Therapy, 1*, 1–10.

Mosey, A. C. (1985). Amonistic or pluralistic approach to professional identity. *American Journal of Occupational Therapy, 39*, 504–509.

Mosey, A. C. (1986). *Psychosocial components of occupational therapy*. New York: Raven.

Mosey, A. C. (1989). The proper focus of scientific inquiry in occupational therapy: Frames of reference. *Occupational Therapy Journal of Research, 9*, 195–201.

Mosey, A. C. (1992). Partition of occupational science and occupational therapy. *American Journal of Occupational Therapy, 46*, 851–855.

Nelson, D. L. (1988). Occupation: Form and performance. *American Journal of Occupational Therapy, 42*, 633–641.

Reilly, M. (1962). Occupation can be one of the great ideas of 20th-century medicine. *American Journal of Occupational Therapy, 16*, 1–9.

Rogers, J. (1982). The spirit of independence: The evolution of a philosophy. *American Journal of Occupational Therapy, 36*, 709–715.

Rommetveit, R. (1980). On meanings of acts and what is meant and made known by what is said in a pluralistic social world. In M. Brenner (Ed.), *The structure of action* (pp. 108–149). Oxford: Basil Blackwell.

Shannon, P. D. (1977). The derailment of occupational therapy. *American Journal of Occupational Therapy, 31*, 229–234.

Slagle, E. C. (1922). Training aids for mental patients. *Archives of Occupational Therapy, 1*, 11–17.

Tracy, S. (1910). *Studies in invalid occupations: A manual for nurses and attendants*. Boston: Whitcomb & Barrows.

Upham, E. G. (1918). *Ward occupations in hospitals. Federal Board for Vocational Education Bulletin 25*. Washington, DC: U.S. Government Printing Office.

White, R. W. (1971). The urge towards competence. *American Journal of Occupational Therapy, 25*, 271–274.

Yerxa, E. (1967). Authentic occupational therapy. *American Journal of Occupational Therapy, 21*, 1–9.

Yerxa, E., Clark, F., Frank, G., Jackson, J., Parham, D., Pierce, D., Stein, C., & Zemke, R. (1989). An introduction to occupational science: A foundation for occupational therapy in the 21st century. In J. Johnson & E. Yerxa (Eds.), *Occupational science: The foundation for new models of practice* (pp. 1–18). New York: Haworth.

Authors

Charles Christiansen, EdD, OTR, OT(C), FAOTA
Florence Clark, PhD, OTR, FAOTA
Gary Kielhofner, DrPH, OTR, FAOTA
Joan Rogers, PhD, OTR, FAOTA
with contributions from
David Nelson, PhD, OTR, FAOTA

for

COMMISSION ON PRACTICE
Jim Hinojosa, PhD, OTR, FAOTA, Chairperson

Adopted by the Representative Assembly April 1995

Previously published and copyrighted by the American Occupational Therapy Association in 1995 in the *American Journal of Occupational Therapy, 49*, 1015–1018.

Chapter 37

Statement—The Philosophical Base of Occupational Therapy

Man is an active being whose development is influenced by the use of purposeful activity. Using their capacity for intrinsic motivation, human beings are able to influence their physical and mental health and their social and physical environment through purposeful activity. Human life includes a process of continuous adaptation. Adaptation is a change in function that promotes survival and self-actualization. Biological, psychological, and environmental factors may interrupt the adaptation process at any time throughout the life cycle. Dysfunction may occur when adaptation is impaired. Purposeful activity facilitates the adaptive process.

Occupational therapy is based on the belief that purposeful activity (occupation), including its interpersonal and environmental components, may be used to prevent and mediate dysfunction and to elicit maximum adaptation. Activity as used by the occupational therapist includes both an intrinsic and a therapeutic purpose.

This statement was adopted by the April 1979 Representative Assembly of the American Occupational Therapy Association, Inc. as Resolution C #551–79.

American Occupational Therapy Association. (1979). The philosophical base of occupational therapy. *American Journal of Occupational Therapy, 33,* 785. (Reprinted in 1995 in the *American Journal of Occupational Therapy, 49,* 1026.)

Chapter 38

Statement—Fundamental Concepts of Occupational Therapy: Occupation, Purposeful Activity, and Function

This statement will begin to clarify the definitions of the concepts of occupation, purposeful activity, and function as they are used today in the profession of occupational therapy and to describe the relationship among them. Historically, the core concepts of *occupation, purposeful activity*, and *function* have been used interchangeably in the literature and practice of occupational therapy.

In 1979, *The Philosophical Base of Occupational Therapy* (AOTA, 1979, Resolution 531-79) identified the key concepts of the profession as purposeful activity and adaptation. Occupation was thought to be synonymous with purposeful activity, as the term *occupation* appears in parentheses. The *Philosophical Base* presents adaptation as central to human existence and defines it as "a change in function that promotes survival and self-actualization" (AOTA, 1979, p. 785). In this definition, the term *function* is the ability to accomplish something. Factors that interrupt adaptation at any time in the life of an individual result in dysfunction, implying that function can be changed or be impaired. The *Philosophical Base* states that "purposeful activity facilitates the adaptive process" (AOTA, 1979, p. 785), resulting in positive changes in function.

As the profession has evolved, and partially in response to changes in society, occupational therapy practitioners have come to realize that adaptation is only one way in which function is changed or altered. Adaptation is the way that individuals accommodate to demands or new circumstances. Furthermore, occupational therapy practitioners may adapt tasks or the environment to improve the individual's performance. The ability to function can be interpreted as a product or an outcome of this process. Occupational therapy outcomes are often described in terms of function or ability within a performance area.

Occupation, Purposeful Activity, and Function

Three position papers recently published by AOTA, *Purposeful Activity* (Hinojosa, Sabari, & Pedretti, 1993),

Occupation: A Position Paper (Christiansen, Clark, Kielhofner, & Rogers, 1995), and *Occupational Performance: Occupational Therapy's Definition of Function* (Baum & Edwards, 1995), have presented differing facets of the fundamental concepts of occupational therapy. As the concepts expressed in these papers evolved from a common philosophy and practice, it is not surprising that there are similarities in the meanings given to the terms. Furthermore, occupational therapy practitioners use the terms *occupation, purposeful activity*, and *function* in ways other than they are generally used by the public. These terms are used so frequently by occupational therapy practitioners that it is taken for granted that all occupational therapy practitioners hold common distinctive meanings for each. However, differences have been noted in the ways the terms are used within the profession. Moreover, the terms have been used interchangeably in both the occupational therapy literature and clinical practice. Furthermore, there appear to be multiple perspectives about the relationships among the concepts of occupation, purposeful activity, and function. The purpose of this statement, therefore, is to distinguish these three terms and to further clarify their relationships for the profession of occupational therapy.

Occupation

Occupational therapists use the term *occupation* to organize and define the profession's domain of concern. Occupational therapy practitioners organize life activities into categories of work, self-care, and play/leisure, although definition of an activity as fitting one of these categories varies from one individual to another. "Occupations are the ordinary and familiar things that people do every day" (Christiansen et al., 1995, p. 1015). Occupations are the activities people engage in throughout their daily lives to fulfill their time and give life meaning.

Occupations involve mental abilities and skills and may or may not have an observable physical dimension.

Occupations always have some degree of personal meaning, having contextual, temporal, psychological, social, symbolic, cultural, ethnic, and/or spiritual dimensions. Occupations reflect the unique characteristics of the person. A person is defined, to some extent, by the occupations in which he or she engages. A person's preferred occupations may change over time, depending on differing factors or circumstances in his or her life. An understanding of occupations is still evolving, and there is a need for more research on the relationship between occupations and a person's health and well-being.

Purposeful Activity

"*Purposeful activity* refers to goal-directed behaviors or tasks...that the individual considers meaningful" (Hinojosa et al., 1993, p. 1081). People continually engage in purposeful activities as a part of their occupations. Purposeful activities have personal meaning combined with a goal-directed quality and are encompassed within occupations. Within this view, "goal-directed" does not necessarily imply a physical product or an outcome but does involve active engagement that meets personal goals or needs. Therapeutically, purposeful activities are used to evaluate, facilitate, restore, or maintain an individual's abilities to meet demands in his or her life; in other words, to engage in occupations. Occupational therapy practitioners specifically use purposeful activities that have meaning to the person in two ways. They are used as a media to facilitate improvements in performance components, and they are also used in patterns or groups to help the individual to develop meaningful occupations.

Function

Function always has been a basic concept in occupational therapy and is seen as equivalent to *performance*. When occupational therapy practitioners use *function*, they are referring to the use of "interventions to improve the occupational performance of persons who lack the ability to perform an action or activity considered necessary for their everyday lives" (Baum & Edwards, 1995, p. 1019). However, function is also used as a verb; *to function* is to be able to do an action for a purpose.

The general public looks at function relative to a context of normalcy, the implication being that, to do something, to function, one needs to do it in an acceptable manner. Occupational therapy practitioners use the word *function* to designate when someone performs effectively. This may include using adaptations or alternative means to accomplish the task when the customary methods are not

possible. Occupational therapy practitioners also tend to use the term *functional activities* to designate specific purposeful activities that facilitate ability to engage in occupations. This use indicates that practitioners believe that function is part of the process rather than an outcome alone. While society currently tends to focus on the functional outcomes of intervention, occupational therapists believe that both the process of change (adaptation) and the functional outcomes are critically important. Societal concerns generally relate to the ability to do something (perform) specifically. Alternatively, occupational therapy practitioners are concerned with the various performance components that work together to bring about function. The process of working toward change in the individual's various performance components leads to a functional outcome.

Summary

Deriving from the philosophical basis of the profession, occupation is the core concept of the profession of occupational therapy. However, in the occupational therapy literature, the term *occupation* is used in a variety of ways. Occupation, a collection of activities that people use to fill their time and give life meaning, is organized around roles or in terms of activities of daily living, work and productive activities, or play/leisure. People engage in occupations for pleasure, for survival, for necessity, and for their personal meaning. It is the individualized, unique combination of activities that comprises an individual's occupations.

Purposeful activities have been described in many different ways: as something all people engage in, as tools or media that therapists use to enhance or facilitate performance, and as vehicles for bringing about change. Purposeful activities are seen as part of the process of occupational therapy. Purposeful activities are a subset of occupations in that they are goal-directed and serve as a major tool in the process of occupational therapy.

The term *function*, viewed as the ability to perform activities required in one's occupations, has become increasingly important to society in describing the performance or change in individuals. This societal shift in ideas has prompted the important process of bringing about change. Occupational therapy practitioners typically have viewed the process as being just as important as the product. When working to improve function, occupational therapy practitioners use purposeful activities that are meaningful to the person in relation to his or her occupational history, preferences, personal goals, and needs.

Occupational therapy practitioners need to keep the individual's occupations in the forefront of their thoughts when using any purposeful activity and to plan interventions toward improving the individual's ability to function within his or her occupations. In the interest of the profession, it is important to concentrate on occupation. Furthermore, it is essential that we study our interventions' relationship to occupation and function and how purposeful activities are used toward supporting the individual's ability to engage in occupation.

References

American Occupational Therapy Association. (1979). The philosophical base of occupational therapy. *American Journal of Occupational Therapy, 33,* 785.

Baum, C., & Edwards, D. (1995). Occupational performance: Occupational therapy's definition of function. *American Journal of Occupational Therapy, 49,* 1019–1020.

Christiansen, C., Clark, F., Kielhofner, G., & Rogers, J. (1995). Occupation: A position paper. *American Journal of Occupational Therapy, 49,* 1015–1018.

Hinojosa, J., Sabari, J., & Pedretti, L. (1993). Position paper: Purposeful activities. *American Journal of Occupational Therapy, 47,* 1081–1082.

Suggested Readings

American Occupational Therapy Association. (1985). *A professional legacy: The Eleanor Clarke Slagle lectures in occupational therapy, 1955–1984.* Bethesda, MD: Author.

Christiansen, C., & Baum, C. (Eds.). (1991). Occupational therapy: *Overcoming human performance deficits.* Thorofare, NJ: Slack.

Fidler, G. S., & Fidler, J. W. (1978). Doing and becoming: Purposeful action and self-actualization. *American Journal of Occupational Therapy, 32,* 305–310.

Kielhofner, G. (1983). *Health through occupation: Theory and practice in occupational therapy.* Philadelphia: F. A. Davis.

Meyer, A. (1977/1922). The philosophy of occupational therapy. *American Journal of Occupational Therapy, 31,* 639–642.

Mosey, A. C. (1986). *Psychosocial components of occupational therapy.* New York: Raven Press.

Nelson, D. L. (1988). Occupation: Form and performance. *American Journal of Occupational Therapy, 42,* 633–641.

Reed, K. L., & Sanderson, S. N. (1992). *Concepts of occupational therapy.* Baltimore, MD: Williams & Wilkins.

Reilly, M. (1962). Occupational therapy can be one of the great ideas of the 20th-century medicine. *American Journal of Occupational Therapy, 16,* 1–9.

Royeen, C. B. (Ed.). (1995). *AOTA Self-Study Series: Human occupation.* Bethesda, MD: American Occupational Therapy Association.

Yerxa, E. J. (1967). Authentic occupational therapy. *American Journal of Occupational Therapy, 21,* 1–9.

Authors

Jim Hinojosa, PhD, OT, FAOTA
Paula Kramer, PhD, OTR, FAOTA

for

THE COMMISSION ON PRACTICE
Linda Kohlman Thomson, MOT, OT(C), FAOTA—Chairperson

Adopted by the Representative Assembly 4/97

Previously published and copyrighted by the American Occupational Therapy Association in 1997 in the *American Journal of Occupational Therapy, 51,* 864–866.

Chapter 39

Commission on Education Position Paper: The Viability of Occupational Therapy Assistant Education

The Commission on Education affirms its support of occupational therapy assistant education at the technical level. The move to advance occupational therapy education to the post-baccalaureate level has raised concerns regarding the continued viability and appropriateness of occupational therapy assistant education. The Commission on Education asserts that the skill sets of the occupational therapy assistant are most effectively and efficiently taught at the technical level.

Continued preparation of the occupational therapy assistants at the technical level is crucial to meeting society's needs for accessible and affordable health and human service care. Health care is shifting to home and community environs. Maldistribution of providers limits access to services for rural residents and urban poor. The focus of health care is changing from short-term medical treatment to management of chronic conditions and promotion of wellness and quality of life. Occupational therapy assistants have historically served persons with chronic handicapping conditions. The use of occupational therapy assistants in delivery of services allows for expanded distribution and access to occupational therapy services for all populations.

An associate degree is an accessible degree for adult learners and individuals from diverse backgrounds. Continued support of this level of education will help to diversify the backgrounds of occupational therapy service providers and contribute to the serving of diverse populations. Availability of this level of education attracts returning adult students who bring rich life and work experiences to the field of occupational therapy. The presence of occupational therapy assistant education programs offers opportunities for the profession to directly influence the development of programs designed to meet local community needs and to support individuals' participation in everyday life activities and occupations. Occupational therapy assistant educators and students are positioned to cultivate an awareness of the importance of engaging in occupations and its relationship to health.

The Commission of Education reaffirms that occupational therapy assistant education adds an important and valued dimension to the provision of occupational therapy services. The Commission of Education is committed to support the continuing contribution of occupational therapy assistant education by promoting the differentiation as well as strengths of both technical and post-baccalaureate levels of education in occupational therapy.

Authors

THE COMMISSION ON EDUCATION

Charlotte Brasic Royeen, PhD, OTR, FAOTA
Chairperson

Chapter 40

The Need for OTA Involvement in the AOTA: "Now Is the Time"

Why be involved? Who has the time or money to do it? Isn't being a member enough? "Well," I would answer the last question, "if that is all you can do at this time, then yes, it is enough." But, if you can do more and just don't know how to go about starting, this is the place to look.

For many years, occupational therapy assistants have voiced feelings of being disenfranchised with the American Occupational Therapy Association (AOTA). For many, this may in fact be true. Changes in administration over the years have left many occupational therapy assistants feeling that AOTA membership or involvement is not necessary. I understand that feeling, and at times I and others were very disappointed with the way in which occupational therapy assistants were represented. In 2003, a small group of occupational therapy assistants met at AOTA Conference and made some very critical decisions. We knew we had to do something to improve the involvement of occupational therapy assistants, and we developed a simple plan. Since then we have helped to elect two occupational therapy assistants to the AOTA Board of Directors, two occupational therapy assistants to the AOTA Representative Assembly (RA), assisted in the change from voice to vote for the occupational therapy assistant representative to the RA, nominated successfully two occupational therapy assistants for AOTA awards, initiated the celebration of the history of occupational therapy assistants with presentations in several states, and wrote and published articles regarding the celebration of the history of the occupational therapy assistant. So if we, as a very small group, can make such changes in the visibility and recognition of occupational therapy assistants in such a short time, imagine what could be done with more!

This writer was elected for the term 2004–2006, and during that time I have seen such incredible gains in the awareness of AOTA to the issues facing the occupational therapy assistant. Much has been accomplished, but we need to do more. I truly feel that "This is the time!" Never before have myself and others been so positive about the role of the occupational therapy assistant within the profession and AOTA and never before have we gotten so much value for our membership.

I know that at times it seems overwhelming to do anything other than be a member and just live your busy life. I feel that all too often we just don't know the facts. Whenever I am asked about how I have the time or money to be involved I say the same thing: "I have to walk the walk if I am going to talk the talk." Now in my role as a OTA educator my students would be making fun of me at this point, but I just keep on talking. Let me help you understand how easy it is to be involved. The major questions I get are hopefully outlined below. If they are not clear or you have questions, feel free to contact any of the occupational therapy assistants serving on AOTA commissions, committees, and boards.

TYPES OF INVOLVEMENT

INFORMAL	FORMAL
• Voting for officers of your local or state association • Voting for officers for national association • Informing your state representative regarding your concerns • Responding for requests for feedback • Keeping informed of current issues.	• Attending local and state OT association meetings • Informing your state representative of you desire to volunteer • Responding to the "Call for Volunteers" • Serving on a committee and helping at Conference • Submitting a proposal or "Call for Paper" to make a presentation • Running for local or state office

Where Do I Start?

- I always encourage anyone who asks me this question to start local with what you are interested in. Pick a position that you feel comfortable with and dive in! You could even start within your work environment. Think about getting involved in fieldwork education and sign-up for the fieldwork listserv.
- Some additional first starts could be to speak to your local Special Interest Section, study group, or district within your state. Serve as a mentor to other occupational therapy assistants, and share your expertise. Start a study group for occupational therapy assistants within your community. Promote occupational therapy within your community at school fairs, special events, etc.
- Then I would look for running for a position locally within your state association or look at being the representative to the assembly from your state. These elected positions are a nice introduction to the national level while staying involved with your state association.

How Do I Know If They Need an Occupational Therapy Assistant to Serve on a Commission, Committee, or Board?

- Read your local OT association newsletter, or check your Web site for your state. Often the positions that are needed are advertised in these ways.
- Check the AOTA Web site and read your AOTA literature (*OT Practice, AJOT, 1-Minute Updates,* Special Interest Section newsletters) and the AOTA listservs. All open or requested positions are sent through these sources.

How Do I Know If I Have the Qualifications to Serve on a Commission, Committee, or Board?

- Look at the qualifications they are looking for regarding that specific position. If you are unsure, contact one of the members to discuss their needs, and then apply for the position!

Does AOTA Make My Reservations for Travel?

- No, you will make your own travel reservations and be reimbursed (within set limits) for your fare.
- AOTA will make your hotel accommodations, and you do not have to pay for your room. You will need to have a credit card to secure any incidentals (phone calls, room service, laundry, etc.) that may be charged to your room.

Do I Get Reimbursed for Travel Expenses?

- Yes, you are reimbursed for all reasonable expenses, within a set limit of expenditures for each day, including travel days.

Author

Kathryn Melin Eberhardt,
MAEd, COTA/L, ROH

Index

The Occupational Therapy Assistant: Resources for Practice and Education

About the Editors

Kathryn Melin Eberhardt, MAEd, COTA/L, ROH, is academic fieldwork coordinator at South Suburban College in the Occupational Therapy Assistant Program. Kathryn received an associate degree in applied science from South Suburban College, a BS from Governors State University, and a master's in adult education from National Louis University. She currently is a director on the Board of Directors for the American Occupational Therapy Association (AOTA) and is director of advocacy for the Illinois Occupational Therapy Association. She also has been involved with the National Board for Certification in Occupational Therapy (NBCOT) as an item writer, Certification Examination Development Committee member, and vice-chair. Her practice interests are adult rehabilitation, home modification, and aging-in-place.

As an occupational therapy assistant educator for 17 years, Kathryn is committed to the quality of education and the role of occupational therapy assistants within occupational therapy. She received AOTA's Recognition of Achievement Award for exemplary dedication to the education and development of occupational therapy assistants; the AOTA Roster of Honor Award for being an advocate for assistants in education, regulation, and clinical excellence; and the AOTA Terry Brittell OTA/OT Partnership Award. She also has been listed in the *Who's Who Among American Teachers,* 1996, 1998, 2004, and 2005 editions.

Teri L. Black, COTA, ROH, has been on the faculty of Madison Area Technical College for 23 years. Previously, she worked at Sauk County Health Care Center in Reedsburg from 1989 to 1998 as an on-call COTA and is currently working in Muscoda for Aegis in the school system and skilled-nursing facilities, in addition to full-time teaching.

Teri served a 3-year term as the OTA representative on the AOTA Board of Directors and was just re-elected as a Board member. Before that, she served for 9 years on the NBCOT Board of Directors, including the Disciplinary Action Committee. She was legislative chair for the Wisconsin Occupational Therapy Association (WOTA) for 11 years and led the effort to get rule changes that allowed occupational therapy to become a licensed profession. Teri has been a keynote speaker for several occupational therapy conferences and done many workshops and an institute at AOTA's Annual Conference & Expo. She also has published articles in *OT Practice* and *Advance,* as well as in the WOTA newsletter.